Pediatric Respiratory Disorders
Clinical Approaches

Pediatric Respiratory Disorders
Clinical Approaches

Edited by

Eliezer Nussbaum, M.D.

Associate Professor
Department of Pediatrics
University of California
Irvine, California

Director, Children's Lung Center and
*   Pediatric Intensive Care Units*
Miller Children's Hospital
Medical Center of Long Beach
Long Beach, California

Stanley P. Galant, M.D.

Clinical Professor of Pediatrics
University of California
Irvine, California

GRUNE & STRATTON

A Subsidiary of Harcourt Brace Jovanovich, Publishers

Orlando   San Diego   San Francisco
New York   London   Toronto   Montreal
Sydney   Tokyo   São Paulo

Library of Congress Cataloging in Publication Data
Main entry under title:

Pediatric respiratory disorders.

   Bibliography
   Includes index.
   1. Pediatric respiratory diseases   I. Nussbaum,
Eliezer.   II. Galant, Stanley P. [DNLM: 1. Respiratory
tract diseases—In infancy and childhood. WS 280 P3675]
RJ431.P4   1983   618.92´2   83-10740
ISBN 0-8089-1571-1

Grune & Stratton, Inc.
Orlando, Florida 32887

Distributed in the United Kingdom by
Grune & Stratton, Inc. (London) Ltd.
24/28 Oval Road, London NW 1

Library of Congress Catalog Number 83-10740
International Standard Book Number 0-8089-1571-1

Printed in the United States of America

Dedication

To Sara, Shai,
Tzvi, and Michelle.

Contents

Preface

Pediatric Respiratory Disorders: Clinical Approaches provides a comprehensive state-of-the-art review of infant, childhood, and adolescent respiratory diseases. The material in this volume was written by leading pediatric specialists in the fields of pulmonary diseases, physiology, allergy, clinical immunology, radiology, infectious diseases, and neonatology.

The multidisciplinary approach emphasizes the clinical aspects of bronchial asthma, cystic fibrosis, bronchopulmonary dysplasia, immune deficiency, and pulmonary infections. This volume addresses new pathophysiologic, technologic, and therapeutic concepts of gastroesophageal reflux, exercise-induced asthma, immotile cilia syndrome, pulmonary hemosiderosis, pharmacology of respiratory disorders, and allergic bronchopulmonary aspergillosis. The chapters dealing with gas transport, pulmonary function testing, respiratory failure, and pulmonary radiology are especially appealing to physicians and related health personnel from many pediatric specialties.

As it is informative and practical on many levels, this book should be of great assistance to all those interested in the field.

Contributors

James W. Bass, M.D.   Colonel, Medical Corps; Chairman, Department of Pediatrics, Tripler Army Medical Center, Oahu, Hawaii.

William E. Berquist, M.D.   Assistant Professor of Pediatrics, Division of Pediatric Gastroenterology, School of Medicine, University of California, Los Angeles, California.

Thomas F. Boat, M.D.   Professor of Pediatrics and Chairman, Department of Pediatrics, School of Medicine, University of North Carolina, Chapel Hill, North Carolina.

Margaret C. Bruce, M.D.   Assistant Professor of Medicine, Case Western Reserve University and Rainbow Babies and Children's Hospital, Cleveland, Ohio.

Hyman Chai, M.D.   Assistant Professor of Medicine, University of Colorado Health Sciences Center; Senior Staff Physician, National Jewish Hospital and Research Center, National Asthma Center, Denver, Colorado.

Gerd J. A. Cropp, M.D., Ph.D.   Professor of Pediatrics, State University of New York at Buffalo; Director, Children's Lung Center, Children's Hospital of Buffalo, Buffalo, New York.

Carl F. Doershuk, M.D.   Professor of Pediatrics, Case Western Reserve University; Director of Pediatric Pulmonary Division, Rainbow Babies and Children's Hospital, Cleveland, Ohio.

Elliot Ellis, M.D.   Professor of Pediatrics, State University of New York at Buffalo; Chairman, Division of Pediatrics, Children's Hospital of Buffalo, Buffalo, New York.

Avroy A. Fanaroff, M.D.   Professor of Pediatrics, Case Western Reserve University; Director, Division of Neonatology, Rainbow Babies and Children's Hospital, Cleveland, Ohio.

Barry Fisher, M.D.   Director of Sleep Disorders Center, Associate Director of Pediatric Pulmonary Medicine, Associate Director of Cystic Fibrosis Center, Phoenix Children's Hospital, a Division of Good Samaritan Medical Center, Phoenix, Arizona.

Stanley P. Galant, M.D.   Clinical Professor of Pediatrics, University of California, Irvine, California.

Christopher G. Green, M.D.   Pediatric Pulmonary Fellow and Instructor in Pediatrics, Case Western Reserve University and Rainbow Babies and Children's Hospital, Cleveland, Ohio.

Michael T. Gyepes, M.D.   Clinical Professor of Radiology, University of California, Los Angeles; Radiologist, Miller Children's Hospital Medical Center of Long Beach, California.

Zack Haddad, M.D.   Professor of Pediatrics, University of Southern California; Director of Allergy and Immunology, Los Angeles County USC Medical Center, Los Angeles, California.

Richard F. Jacobs, M.D.   Fellow, Division of Infectious Diseases, Children's Orthopedic Hospital and Medical Center, University of Washington, Seattle, Washington.

Carolyn R. Kercsmar, M.D.   Instructor, Department of Pediatrics, Case Western Reserve University; Rainbow Babies and Children's Hospital, Cleveland, Ohio.

Kumar N. Kulkarni, M.D.   Clinical Instructor in Pediatrics, School of Medicine, University of Southern California; Attending Allergist, Los Angeles County USC Medical Center. Los Angeles, California.

Jack Levy, M.D.   Fellow, Division of Infectious Disease, Children's Orthopedic Hospital and Medical Center, University of Washington, Seattle, Washington.

Richard J. Martin, M.D.   Associate Professor, Case Western Reserve University and Rainbow Babies and Children's Hospital, Cleveland, Ohio.

Paul M. Mendelman, M.D.   Fellow, Division of Infectious Diseases, Children's Orthopedic Hospital and Medical Center, University of Washington, Seattle, Washington.

Eliezer Nussbaum, M.D.   Associate Professor, Department of Pediatrics, University of California, Irvine; Director, Children's Lung Center and Pediatric Intensive Care Units, Miller Children's Hospital Medical Center of Long Beach, Calfiornia.

Gary S. Rachelefsky, M.D.   Clinical Professor of Pediatrics, School of Medicine, University of California, Los Angeles, Allergy Medical Clinic, Los Angeles, California.

Sheldon C. Siegel, M.D.   Clinical Professor of Pediatrics, School of Medicine, University of California, Los Angeles; Director Allergy Medical Clinic, Los Angeles, California.

Arnold L. Smith, M.D.   Professor of Pediatrics, School of Medicine, University of Washington; Chief, Division of Infectious Disease, Children's Orthopedic Hospital and Medical Center, Seattle, Washington.

William T. Speck, M.D.   Professor and Chairman of the Department of Pediatrics, Case Western Reserve University and Rainbow Babies and Children's Hospital, Cleveland, Ohio.

Terrence L. Stull, M.D.   Acting Assistant Professor, University of Washington, Seattle, Washington.

Kathy E. Wedig, M.D.   Pediatrics Fellow, Case Western Reserve University and Rainbow Babies and Children's Hospital, Cleveland, Ohio.

Miles M. Weinberger, M.D.   Professor of Pediatrics, University of Iowa; Chairman, Pediatric Allergy and Pulmonary Division, University of Iowa Hospitals, Iowa City, Iowa.

Paul F. Wehrle, M.D.   Hastings Professor of Pediatrics, School of Medicine, University of Southern California; Director of Pediatrics, Los Angeles County MSC Medical Center, Los Angeles, California.

Christopher B. Wilson, M.D.   Assistant Professor of Pediatrics, Division of Infectious Diseases, School of Medicine, University of Washington, Seattle, Washington.

Pediatric Respiratory Disorders

Clinical Approaches

Epidemiology of Acute Respiratory Tract Infections

Carolyn M. Kercsmar
William T. Speck

Acute infections of the respiratory tract inflict substantial morbidity on the pediatric population. A child normally develops between 6 and 8 upper respiratory tract infections per year. Moreover, lower respiratory tract infections produce considerable mortality in infants and children under 5 years of age with bronchiolitis, and pneumonia, the infectious diseases most often responsible for respiratory deaths. Although many different bacteria cause both upper and lower respiratory tract infections, viruses and *Mycoplasma* organisms produce a majority of these illnesses. Whatever the cause, it is often difficult to conclusively identify a pathogen in pediatric respiratory tract infections. Adequate specimens for culture, such as sputum, tracheal aspirates, or lung fluid, frequently are not readily available. Knowledge of the epidemiology of acute respiratory tract infections therefore can provide valuable information to aid in establishing diagnoses and understanding pathogenesis.

This chapter summarizes the epidemiology of those respiratory pathogens responsible for the greatest morbidity and mortality in the pediatric population.

VIRUSES

Respiratory Syncytial Virus

Although first recognized as an agent of disease at the turn of the century, respiratory syncytial virus (RSV) was not differentiated from measles, influenza, and pertussis until 1940. Today it remains the single most important viral respiratory pathogen in infants and young children. RSV is the major cause of bronchiolitis and pneumonia in the first few years of life. Moreover, the most severe disease occurs in infants less than 6 months of age. Although illness is relatively uncommon during the first 4 weeks of life, sporadic outbreaks producing atypical, but severe, neonatal disease do occur.

A member of the paramyxovirus group, RSV is an enveloped RNA virus. The organism is extremely thermolabile and deteriorates rapidly at 55°C. Although the virus readily grows and produces syncytia in HeLa and Hep-2 cells, the cell culture lines vary in susceptibility to infection. Moreover, with time certain cell lines lose their ability to become infected. Recovery attempts therefore may be hampered by such technical difficulties.

Clinical Manifestations

Bronchiolitis accounts for the majority of RSV-induced illness. The syndrome consists of fever, cough, tachypnea, and dyspnea. Affected infants exhibit hyperinflated chest, occasional rales, and wheezing. Although the illness is usually self-limited and resolves in several days, severe pneumonia may ensue. Alternatively, pneumonia may occur as a separate entity; occasionally destructive disease (bronchiolitis obliterans) develops with attendant respiratory failure. RSV infection may also cause croup, but is a relatively uncommon etiologic agent for the disease. In the Washington, D.C. study, 4 percent of patients with croup yielded RSV.[1] Upper respiratory tract infection is the primary manifestation of RSV in older children and adults. Otitis media may also arise secondary to RSV. Asymptomatic infections rarely occur.

Epidemiology

Incidence. RSV epidemics occur yearly with onset in midwinter and persistence through early spring. Intervals between outbreaks often alternate between long (13–16 months) and short (7–12 months) duration.[1] The virus exhibits greatest activity during late December through early April and is notoriously absent in August and September.[1] Outbreaks often last from 1 to 5 months.

Age. RSV spares few age groups, with infections occurring in patients from ages 3 weeks through adulthood. The majority of infections occur in individuals ages 3 weeks to 24 months; infants less than 1 year have the highest infection rate (29 percent).[2,3] Although the younger age groups (less than 2 years) have the highest frequency of infection, susceptibility to and incidence of RSV disease remains significant at all ages. Antibody to RSV is detectable in the serum of 95 percent of 5-year-old children; virtually 100 percent of adults have serologic evidence of RSV infection.

In families with a single infected individual, 46 percent of all members subsequently become infected.[2] Again, the highest rate is in infants under 1 year of age, however, no index cases are found in this age group. Consequently, older siblings (greater than 1 year) are the most probable introducers of virus into families. Children less than 2 years of age shed the virus for significantly longer periods of time than do older children. This phenomenon may then contribute to the high infection rate seen in families with young children.

Reinfections are common in children and adults. Henderson et al.[4] suggest that single infections produce a small but statistically significant protective immunity which lasts up to 1 year. Further infections appear to offer cumulative resistance to, as well as decreased severity of, subsequent illness. It is difficult, however, to identify the effects of increasing age independent of immunity on the pattern of the disease; both parameters appear to play a role.

Although presumed to be uncommon, RSV infection can readily occur in neonates. Because the appearance may be atypical, the disease often is missed. In a recent study[5] 28 percent of 82 neonates became infected with RSV during hospitalization at the time of a community outbreak. Of this group, 87 percent were under 1 month of age, and 14 percent were less than 3 weeks old. Although 61 percent of the infants exhibited signs of respiratory tract infection, 35 percent of patients had only nonspecific findings, such as lethargy, poor appetite, irritability, and apnea. Such nonspecific signs occurred more frequently in infants younger than 3 weeks). These differences were not related to prematurity or underlying disease. Mortality associated with RSV infections in this series was 17 percent.

Sex. The infection rate in males is slightly greater than that in females as reported in some series. These differences are small, exist primarily in infancy, and are probably not significant. When only minor illness or inapparent infection is considered, there is indeed no difference in attack rate between the sexes. Severe bronchiolitis and other lower tract diseases, that is, diseases severe enough to seek medical attention, do exhibit a 2:1 male/female predominance.

Morbidity and mortality. RSV infections result in bronchiolitis, croup, pneumonia, and upper respiratory tract illness. Infants less than 2 years of age make up the population that develops bronchiolitis and pneumonia; approximately 1 in 100 of such patients will require hospitalization. Mortality for hospitalized infants under 1 year of age is 1–3 percent. Neonatal mortality may be much higher. Adults infected with RSV largely suffer upper respiratory tract symptoms. When compared to adults with rhinovirus illness, those with RSV have significantly more discomfort and time lost from work.[3]

Socioeconomic factors. The role of socioeconomic factors on the development and severity of RSV illness remains somewhat unclear. In some populations more severe illness occurred in low-income and rural families.[3] In other studies, however, regarding family size, crowding, and education,[2] households that had no RSV infection did not differ significantly from those who did.

Nosocomial infection. RSV is a severe and major cause of respiratory tract infection among hospitalized infants and neonates. Nosocomial infections largely reflect the pattern of disease seen in the community with respect to frequency, season, and age. In one series, 32 percent of the people in contact with the hospitalized infant developed illness; 42 percent of the hospital staff caring for the infants acquired RSV.[6] Masks and gowns were not useful in controlling spread of the disease when other measures, such as good handwashing and cohorting of staff and patients, were used. Transmission occurred largely via large-particle aerosols; contaminated secretions acquired during close contact with infected infants were either transmitted to other common surfaces or self-innoculated through contact with the eyes or nose. In addition to handwashing, masks may be of value if infected personnel must care for noninfected infants.

Parainfluenza Virus

Parainfluenza viruses were recognized in 1954 as causes of upper and lower respiratory tract disease in children. A member of the paramyxovirus group, this relatively large RNA-containing virus occurs in at least four serologic types, all of which cause illness in humans. Types 1 and 3 are the most frequent serotypes associated with human disease. Type 2 infections produce much milder and less frequent clinical manifestations, whereas type 4 infections are largely asymptomatic or cause only trivial illness. Although the virus is readily recovered from the human pharynx, its actual modes of transmission are unknown. The virus is stable in aerosolized preparations, but the role of such small-particle aerosols in addition to direct contact with secretions is unclear. Isolation of virus from secretions may be achieved on human or monkey kidney cell cultures.

Clinical Manifestations

Infections with parainfluenza virus are rarely asymptomatic, and a high proportion involve the lower respiratory tract. Upper respiratory tract infections often include fever and laryngeal or tracheal involvement. Type 1 parainfluenza is largely responsible for most cases of croup. In slightly older age groups (greater than 4–5 years) this serotype produces tracheobronchitis and febrile upper respiratory tract illness. Type 2 infections cause the same symptoms; however, the illnesses are generally less severe and infrequent. Parainfluenza type 3 infection resembles RSV in that is causes a significant proportion of bronchiolitis and pneumonia in infants, whereas in older

children, croup and tracheobronchitis are common manifestations. Type 4 infection results in an asymptomatic state or a mild afebrile illness such as rhinitis, hoarseness, or pharyngitis.

Epidemiology

Incidence. Parainfluenza is largely a ubiquitous virus; however, among the serotypes some seasonal variation does exist. Type 1 activity predominates in the autumn; large outbreaks occur usually every other year (even numbered). Epidemics of type 2 parainfluenza also peak in the fall months of odd-numbered years; these outbreaks are much less predictable, however. Type 3 virus is essentially endemic and may persist in the community even during epidemics of other agents. All serotypes of parainfluenza virus account for 8–12 percent of pediatric respiratory tract illnesses.

Age. Parainfluenza viruses produce disease in all age groups. Type 1 tends to predominate in slightly older children and along with type 2 is the major cause of croup in children ages 8–30 months.[3] Primary infection with type 3 has a peak occurrence in infancy; up to 50 percent of infants less than 12 months of age will have type-specific serum antibodies.[7] Types 1 and 2 occur predominantly in older infants and children 6–9 years of age.[7,8]

All types of parainfluenza spread readily among family members. In the Seattle Virus Watch study, 41 percent of all members of families in which at least one person shed virus developed seroconversion.[7] The highest infection rates occurred in children under 6 years (84 percent).

Sex. In children less than 6 years of age with types 1 and 2 infection, almost twice as many patients are males. The male predominance applies only to illnesses severe enough for the family to seek medical attention. There is no appreciable difference between the sexes for minor illnesses due to these serotypes or to infections occurring in children over age 6 years. Parinfluenza type 3 produces identical infection rates in both sexes. Similarly, more young boys develop serious croup secondary to types 1 and 2 parainfluenza than do girls.

Morbidity and mortality. Most infectious croup is self-limited and resolves within 5 days. Illness may be protracted to as long as 10–14 days. Parainfluenza infection that spreads to the lower respiratory tract accounts for increased hospitalization. Croup-associated deaths are rare and occur almost entirely as a result of complete airway occlusion or tracheostomy complications.

Nosocomial infection. Hospital-acquired parainfluenza infection poses a threat to hospitalized infants and children. Nosocomial infection due to the virus is less common than that associated with RSV and is often asymptomatic.

Adenovirus

Adenoviruses are nonenveloped, double-stranded, DNA-containing organisms that exist in numerous different serotypes. Infectious particles are readily recovered from the conjunctiva, throat, and stool; recovery rates from asymptomatic and ill patients are often similar. Transmission occurs by aerosolized small and large droplets. Portals of entry include the nose, conjunctiva, throat, and gastrointestinal tract.

Clinical Manifestations

Mild upper respiratory tract infections, with or without fever constitute the majority of illness produced by adenoviruses. More specifically, types 1, 2, 3, 5, 6 and 7 are frequently isolated from children with such infections.[9] The triad of conjunctivitis, pharyngitis, and fever comprises a common adenovirus syndrome, which may occur in epidemic proportions. Croup is rarely secondary to adenovirus infection. In one large series adenovirus was isolated from up to 10 percent of children with mild pneumonia, but its role as the sole etiologic agent remained questionable. Although bronchiolitis is also infrequently caused by adenovirus, this pathogen may be associated with bronchiolitis fibrosa obliterans or bronchiectasis. Nearly all the cases of severe progressive adenoviral pneumonia occur as outbreaks in select populations. Polynesians from New Zealand, native Canadian Indians, and Scandinavians constitute the most commonly affected peoples. Types 7 and 21 are the usual agents responsible for destructive pneumonia or bronchiolitis.

Epidemiology

Incidence. Adenoviruses cause between 2–10 percent of all respiratory illnesses in children; actual incidences vary widely among studies. The highest rates of virus recovery occur in upper respiratory syndromes, pharyngitis, and bronchitis.

Surveillance studies show that adenovirus is present in the community in nearly all months. It is most prevalent during November through July; epidemics occur in winter, spring, and early summer. Warm-weather outbreaks are usually secondary to public swimming pool contamination with strains producing pharyngoconjunctival fever and epidemic keratoconjunctivitis.

Age. Most newborns have both complement-fixing and neutralizing antibodies, the latter of which appear protective. As with many respiratory illnesses, the highest infection rate is in infants 7–12 months old. Children 3–18 months old are the most susceptible to destructive pneumonia and bronchiolitis. Children ages 1–5 years living in closed environments (e.g., day-care centers or boarding schools) demonstrate a greater than average predilection for adenovirus illness. By age 5 years 70–80 percent of children have neutralizing antibodies to types 1 and 2, whereas over 50 percent have antibodies to type 5. Infection rates diminish precipitously by young adulthood, in which only 1 percent of all respiratory tract infections are associated with adenovirus.[9] No differences in infection rates between the sexes are noted.

Influenza

Influenza provides perhaps the ultimate paradigm of an epidemic disease. The virus produces illness of all magnitudes, with localized, nationwide, and global outbreaks. Sporadic occurrences are rare. Although the mortality from influenza is now greatly diminished, it continues to inflict considerable morbidity.

Influenza is a negative-stranded RNA virus. It occurs in three serotypes: A, B, and C. Types A and B are the most important causes of disease in humans; all types cause hemagglutination.

Clinical Manifestations

Influenza A characteristically produces abdominal pain, nausea, vomiting, and a dry hacking cough within 1–4 days of exposure. The illness is usually of sudden onset and accompanied by fever. In younger children, several manifestations of respiratory illness occur, such as laryngotracheobronchitis, bronchiolitis, pneumonia, and upper respiratory tract infections. The latter often is characterized by fever, a cough, a clear nasal discharge, pharyngitis, and irritability. In infants the infection may simulate bacterial sepsis. Complicating bacterial infections, such as pneumonia, sinusitis, or otitis media may occur in approximately 10 percent of all influenza infections. These secondary infections usually occur during the early convalescent stage. The most common secondary bacterial pathogens are the pneumococcus and staphylococcus.

Influenza B more typically produces milder illness; many children with serologic evidence of infection remain asymptomatic.[10] Serious morbidity is rare in children, and less than 10 percent of all infected patients will have signs of lower respiratory tract disease. Influenza B probably contributes little to the incidence of pneumonia.

Epidemiology

Incidence. Influenza epidemics exhibit distinct seasonality. In temperate climates influenza outbreaks occur almost exclusively in the winter months with peak rates late in January. Epidemics typically extend over 4–6 weeks. The infection is spread via contaminated large droplets and fine aerosols. The secondary attack rate among family members approaches 30 percent.[11]

Age. As many as 15–25 percent of all school-age children sustain infection during epidemics of influenza A. Adolescents account for up to 50 percent of the affected childhood population.[11] Although rates of pneumonia during influenza epidemics are highest in children less than 5 years of age, it is difficult to assign a causative role solely to influenza. Changes in the incidence of pneumonia due to influenza could easily be masked by the high number of pneumonic illnesses caused by RSV and parainfluenza in this age range.[12] Nevertheless, during epidemics, respiratory diseases associated with influenza may exceed those caused by all others. Persons with underlying chronic illness, such as pulmonary, cardiac, and neuromuscular diseases, are at greatest risk for developing severe life-threatening disease.

Sex. Infection rates are similar in both sexes over the age range of 5–60 years. In those less than 5 years and greater than 60 years, however, male predominance in susceptibility occurs.

Morbidity and mortality. Previously healthy children living in modern societies rarely die as a result of influenza. Certain subgroups, such as those with chronic lung, cardiac, or neuromuscular diseases, incur considerable morbidity and mortality. Individuals with such underlying conditions warrant immunization yearly with influenza vaccine. Although immunity to influenza A involves interplay of humoral, secretory, and cell-mediated mechanisms, vaccination can produce an adequate protective antibody response in as high as 80 percent of the recipients. Approximately 10 days are required after vaccination to achieve protective titers. Amantadine hydrochloride offers approximately 70 percent efficacy in the prevention of influenza A infections when administered prophylactically. Moreover, if the drug is taken within 48 hours of onset of symptoms, the resulting illness is both ameliorated and shortened in duration. Amantadine has no effect on influenza B.

MYCOPLASMA INFECTIONS

Mycoplasma pneumoniae is a human pathogen belonging to the group of smallest free-living microorganisms. These slow-growing microbes lack cell walls and require sterol for growth. *M. pneumoniae* remains the only mycoplasma clearly documented to cause respiratory tract disease; *M. hominis* and *Ureaplasma urealyticum* are suspect respiratory pathogens.

M. pneumoniae spreads relatively slowly in both closed populations and open communities. Contaminated small-particle aerosols or large droplet secretions constitute the modes of transmission. Only symptomatic individuals appear capable of effective spread. Incubation times remain uncertain. Experimentally induced illness may occur in 10 days, whereas community-acquired disease may take up to 3 weeks to emerge.

Clinical Manifestations

Most infections with *M. pneumoniae* produce fairly insignificant illness, such as upper respiratory tract infection or tracheobronchitis. Cough, headache, sore throat, and malaise are frequent. Nevertheless, the symptoms are rarely severe enough to cause the patient to seek medical attention. Bullous myringitis and other nonspecific ear complaints occur in approximately 12–20 percent of infected patients. Clinically detectable pneumonia occurs in 3–15 percent of all infected persons; however, less than 2 percent are severe enough to require hospitalization. Severe pneumonia with attendant respiratory distress, pleural effusion, or abscess formation develops on rare occasions.

Clinical studies indicate that a substantial percentage of *M. pneumoniae* infections cause no apparent disease. In a family study, asymptomatic *Mycoplasma* infections predominated in younger age groups, that is, 27 percent of those less than 5 years old and only 8 percent of those greater than 15 years remained asymptomatic.[13] When children in a day-care setting were examined, 74 percent of those with serologic evidence of infection had no signs of respiratory disease.[14]

Epidemiology

Incidence. *M. pneumoniae* usually is endemic with occasional superimposed epidemics. Such outbreaks may be protracted many months before subsiding to endemic levels. Infection rates vary from 2–35 percent in endemic and epidemic periods respectively.[15]

Age. School-age children (ages 5–9 years) account for the majority of primary infections. The highest incidence of pneumonia, 1 in 10 of those infected, also occurs in children 5–9 years old. Individuals 10–14 years have the next highest pneumonia rates, with adults over 40 years the lowest. Although children under 5 years old are commonly believed to have only infrequent occurrences of *M. pneumoniae* pneumonia, they develop pneumonia at a rate twice that of adults and half that of the school-age group. Infants under 6 months rarely develop *Mycoplasma* infection.

Sex. Males experience more *M. pneumoniae* infection than females in the age group under 5 years. Little difference in sex predominance is seen otherwise.

Morbidity and mortality. *M. pneumoniae* infections are generally benign, self-limited, and have minimal morbidity. Nevertheless, the disease can be severe in some instances. More specifically children with underlying illnesses, such as sickle cell anemia, asthma, and chronic respiratory disease, may be at greater risk for serious illness. Data are as yet equivocal, however.

BACTERIA

Legionnaire's Disease

During the summer of 1976, nearly 200 individuals attending a convention in the Philadelphia Bellevue Stratford Hotel developed a pneumonic illness. The disease had many systemic manifestations and was fatal in 29 patients. The etiologic agent was identified 17 months later as a unique gram-negative bacterium, *Legionella pneumophila*. This 2–3μ long aerobic coccobacillus grows on enriched Mueller-Hinton agar. The organism exists in at least four serotypes and occurs naturally in soil and water. Current estimates place *L. pneumophila* as the cause of up to 1 percent of all adult pneumonias; the microbe also produces opportunistic infection in immunocompromised hosts. Little is yet known, however, regarding its etiologic role in childhood pneumonias.

Clinical Manifestations

The primary manifestation of *Legionella* infection is a diffuse pneumonitis. Within 2–7 days after exposure, the patient develops a cough and fever. Sputum production or hemoptysis occurs in approximately half of the patients.

Physical examination reveals diffuse rales and rhonchi; a chest roentgenogram shows alveolar or interstitial infiltrates progressing to lobar consolidation. Numerous systemic manifestations occur, including diarrhea, hepatic dysfunction, hematuria, proteinuria, and neurologic deterioration. Mortality in adults is usually approximately 15 percent. *L. pneumophila* has been associated with pneumonia in pediatric patients, but evidence of systemic involvement is lacking.[16,17]

Epidemiology

Incidence. The true incidence of *Legionella* infection in children remains uncertain. The number of documented cases thus far reportd remains extremely small. Diagnosis of *Legionella* infection requires isolation of the organism, direct immunofluorescence, or a fourfold or greater rise in antibody titer to greater than or equal to 128. A single serum titer of greater than or equal to 256 provides presumptive evidence of infection at an undetermined time. Several serologic surveys suggest that a large number of children may experience asymptomatic infection with *Legionella* organisms. In one series, up to 52 percent of children less than 4 years old showed a greater than fourfold titer rise; however, no serologic response occurred in conjunction with acute illness.[18] Such responses may indicate past infection with *Legionella* organisms or some closely related or cross-reacting organism. Only a mild upper respiratory tract illness presumably occurs in such cases.

Age and Sex. In adults, *L. pneumophila* most commonly affects males in their middle fifties. In the limited experience in children, age and sex have no apparent role.

Morbidity and mortality. Fatalities in the pediatric age group have not yet been reported for Legionnaire's disease. Most infections appear to cause only mild illness. Immunocompromised patients may be susceptible to more fulminant disease, as are smokers and those who consume alcohol.

Pertussis

Pertussis was a major cause of childhood morbidity and mortality in the United States at the turn of the century. As many as 450 of every 100,000 affected infants less than 1 year old died of the disease. The incidence of pertussis declined spontaneously in the 1930s, but introduction of pertussis vaccines during the 1940s probably contributed to the further dramatic decrease. Although pertussis continues to be a major health problem in certain parts of the world, it currently accounts for less than 1 death per 100,000 infants in North America.

Bordetella pertussis is a small, fastidious gram-negative rod. It requires special media and handling to recover it from nasopharyngeal secretions. Under optimal circumstances the organism is recovered in only 50–60 percent of the patients. This pathogen is most prevalent in secretions during the first week of illness. Other pathogens, such as *B. parapertussis* and adenovirus types, 1, 2, and 3, can occasionally produce an illness clinically similar to pertussis.

Clinical Manifestations

Typical pertussis occurs in three phases. After a 6–20 day incubation period, the catarrhal stage begins. During this phase the patient develops a mild fever, rhinorrhea, conjunctival infection, and some sneezing. The paroxysmal stage ensues

1–2 weeks later. During this phase, paroxysmal episodes of severe coughing begin. The patient is usually afebrile unless this phase is associated with pneumonia or atelectasis. When pneumonia occurs, it is either a primary infection or secondary to a bacterial pathogen. Within 1–4 weeks, the convalescent stage follows; the cough subsides and the illness resolves.[19]

Epidemiology

Incidence. Pertussis is endemic with no seasonal preference. Epidemics do occur, however, and attack rates may reach 100 percent in susceptible populations.

Several thousand cases per year are reported in the United States. Mortality approximates 0.003 deaths/1000 children under 1 year of age.[20] Immunity after infection with *B. pertussis* appears to be complete and persistent. There are few, if any, asymptomatic infections, and no known carrier state exists.

Age. All age groups are susceptible to pertussis, but the greatest incidence is among infants and small children.

Sex. As opposed to many other respiratory tract infections, pertussis affects substantially more females than males.

Morbidity and Mortality. Pertussis produces significant illness in both adults and children. Mortality is highest in infancy; over 70 percent of all deaths occur in those under 1 year of age. Both erythromycin and ampicillin are effective against *B. pertussis*. Neither antibiotic shortens the duration of the paroxysmal stage, however. Erythromycin may eliminate nasopharyngeal carriage and shorten or terminate the catarrhal stage.[20]

Prevention is the ultimate "treatment" for pertussis. Although vaccines have been in use since the 1930s, controversy as to their efficacy still exists. Vaccines are made from whole killed organisms and vary substantially from lot to lot. Immunity is incomplete at best and probably not of lifelong duration. Side effects of the vaccine are common and consist of transient fever and irritability; more severe but less frequent problems such as prolonged crying, drowsiness, and convulsions also occur.[20] Nevertheless, the vaccine appears responsible in large part for the substantial reduction in the number of annual cases, and the benefits of administration far outweigh the risks.

Chlamydia Infections

Shortly after the turn of the century the first observations were made of intracytoplasmic inclusion bodies in conjuctival cells from patients with trachoma. Further investigation identified these structures as microorganisms of the genus *Chlamydia*. Although these small, obligate intracellular parasites were originally believed to be viruses, several characteristics indicated that they are bacteria. *Chlamydia* organisms have a cell wall, contain RNA and DNA, reproduce by binary fission, and are killed by antimicrobial agents. Unlike bacteria, however, *Chlamydia* organisms replicate only intracellularly and must commandeer the host cell's synthetic machinery (ATP) for its own metabolic needs.

The genus *Chlamydia* contains two species, *C. trachomatis* and *C. psittaci*. The latter is a sulfonamide-resistant pathogen in which animals are the principal host. It produces disease in humans only as zoonoses, such as psittacosis. *C. trachomatis* exists in several serotypes, is susceptible to sulfonamides, and produces illness primarily in humans.

Clinical Manifestations

C. trachomatis produces inclusion conjunctivitis, trachoma, genital tract infection (including lymphogranuloma venereum), and pneumonitis in infants. The latter is the primary respiratory illness caused by *C. trachomatis*. Infants with this syndrome typically are between 3 and 12 weeks of age and gradually develop an afebrile illness associated with congestion and a prominent staccato cough. Physical examination reveals mild respiratory distress with tachypnea and scattered rales. A chest roentgenogram is characterized by hyperinflation and bilateral interstitial infiltrates. Laboratory investigations frequently show eosinophilia (greater than $400/mm^3$) and elevated serum immunoglobulins, notably IgG and IgM. Although the pneumonia is not typically life threatening, its course may be protracted.

Epidemiology

Incidence. Pneumonia caused by *Chlamydia* organisms is acquired perinatally by passing through an infected birth canal. Chlamydial infection of the uterine cervix occurs in from 2 to 18 percent of pregnant women.[21,22] Infected women tend to be younger and unmarried as compared to uninfected women. Transmission rates ranging from 23 to 70 percent have been reported. When large series of infants were examined and recovery of the organism from the conjunctivae or nasopharynx was considered evidence of infection, a 28 percent infection rate was obtained.[21] If the presence of tear or serum antibodies is used to identify infection, higher rates of transmission are found.[22] A high percentage of infected infants develop conjunctivitis, as many as 95 percent in some large series.[21] Only 77 percent of infected infants develop respiratory tract diseases, however. Conjunctival infection may precede nasopharyngeal or lower respiratory tract infection but is not a prerequisite.

Age and sex. There appears to be no predisposition to infection based on sex. The age of infection, however, seems quite specific. Nearly all conjunctival infections will be detected by the time affected infants are 2 weeks old. In contrast, nasopharyngeal infections manifest later, and it is not until 6 weeks of age that most are identified. Although the majority of chlamydial infections are acquired perinatally, postnatal infection may occur through contact with contaminated secretions.

Morbidity and mortality. Pneumonia caused by *Chlamydia* organisms does not produce life-threatening illness but can cause significant morbidity. Infants often have persistent paroxysms of cough for weeks. Although treatment with erythromycin may shorten the course of the acute illness, recurrences are not prevented. Biopsy studies reveal that bronchial and parenchymal injuries are mild, but such damage may predispose to other future respiratory tract infections.

The optimal method of interrupting the spread of neonatal chlamydial infection remains unclear. Eradication of maternal genital tract carriage and the use of prophylactic conjunctival or systemic antibiotics both have limitations and require further study.

Streptococcus pneumoniae Infections

Streptococcus pneumoniae (pneumococcus) is a gram-positive lance-shaped microbe that grows aerobically. The pneumococcus exists in many different serotypes, as identified by the capsular polysaccharide present. It is this capsular material which is responsible for the virulence of the organism. Types most commonly causing childhood infections include 1, 3, 4, 6, 7, 9, 14, 18, 19, and 23.[23]

Clinical Manifestations

S. pneumoniae produces numerous illnesses in children, most frequently otitis media, bacteremia, pneumonia, and meningitis. The organism causes the majority of pediatric bacterial pneumonias in infants and older children. The incubation period is 1–3 days, and the onset of the pneumonic illness is heralded by fever, malaise, nausea, and sometimes a single shaking chill. Coughing, when present, is likely to produce greenish or rusty-colored sputum. Roentgenographic studies typically show lobar or segmental disease with consolidation of lung parenchyma. Multiple lobes are not usually involved, but pleural effusion is not uncommon. In uncomplicated pneumonia therapy with penicillin usually produces clinical improvement within 24 hours.

Epidemiology

Incidence. The best estimates suggest that the rate of pneumococcal pneumonia is approximately 1 or 2 cases a year for every 1000 individuals. It accounts for over 50 percent of all pediatric bacterial pneumonias, and the actual incidence may be much higher. Pneumonia is relatively uncommon, however, accounting in one study for less than 4 percent of all pneumococcal infections.[23] Among bacteremic patients, 25–35 percent demonstrate pneumonia.[23,24] Major peaks of illness occur in the midwinter months superimposed on a low endemic level.

Studies on carriage and acquisition of pneumococcal strains demonstrate that greater than 96 percent of all children acquire at least one type by 24 months of age.[25] The mean age of acquisition is 6 months, with a second strain most typically noted in the ensuing 6 months. Infection often follows acquisition of a new strain, although prolonged carriage of a given serotype rarely accounts for illness. Children with older siblings or viral upper respiratory tract illness more readily acquire pneumococcal infections. There is no evidence of epidemic spread, however, since clusters of illness produced by the same serotype are not noted.

Age and sex. Most pneumococcal infections occur in children under 2 years of age. Although the disease strikes those under 5 years of age most frequently, pneumonia affects a broad age group. Males appear to be infected slightly more often than females.

Morbidity and mortality. Uncomplicated pneumonia responds readily to penicillin therapy without incurring prolonged morbidity. Penicillin-resistant pneumococci do occur but as yet remain most infrequent. Pneumococcal pleural effusions rarely require drainage. Multiple lobe involvement heralds a poorer prognosis, however. Additional risk factors associated with more severe disease include bacteremia, underlying illness with splenic dysfunction, leukopenia, extremes of age, and infection with serotype 3.

Haemophilus influenzae Infections

Haemophilus influenzae is a small pleomorphic gram-negative rod that grows aerobically. Many serotypes based on the capsular carbohydrate are known. Nearly all serious *H. influenzae* infections are produced by type B, a strain capable of producing β-lactamase.

Clinical Manifestations

H. influenzae produces a multitude of childhood illnesses, including otitis media, bacteremia, meningitis, and epiglottitis. Although pneumonia was previously believed to be an uncommon entity, it is now recognized with increasing frequency. Pneumonia caused by *H. influenza* is often indistinguishable from other bacterial pneumonias, particularly those of pneumococcal origin. Pneumonia caused by *Haemophilus* organisms begins with fever, tachypnea, and cough after an incubation period of slightly greater than 72 hours. Roentgenographic findings are nonspecific, and segmental consolidation in one or more lobes is a common feature. Pleural effusions are not rare and exist in 40–75 percent of the cases. Children with *H. influenzae* pneumonia often have additional systemic manifestations of the disease, most notably otitis media and meningitis.[26] Although epiglottitis is a frequent result of *H. influenzae* infection, it rarely occurs concurrently with pneumonia. Bacteremia is present in most patients with pneumonia or epiglottitis.

Epidemiology

Incidence. The actual frequency of *H. influenzae* pneumonia is unknown, but it approximates 15 percent of all systemic *H. influenzae* infections.[27] Although most studies indicate that type B is responsible for under 10 percent of all pediatric pneumonias, some series report an incidence of 30–50 percent.[26,28] Epiglottitis occurs slightly more frequently than pneumonia.

Most *H. influenzae* infections occur in the early winter (November to December) and spring.

Nasopharyngeal carriage is not uncommon among children, with as many as 50 percent affected in some series.[27] Although carriage does not appear to predispose to infection, it does contribute to spread of disease. Children in younger age groups (less than 5 years) are the most susceptible. Antibiotic therapy for eradication of the carrier state or prophylaxis against disease development remains controversial. Rifampin, 20 mg/kg as a single daily dose for approximately 4 days, offers some promise; subsequent development of resistant strains or recolonization may be a problem.

Age. The majority of patients with *H. influenzae* pneumonia are under 2 years of age, and greater than 80 percent are under 4 years.[28] Epiglottitis affects slightly older children, with the average age of incidence being 4 years; the disease is not uncommon in the 6- to 8-year-old range.

Sex. Males develop *H. influenzae* pneumonia almost twice as frequently as females. There is no appreciable male/female predominance in the incidence of epiglottitis.

Morbidity and mortality. Pneumonia caused by *Haemophilus* organisms largely resolves without sequelae when treated with appropriate antibiotics. Unfortunately, when drug therapy for *H. influenzae* infections is necessary, it may be challenging. Ampicillin-resistant strains account for greater than 10 percent of all isolates, and chloramphenicol resistance has also been reported. Nevertheless, chloramphenicol should be used when *H. influenzae* is suspected. Additionally other organ system involvement should be sought; 15–17 percent of children with pneumonia also have meningitis. Infectious complications such as pericarditis may also occur. Mortality from *H. influenzae* pneumonia ranges from 5 to 7 percent.

Staphylococcus Aureus Infections

Staphylococcus aureus is a gram-positive coccus that appears as golden-colored colonies on blood agar plates. This pathogenic organism is coagulase positive and ferments mannitol; the cell wall has ribital techoic acid, a compound to which serum antibodies may be formed.

Clinical Manifestations

Normal individuals harbor *S. aureus* in the nares, with as many as 20–40 percent of adults serving as asymptomatic carriers. Although the *Staphylococcus* organism can cause a multitude of disease states, the primary respiratory illness is pneumonia. The illness is characterized initially by nonspecific symptoms such as irritability, anorexia, gastrointestinal upset, and fever. As the disease progresses, the patient appears toxic and develops a productive cough and dyspnea. A rapid deterioration may follow development of pleuritic involvement. Chest roentgenograms reveal either diffuse or localized infiltrate; segmental involvement is not typical. Pneumatoceles and a pyopneumothorax occur frequently in pediatric patients.

Epidemiology

Incidence. Staphylococcal pneumonia is the result of two different mechanisms. Primary pneumonias presumably arise via aspiration of contaminated upper airway secretions. Once infection is established in the bronchi, rapid extension to the periphery of the lung ensues. Previous viral infections, particularly influenza, predispose older patients and less frequently infants to staphylococcal invasion. The incidence in this continent of such primary infections has declined in recent years. Since the actual number of staphylococcal infections has increased, the reasons for the decline in pneumonia remain somewhat obscure. Although staphylococcal pneumonia has been reported to account for up to 15 percent of all patients hospitalized with bacterial pneumonias, the incidence is generally less than 10 percent.[28] Most infections are acquired during hospitalizations.[29] Bacteremia occurs in only 20–25 percent of patients.

Secondary, or bacteremic, pneumonia arises as a result of metastatic spread of *Staphylococcus* infection from a previously identified site. Such disseminated disease is uncommon in otherwise healthy children; those who are chronically ill or immunosuppressed have a greater susceptibility.

Age and sex. The highest incidence of primary staphylococcal pneumonia is in children under 2 years of age. Moreover, the majority of cases occur in infants less than 6 months.[30] Bacteremic pneumonia affects a much wider age group; most patients with disseminated staphylococcal disease are older children and adolescents. There is no difference in infection rate between the sexes.

Morbidity and mortality. Staphylococcal pneumonia carried an 80–90 percent mortality in the preantibiotic era. The appropriate use of antistaphylococcal penicillins combined with vigorous medical-surgical management has lowered the mortality to approximately 10–30 percent. Although chest roentgenographic abnormalities are often profound (pyopneumothorax and pneumatoceles) nearly all children who survive regain normal lung function.[31]

REFERENCES

1. Kim HW, et al: Epidemiology of RSV infection in Washington, D.C. *Am J Epidemiol* 98:216, 1973.
2. Hall C, et al: RSV infections within families. *N Engl J Med* 294:414, 1976.
3. Glezen PW, Denny FW: Epidemiology of acute lower respiratory disease in children. *N Engl J Med* 288:498, 1973.
4. Henderson FW, et al: Respiratory syncytial virus infections, re-infections and immunity: a prospective longitudinal study in young children. *N Engl J Med* 300:530, 1979.
5. Hall CB, et al: Neonatal RSV infection. *N Engl J Med* 300:393, 1979.
6. Hall CB, Douglas RG Sr: Nosocomial RSV infections. *Am J Dis Child* 135:512, 1981.
7. Cooney MK, Fox JP, Hall CE: The Seattle virus watch: VI. Observations of infections with an illness due to parainfluenza, mumps and respiratory syncytial viruses and *Mycoplasma pneumoniae. Am J Edidemiol* 101:532, 1975.
8. Monto AS, Cavallaro JJ: The Teaneck study of respiratory illness. *Am J Epidemiol* 94:280, 1971.
9. Brandt CD, Kim HW, Vargosko AJ, et al: Infections in 18,000 infants and children in a controlled study of respiratory tract disease: I. Adenovirus pathogenicity in relation to serologic type and illness syndrome. *Am J Epidemiol* 90:484, 1964.
10. Klein JD, Collier AM, Glezen WP: An influenza B epidemic among children in day care. *Pediatrics* 58:340, 1976.
11. Foy HM, Cooney, MK, Allan I: Longitudinal studies of types A and B influenza among Seattle schoolchildren and families: 1968–1974. *J Infect Dis* 134:362, 1976.
12. Foy HM, Cooney MK, Allan I, et al: Rates of pneumonia during influenza epidemics in Seattle: 1964–1975. *JAMA* 241:253, 1979.
13. Foy HM, Grayston JT, Kenny GE, et al: Epidemiology of *Mycoplasma pneumoniae* infection in families. *JAMA* 197:137, 1966.
14. Fernald GW, Collier AM, Clyde WA: Respiratory infections due to *Mycoplasma pneumoniae* in infants and children. *Pediatrics* 55:327, 1975.
15. Foy HM, Kenny GE, Cooney MK, et al: Long-term epidemiology of infections with *Mycoplasma pneumoniae. J Infect Dis* 139:681, 1979.
16. Sturm R, Staneck JL, Myers JP, et al: Pediatric Legionnaires' disease: diagnosis by direct immunofluorescent staining of sputum. *Pediatrics* 68:539, 1981.
17. Muldoon RL, Jaecker DL, Kiefer HK: Legionnaires' disease in children. *Pediatrics* 67:329, 1981.
18. Anderson RD, Lauer BA, Fraser DW, et al: Infections with *Legionell pneumophila* in children. *J Infect Dis* 143:386, 1981.
19. Olson LC: Pertussis. *Medicine* 54:427, 1975.
20. Mortimer EA: Pertussis immunization: problems, perspectives, prospects. *Hosp Pract* 80:103, 1979.
21. Heggie AD, Lumicao GG, Stuart LA, et al: *Chlamydia trachomatis* infections in mothers and infants: a prospective study. *Am J Dis Child* 135:507, 1981.
22. Frommell GT, Rothenberg R, Wang S, et al: Chlamydial infection of mothers and their infants. *J Pediatr* 95:28, 1979.
23. Grey BM, Converse GM, Dillon HC: Serotypes of *Streptococcus pneumoniae* causing disease. *J Infect Dis* 140:979, 1979.
24. Jacobs NM, Lerdkeshonsuk S, Metzger WI: Pneumococcal bacteremia in infants and children: a ten-year experience at the Cook County Hospital with special reference to the pneumococcal serotypes isolated. *Pediatrics* 64:296, 1979.
25. Gray BM, Converse GM, Dillon HC: Epidemiologic studies of *Streptococcus pneumoniae* in infants: acquisition, carriage and infection during the first 24 months of life. *J Infect Dis* 142:923, 1980.
26. Ginsberg CM, Howard JB, Nelson JD: Report of 65 cases of *Haemophilus influenzae* B pneumonia. *Pediatrics* 64:283, 1979.
27. Dajani AS, Osman BI, Therumoorthi MC: Systemic *Haemophilus influenzae* disease: an overview. *J Pediatr* 94:355, 1979.
28. Jacobs NM, Harris VJ: Acute *Haemophilus* pneumonia in childhood. *Am J Dis Child* 133:603, 1979.
29. Tuazon CV: Gram-positive pneumonias. *Medical Clin North Am* 64:343, 1980.
30. Oliver TK, Smith B, Clatworthy HW: Staphylococcal pneumonia, *Pediatr Clin North Am* 6:1043, 1959.
31. Ceruti E, Contreras J, Neira M: Staphylococcal pneumonia in childhood. *Am J Dis Child* 122:386, 1971.

2

Infantile and Childhood Asthma

Sheldon C. Siegel

Asthma is a disease characterized by increased responsiveness of the trachea and bronchi to various stimuli. It is manifested by widespread narrowing of the airways that changes in severity either spontaneously or as a result of therapy.[1] Despite the fact that the cause of this exaggerated responsiveness remains unknown, the mechanisms involved are probably the same in both children and adults. Nevertheless, a number of age-related factors (e.g., disproportionally smaller peripheral airways, increased susceptibility to viral respiratory tract infections, prognosis, differential diagnosis, and types of complications) make the diagnosis and management of bronchial asthma in infancy and childhood quite different. This chapter will feature those aspects of asthma which are characteristic in infancy and childhood.

EPIDEMIOLOGY

Although asthma is a common disease of both children and adults, its true incidence and prevalence have not been well defined. The reported prevalence rates reported vary from a low of 0.06 percent reported in the Scandinavian countries to 6.6 percent in the United States.[2] It is unlikely that the significant variations observed in the prevalence of asthma throughout the world are due to differences in environment or ethnic origins; more likely these differences are due to lack of uniform diagnostic criteria, interpretation of age of onset, and methodologic variations used in the statistics. Despite these variations, even the most conservative estimates affirm that asthma in children is common and affects all age groups. Recent studies in the United States

indicate that the prevalence for asthma in children is in the range of 5–7 percent. When children who only wheeze with infection are included, a prevalence of 14.4 percent has been reported.[3]

Asthma usually has its onset within the first few years of life. Half of childhood asthma begins before 2 years of age. Individuals developing asthma during the first two decades of life are more likely to have demonstrable allergies as etiologic factors and often have other associated atopic disorders such as allergic rhinitis and atopic dermatitis. Until puberty asthma is twice as common in boys as in girls. With increasing age there is a reversal of this trend; in the older age groups the sex ratio is even reversed.

MORBIDITY AND MORTALITY

Asthma in children is a major cause of school absenteeism, physician visits, and hospitalization. In addition to producing physical disability and debilitation, it has a disruptive effect on the child's intellectual and emotional development and quality of life and often a devastating effect on the economic and psychologic stability of the family.

It is reliably estimated that 2000 to 4000 Americans die annually from asthma. Although most of these deaths occur in adults, a significant number occur in children and young adults. These deaths are tragic in that some might have been prevented. The following factors might help identify patients who are at high risk for life-threatening asthma: (1) a history of early onset of severe asthma, especially under 1 year of age; (2)

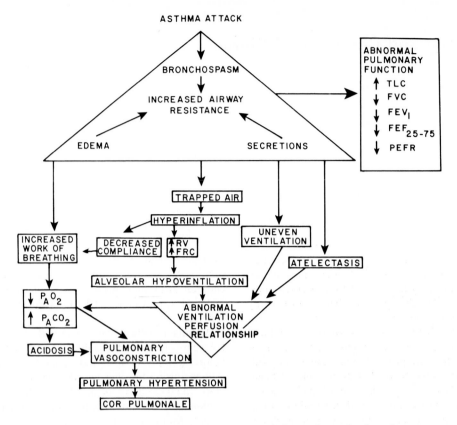

Figure 2-1. Pathophysiologic consequences of airway obstruction in asthma.

frequent bouts of wheezing, necessitating hospitalization; (3) oral or inhaled steroid dependence; (4) excessive use of adrenergic aerosols; and (5) noncompliant patients with severe asthma. Recently, an increase in sudden deaths in young patients with acute asthma in Auckland, New Zealand, was attributed to addictive toxicity of sustained-action theophylline preparations and inhaled β-agonists, which produced cardiac arrest.[4] Although some questions have been raised regarding the validity of this latter study, it does serve to emphasize that acute asthma can lead to death in young people.

PATHOPHYSIOLOGIC PROCESS

The essential disorder in asthma is widespread obstruction of the airways primarily due to bronchospasm, mucosal edema, and inspissation of viscid intraluminal secretions. Bronchospasm is the major cause of obstruction during acute attacks of asthma, whereas edema associated with inflammatory cellular infiltrates and mucus plugging play a greater role in chronic asthma and status asthmaticus. The physiologic abnormalities observed in any given patient will vary with the severity and type of airway obstruction. The abnormalities can vary from severe obstruction with alveolar hypoventilation and respiratory failure to minimal blockage in the small airways so that the patient remains essentially asymptomatic. The pathophysiologic consequences of impedance of airflow are an increased resistance to airflow, increased lung volumes (hyperinflation), and nonuniform distribution of ventilation, leading to abnormalities of gas exchange (Figure 2–1).

During an asthma attack, airway resistance is increased with a reduction in flow rates. To maintain adequate airflow and minute ventilation two compensatory mechanisms are called into play. First, accessory muscles (which increase the work of breathing) are used to achieve the necessary positive expiratory pressures and negative inspiratory pleural pressures. Second, breathing at a higher lung volume reduces airway resistance by increasing the airway diameter. As additional forces of expiration are required and hyperinflation increases, an increase in pressure surrounding the small airways causes them to be compressed and produces additional outflow obstruction.

Varying degrees of obstruction, atelectasis, and decreased compliance (greater stiffness of the lung) cause regional differences in ventilation and perfusion (uneven ventilation-perfusion ratios). Consequently, the carbon dioxide tension rises, and the oxygen tension falls in the blood perfusing the obstructed alveoli. Because of the compensatory hyperventilation and linear relationship of the carbon dioxide content to tension, the less affected alveoli are able to eliminate an increased amount of carbon dioxide. Early in acute attacks of asthma (and in most patients with chronic asthma), carbon dioxide tensions are frequently below normal. Because of the sigmoid shape of the oxygen dissociation curve, similar compensation for low blood oxygen does not occur. Very little oxygen is added to the arterial blood derived from the hyperventilated areas, resulting in arterial hypoxemia. As more airways become obstructed, the total volume of ventilation may no longer be maintained, and hypercapnia and respiratory acidosis ensue.

Both hypoxia and hypercapnia play a role in producing respiratory acidosis. The former causes metabolic acidosis by accumulation of organic acids (primarily lactic acid), whereas the latter produces respiratory acidosis by conversion of carbon dioxide to carbonic acid. The acidosis may be further complicated by other fluid and electrolyte disturbances produced by increased respiratory water loss, fever, sweating, poor intake, and vomiting.

CLASSIFICATION OF ASTHMA

Historically asthma has been classified as being either extrinsic or intrinsic or both. *Extrinsic asthma* implies that the symptoms are provoked by factors outside the body, and the term is often used to indicate an underlying allergy. *Intrinsic asthma* connotes that the symptoms are provoked by factors within the body, and this designation has been used synonymously with the term

Table 2-1 *Classification of Asthma*

- Allergic (extrinsic)

    Type I (immediate)
    Type III (immune complex mediated)

- Idiopathic (intrinsic, infectious)

- Mixed

- Aspirin induced

- Exercise induced

- Occupational

infectious, or *idiopathic, asthma.* A more reasonable classification of asthma, as shown in 2–1 is based on our present knowledge of its etiologic factors. It must be kept in mind, however, that this classification is somewhat arbitrary because the precise mechanisms of how the airways become hyperactive and symptoms are provoked have not been clearly delineated, and often multiple factors are known to precipitate symptoms. Nevertheless, the classification does serve as a framework to direct the patient's treatment in a more rational manner.

ETIOLOGY

Allergic Asthma—Type I

Allergic asthma is that type of asthma caused by an immediate-type (type I) hypersensitivity reaction to allergens. It is mediated primarily by IgE, the major antibody with reaginic activity. A subgroup of homocytotropic IgG antibodies that fixes to mast cells and releases mediators after union with specific allergens has been described, but its importance in human allergic disorders has not been clearly determined.

The majority of asthmatic children have clear-cut evidence for an underlying type I, IgE-mediated hypersensitivity. Adult-onset asthma, on the other hand, is more likely to be idiopathic. Nevertheless, it should be emphasized that even adults may have their first symptoms of allergic asthma late in life. Frequently the onset of allergic asthma is preceded or accompanied by other atopic manifestations (atopic dermatitis or allergic rhinitis). Allergic asthma is commonly caused by exposure to inhalant allergens. The most frequent offenders are pollens of grasses, weeds, and trees; mold spores and hyphae; house dust; house dust mites; and dander and secretions from animals. Foods may also be offenders, especially in children under the age of 2, but they play a decreasing role as provocative agents in the older age groups. Those foods which commonly have been reported to cause asthma are milk, eggs, peanuts, nuts, fish, shellfish, and soy. A recent study suggests that there is a tendency to "outgrow" a food sensitivity to cow's milk, eggs, and soy diagnosed during the first 2 years of life, whereas sensitivity to peanuts persists.[5] Children with a food sensitivity diagnosed at older ages by a positive food challenge and skin testing tended not to "outgrow" their food allergy.

Allergic Asthma—Type III

Type III reactions are the result of antigen-antibody complex formation with complement activation, which in turn causes a diversity of inflammatory reactions when the complexes are deposited in tissues. Classic examples of immunologic injury produced by this type of immune reaction are the Arthus reaction and serum sickness. Type III reactions have also been implicated in "late" or "delayed" asthmatic reactions (reactions occurring 2 to 6 hours after exposure to an allergen) that are blocked by corticosteroids and cromolyn sodium.[6] More recent evidence suggests that many of the delayed reactions are probably secondary to a chain of primary and secondary biochemical changes initiated by type I reactions. It has long been believed that type III reactions also play a significant role in the pathogenesis of various hypersensitivity pneumonias.[7]

Idiopathic Asthma

Idiopathic asthma (intrinsic, infectious) is a form of the disease in which no definite cause can be identified, and there is no convincing relationship between the allergy and respiratory symptoms. In some instances attacks of asthma occur after known or suspected respiratory tract infections, suggesting that infection may be an important factor; however, respiratory tract infections commonly precipitate attacks of wheezing in almost all types of asthma, including those known to be allergic in origin. Because of this possible relationship to infection, the term *infectious asthma* has been used by some physicians in place of the designations idiopathic or intrinsic.

In the pediatric age group, the term *asthmatic bronchitis* (or wheezy bronchitis) is employed by some pediatricians and allergists to designate single or recurrent attacks of wheezing associated only with respiratory infections. Children under 3 years of age are more commonly affected. The attack characteristically begins with signs of a "cold" (rhinorrhea and nasal congestion), followed by coughing and within approximately 24 hours by wheezing. Fever and other signs of infection (inflammatory changes of nasal mucous membranes or coarse rales) may be present. Children may respond to the administration of bronchodilators. Followup studies of children with asthmatic bronchitis have revealed that a significant number develop asthma.[8] Children over 18 months of age who wheeze repeatedly with respiratory tract infections and have a positive family history for allergy are particularly likely to be allergic asthmatic individuals and should be investigated thoroughly for other possible allergic etiologic factors. On the other hand, in adults over age 40 who have onset of wheezing after a respiratory tract infection, it is unlikely to find an underlying IgE mechanism as a cause of the wheezing.

Aspirin-induced Asthma

Aspirin-induced asthma is a clinical syndrome characterized by a triad of symptoms consisting of hyperplastic rhinitis with or without polyp formation, bronchial asthma, and exacerbation of symptoms after oral challenge with aspirin. Associated sinusitis is common. This syndrome occurs more frequently in adults than in children, females being more often affected than males by a ratio of 3:2. As a rule, the initial symptoms of asthma appear between the third and fifth decades of life. The syndrome also may begin in childhood, however, and is probably more common in this age group than heretofore realized.

In a double-blind, placebo-controlled study, 14 of 50 children ages 6 to 18 years with severe chronic asthma developed significant bronchospasm when challenged with 60 mg of aspirin.[9] As with previous reports of aspirin intolerance in adults, there was also a female preponderance. These patients had evidence of atopy as determined by the history and positive skin tests, raising a question about the validity of classifying aspirin-sensitive asthma as a distinct clinical syndrome in which allergy plays little or no role. It was also of interest that sinusitis was diagnosed more frequently in the 14 patients with aspirin intolerance than in the aspirin-tolerant group.

In a subsequent study, Vedanthan et al.[10] also demonstrated a high incidence of aspirin intolerance in asthmatic children. These authors found significant adverse pulmonary responses in 5 of 56 moderately severe 10- to 17-year-old chronic asthmatic patients challenged with aspirin. Two additional patients included in this sample had an adverse response to aspirin on the history and were consequently not challenged. They concluded that aspirin intolerance is sufficiently common in children with chronic severe asthma to warrant aspirin avoidance unless the drug is needed for another condition, such as rheumatoid arthritis, in which case, careful provocation tests with aspirin should be considered. Unfortunately, other nonsteroidal anti-inflammatory agents, as well as tartrazine (FDA yellow dye No. 5), may also cause airway obstruction in aspirin-intolerant patients. Acetaminophen does seem to be tolerated in these patients, but further studies are necessary to better define its safety.

The mechanism by which aspirin induces bronchospasm ramains unknown. Although some urticarial reactions to aspirin may involve a classic hapten-mediated allergic mechanism, there is no convincing evidence that aspirin-induced asthma is due to an immunologic mechanism. The most plausible theory of its pathogenesis is that aspirin and the nonsteroidal agents, by blocking the cyclooxygenase or peroxidases in the lung, inhibit the synthesis and release of endogenous prostaglandins and at the same time direct the metabolism of arachidonic acid via the lipoxygenase pathway into the formation and accumulation of slow-reacting substance of anaphylaxis (SRS-A) (leukotrienes).[11] The leukotrienes in addition to inducing bronchospasm directly also may sensitize receptors to other mediators and spasmogenic stimuli.

Treatment of patients with aspirin intolerance requires the strict avoidance of aspirin, nonsteroidal anti-inflammatory drugs, and various offending dyes. Because aspirin and other agents are frequently present in proprietary drug preparations, education of patients is essential so that they can consistently avoid their use. In patients who are intolerant to tartrazine and to a lesser extent other dyes, avoidance of these substances is more difficult. Because tartrazine, a yellow azo dye, is extensively used as a coloring agent in a variety of foods and drugs, the opportunities for exposure are considerable. A few of the foods that may contain tartrazine and other dyes are as follows: butter substitutes, oleomargarine, candies, ice cream, yogurts, prepared meats, multiple prepared beverages, cheeses, gelatins, puddings, mustard, and canned fruits. Fortunately, only a small percentage of patients with aspirin intolerance will also react to tartrazine and other dyes.

Recently successful desensitization to aspirin has been reported.[12] Further studies will be necessary before this technique is widely accepted as treatment for children who are intolerant to aspirin.

Exercise-induced Asthma

Exercise-induced asthma (EIA) is a phenomenon that occurs in approximately 90 percent of childhood asthmatics and in 40 percent of children with allergic rhinitis. Characteristically EIA occurs after 5–6 minutes of heavy exercise. Initially there is a short period of bronchodilation during the exercise period, followed by the onset of bronchoconstriction after the exercise has stopped. Usually the EIA is short lived (approximately 20 minutes) but may last up to several hours.

Many theories have been proposed to explain the mechanisms involved in EIA. Recently airway cooling caused by hyperventilation with ambient air that has to be warmed and humidified has been suggested as the major triggering mechanism. The heat loss in turn causes release of mediators that act locally through neural reflexes to produce bronchoconstriction. Although the heat loss theory is supported by much data, it does not satisfactorily explain all of the experimental observations made with EIA. Nevertheless, although the precise mechanism by which bronchospasm is produced by exercise remains obscure, its occurrence and severity is known to be affected by many factors, such as the direction and extent of physical stress, the nature of the exercise (e.g., swimming versus free running), humidity, irritants (e.g., air pollution), and allergen exposure.

Fortunately EIA can generally be controlled

by premedication with various pharmacologic agents. Cromolyn sodium (Intal), a nonbronchodilating drug, inhibits EIA to a considerable degree in most asthmatics and is particularly useful in patients who experience side effects with other medications. Premedication with inhalation of a β-adrenergic agent shortly before exercising will, in most instances, completely inhibit EIA. Appropriate doses of oral theophylline and β-adrenergic bronchodilators will also prevent or modify EIA. Although atropine and its isomer, SCH-1000 (Ipatropium, Atrovent—not available in the United States) are bronchodilators, their effect on EIA is less clear. Corticosteroids administered by any route have virtually no effect on EIA.

In general, children who experience EIA should recognize the need for certain adjustments in daily medication or a change in the routine of their exercise program. With our present understanding of the mechanisms involved in EIA and methods to prevent it, there is no reason why most asthmatic children cannot actively participate in most types of physical activity and even be active in sports programs.

Occupational Asthma

Classification of occupational asthma is included for the sake of completeness. Placing it into a separate category is of no help in indicating allergic or nonallergic mechanisms, but is useful in highlighting the occupation-related nature of the problem. For obvious reasons it is unlikely that a child's asthma would be classified in this category; however, children can be exposed to various dusts, gases, and vapors that can cause asthma and other types of lung diseases. For example, children living on farms can be at risk to developing acute or chronic lung dysfunction as a result of exposure to a variety of inhaled substances. These include antigens such as pollen; fungal spores; animal danders and excretions; grain dust and mites; synthetic chemicals including fertilizers, insecticides, and herbicides; and toxic gases associated with decomposing plant or animal material. In addition to asthma, respiratory manifestations from the inhalation of these substances include hypersensitivity pneumonitis, mycotoxicosis, acute laryngotracheobronchitis, and acute noncardiogenic pulmonary edema.

Hyperirritability of Airways

The basic mechanism underlying the exaggerated responsiveness in asthma remains poorly understood. Undoubtedly, genetic mechanisms predispose the atopic individual to various immune and physiologic responses, and host-environment interactions experienced by the individual is a crucial conditioner of the phenotypic expression of the disease state.

Several theories have been advanced to account for the heightened responsiveness of airways to various specific and nonspecific precipitating factors (2–2). One unifying concept to explain this phenomenon is the β-adrenergic blockade theory. This hypothesis states that there is a congenital or acquired diminished responsiveness of β-adrenergic receptors in patients with asthma. Although there is indirect evidence consistent with this theory, direct evidence is still lacking. Another attractive concept, which is also supported by much experimental evidence, is the neurogenic hypothesis. This theory implies that the most important factor leading to bronchoconstriction is increased cholinergic activity because of some intrinsic or acquired abnormality in irritant receptors. Recently an impaired nonadrenergic inhibitory nervous system and a "calcium hypothesis" have been proposed as possible explanations for the airway hyperactivity characteristic of asthma.[13]

Regardless of which basic underlying etiologic and pathogenic factors of asthma may be operative, certain factors play a greater role in the development of asthma in small infants and children.

A principal factor is infection. Recent studies have confirmed that viral respiratory agents are the most common precipitating factor of wheezing in children. Early in life, respiratory syncytial virus (RSV) and parainfluenza are most often involved; in older children and adults rhinovirus and influenza A are more often associated with exacerbations of asthma.

The mechanisms by which infection triggers wheezing remains unclear. It is quite evident that the viral agents do not act as allergens. More likely, the inflammation produced by their invasion of the respiratory mucosa results in exposures and enhanced sensitivity of the irritant receptors. This in turn potentiates vagally mediated bronchoconstriction to various nonspecific stimuli. Other studies have suggested that viral infections may exacerbate or initiate wheezing by other mechanisms. It has been demonstrated that interferon produced as a consequence of the infection enhances endogenous histamine release from the mast cells. Higher RSV-IgE titers and detectable histamine have been found in the secretions of wheezing infants versus nonwheezing infants infected with RSV. An earlier and greater development of cell-mediated responsiveness to RSV antigens has also been noted in the infected wheezing infants. Frick,[14] in a prospective study of babies born to parents with atopic diseases, observed that the onset of symptoms of asthma was often preceded by a viral infection. Markers of IgE-mediated immunologic responsiveness also increased shortly after a viral respiratory illness.

Another important factor in the pathogenesis of wheezing in infants and young children is their increased susceptibility to viral respiratory tract infections. Normally a child will have on the average three to six "colds" a year up until 6 or 7 years of age. The number of "colds" will be increased in children who attend nursery school. In contrast, an adult will suffer no more than one to three upper respiratory tract infections a year.

Clearly mechanical factors increase the risk of babies and young children developing disorders causing wheezing. Until approximately age 5, children have disproportionately small peripheral airways compared to adults. Fifty percent of an infant's total resistance is contributed by the peripheral airways; in contrast, adult peripheral airways contribute 20 percent or less of the total lung airway resistance. Furthermore, because of the small size of the bronchioles in infants, edema, cellular debris, and secretions are more likely to cause airway obstruction. Since the resistance of airflow varies inversely with the fourth power of the radius of the bronchioles, it is easy to see how any obstruction of the bronchioles significantly increases the resistance to airflow. The airways of infants, in addition to being smaller, are also softer and more pliable than in adults and accordingly may more readily collapse.

Another factor that may play a role in the development of asthma in infants is the increased exposure to food antigens via the gastrointestinal tract. Considerable evidence has accumulated to suggest that during the first few months of life gastrointestinal permeability to food antigens is increased, making it possible for susceptible infants to become easily sensitized to specific ingested proteins. Accordingly, in early infancy and childhood, foods are more likely to provoke asthma; however, as the child increases in age, inhalant allergens more commonly trigger symptoms.

Table 2-2 *Precipitating Factors in Asthma*

- Allergens
- Irritants

  Fumes
  Dusts
  Air pollutants
  Smoke

- Meteorologic factors

- Exposure to cold

- Infection

  Viral respiratory pathogens
  Bacteria
  Fungus
  Parasites

- Exercise

- Psychologic factors

- Endocrine factors

- Gastroesophageal reflux

- Drug-induced factors

  Aspirin and related agents
  Bronchoconstrictor drugs
  Hypersensitivity reactions

CLINICAL MANIFESTATIONS

The clinical picture of asthma in infants and children varies significantly between patients and even in the same patient. The onset of an attack of asthma may be acute or insidious. When airway obstruction develops rapidly within a few minutes, it is most likely due to smooth muscle spasm in large airways. Usually attacks precipitated by a respiratory tract infection are slower in onset; rhinorrhea and coughing often are present for a day or two before the wheezing can be noted. It is important to emphasize that not all patients exhibit the stereotyped picture of intermittent attacks of acute bronchospasm with wheezing. Often asthma will begin merely as a nonproductive cough (or as exertional dyspnea in older children and adults) without any overt wheezing.

The symptoms and signs of asthma will also vary with the severity of the attack. During a severe asthma attack, there is pronounced coughing, dyspnea, wheezing, and the characteristic prolonged expiratory phase of respiration. Usually the patient will be pale and apprehensive, may show some peripheral cyanosis, and sits upright, hunched forward to facilitate the use of respiratory muscles. Use of the sternocleidomastoid muscles and the presence of pulses paradoxus are indicative of severe compromise of pulmonary function. The lips are pursed during the expiration and the chest held in an inspiratory position, both of which allow for maximal bronchial tree dilation and a reduction in airway resistance. Vomiting is not uncommon and may be followed by relief of symptoms.

When the patient is in extreme respiratory distress and in impending respiratory failure, it is important to remember that the cardinal sign of wheezing may be absent. Other symptoms and signs of overt respiratory failure include severe intercostal retraction, pulsus paradoxus, cyanosis in 40 percent oxygen, a decreased response to pain, altered sensorium, diaphoresis, and poor skeletal muscle tone.

DIAGNOSIS

The diagnosis of asthma is based on the history, characteristic physical findings, and laboratory tests. The diagnosis of asthma is usually easily made. Although patients with asthma may present with a variety of symptoms, usually the recurrent episodes of coughing and wheezing are so characteristic that the diagnosis can be established by the history alone. The wheezing associated with asthma is usually expiratory, although in young children especially, it often is heard in both inspiration and expiration. When wheezing is heard only on inspiration the possibility of an upper airway obstruction should be considered. Initial attacks are usually episodic, with symptom-free periods in between the acute attacks. If the disease progresses and becomes more chronic, the symptom-free intervals tend to diminish progressively. If the patient is an atopic

individual, often the history will provide clues to current and future allergens. A history of other previous or concomitant allergic manifestations and a positive family history for allergies (e.g., atopic dermatitis, allergic rhinitis) are also helpful in establishing the diagnosis.

It is important to reemphasize that wheezing, recognized by either history or physical examination, may not be evident in a patient with asthma. The child may merely have a nonproductive, persistent cough, especially at night. If the child is old enough, pulmonary function studies will demonstrate obstruction of the airways that can be significantly reversed with bronchodilators. In rare instances, the airway hyperreactivity can only be established by exercise provocation and the patient's response to bronchodilators.[15] The terms *hidden,* or *variant,* have been used in referring to this type of asthma.

Physical examination of a child with asthma should focus on growth and development, and special attention should be given to the eyes, ears, skin, and respiratory tract. Measurements of weight and height, when compared to norms and prior values, will often provide a clue as to the degree of severity of the asthma. The finding of a round-shouldered posture with an increase in the anteroposterior diameter is indicative of long-standing hyperinflation. Children who have developed asthma in early childhood often will develop a "pseudorachitic" chest deformity. In uncomplicated asthma, wheezing on auscultation is often heard both on inspiration and expiration. Increased secretions along with bronchospasm may alter the breath sounds so that rhonchi (which clear on changing position or after coughing) and moist rales are audible. The latter may lead to a mistaken diagnosis of pneumonia. During asymptomatic periods, the typical wheeze often can be induced by having the child make a forced expiratory effort (easily induced by asking the child to blow out the light of your otoscope). Even in very young children, this can be diagnostic, since manual compression of the chest wall can simulate a forced exertion.

The recognition of signs of upper respiratory tract allergy that coexist frequently with asthma may help in establishing the diagnosis and uncover complications. If nasal polyps are present, cystic fibrosis, immotile cilia syndrome, and aspirin intolerance should be ruled out. Purulent secretions in nasal passages should suggest the possibility of sinusitis. Often the typical findings of allergic rhinitis and atopic dermatitis will be present; this helps to identify the patient as being an atopic individual and alerts one to identify allergic factors as contributing to the patient's asthma. Eardrums should be examined with a pneumatoscope for serous otitis. Patients with severe concomitant atopic dermatitis or who require chronic treatment with corticosteroids require a slit-lamp examination of their eyes for cataracts.

Laboratory Evaluation

Laboratory procedures are essential for the proper evaluation of the asthmatic child.

Complete Blood Counts

Complete blood counts are usually normal, except for a tendency to eosinophilia. Although the latter suggests an allergic cause, there are many other causes of eosinophilia, such as parasitic infections, bronchopulmonary aspergillosis, Loeffler's syndrome, and immune disorders. Idiopathic asthma may also be associated with eosinophilia. Patients receiving corticosteroids will have low eosinophil counts and high total white blood counts. Epinephrine may also temporarily induce leukocytosis.

Sputum and Nasal Secretions

Examination of sputum and nasal secretions also can be a simple helpful procedure. Asthmatic sputum usually is obtained in older children and adults, since younger children tend to swallow it. It is grossly tenacious, rubbery, and whitish or clear. It may contain yellowish plugs (usually containing clumps of eosinophils), and on occasion Charcot-Leyden crystals, creola bodies, or Curschmann's spirals may be found. Sputum eosinophilia is present in both allergic and idiopathic asthma.

Nasal secretions should be obtained and examined for eosinophils as a regular part of the laboratory workup of the asthmatic patient. The secretions are easily obtained and stained either with Hansel's or Wright's stain. An eosinophil count greater than 10 percent is usually indicative of an allergy in children; however, a significant eosinophil count in nasal secretions may also be observed in "nonallergic" rhinitis. A predominance of polymorphonuclear neutrophil leukocytes (PMNs) and ingested bacteria suggests the possibility of sinusitis.[16]

Roentgenograms

Every child suspected of having asthma should have chest roentgenography with posteroanterior and lateral views. This rules out other causes of chronic wheezing and parenchymal disease (e.g., atelectasis, pneumonia, and a pneumomediastinum). Lung marking are commonly increased, and hyperinflation occurs during acute exacerbations and in patients with chronic wheezing. With a persistent cough, purulent rhinorrhea, and symptoms of a sore throat, a Water's view of the sinuses should be obtained to rule out maxillary sinusitis.

Allergy Testing

Skin tests, RAST RadioAllergoSorbent Test or the ELISA Enzyme-Linked ImmunoSorbent Assay test may be indicated in those patients in whom specific allergic factors are considered to be etiologic. Skin tests are rarely necessary for the very young child with asthma.

IgE Level

The determination of a serum IgE level is seldom necessary to establish whether a patient has allergic asthma. It is more useful in infancy and for diagnosing and monitoring the course of bronchopulmonary aspergillosis. Although an elevated IgE level may be helpful in differentiating allergic from nonallergic asthma, it should be remembered that a normal or low IgE level does not rule out allergy. Measurements of IgE levels in infancy have also been shown to be of value in predicting the development of future atopic manifestations.

Provocation Test

Provocation tests may be useful in determining the diagnostic significance of a specific allergen and to demonstrate that the patient does indeed have hyperreactive airways. These tests include the inhalation of cold air or graded concentrations of histamine or methacholine and monitoring the response by pulmonary function. A positive exercise tolerance test may also be useful in establishing the diagnosis of asthma.

Pulmonary Function Tests

Pulmonary function tests are described elsewhere in great detail. Briefly, lung function tests are objective, noninvasive, and cost-effective in diagnosing and monitoring patients with chronic asthma. In addition to determining the degree of airway obstruction, pulmonary function tests are valuable in determining whether the patient has significant reversible airway obstruction. A greater than 15 percent improvement "in forced expiratory volume in 1 second (FEV^1) or 20 percent in forced expiratory flow in the middle half of forced vital capacity." (FEF 25–75) after the administration of a bronchodilator is considered diagnostic of asthma. Economic spirometers and peak flowmeters are now available, so that expiratory flow rates and peak flow can be readily measured in the office and even by the patient at home.

Special Tests

When it is difficult to determine whether the wheezing is due to allergy or some other cause of respiratory tract obstruction, or when a complication is suspected, a number of special tests may be indicated. A sweat chloride test should always be performed in any child with chronic respiratory symptoms, especially with accompanying symptoms of pancreatic insufficiency and nasal polyps. To rule out immunodeficiency disorders in patients subject to frequent or chronic infections, quantitative immunoglobulins should be obtained as one of the initial steps in the patient's workup. Children with recurrent pneumonia and persistent wheezing should be investigated for gastroesophegeal reflux, (See Chapter 12.) Patients with chronic otitis, sinusitis, and bronchitis should have a biopsy of their respiratory tract and the specimen examined under the electron microscope for possible axoneme abnormalities characteristic of the immotile cilia syndrome.

DIFFERENTIAL DIAGNOSIS

Because other chapters are devoted to various pulmonary disorders that must be considered in the differential diagnosis of asthma in infants and children, the most common causes of wheezing are listed in Table 2–3. A comprehensive list and description of various disorders causing wheezing in infants and children can be found in the literature.[17,18]

Since asthma is a common disorder, it may coexist with other conditions that cause wheezing. Wheezing in the infant deserves some special mention because it is common and is fraught with both diagnostic and therapeutic problems. Unfor-

tunately, most physicians are reluctant to consider the diagnosis of asthma in the first year of life, despite the fact that more than 50 percent of children subsequently shown to have asthma have their first symptoms before 2 years of age. The condition most likely to be mistaken with infantile asthma is bronchiolitis. The following points may be helpful in attempting to differentiate the two conditions: 1) bronchiolitis is unlikely to recur, accordingly two or three wheezing bouts in the same infant suggest the diagnosis of asthma; 2) a family history of allergies, the presence of other atopic manifestations, and the onset of wheezing without any evident respiratory tract infection or precipitated by a known allergen strengthen the likelihood of a diagnosis of asthma; 3) bronchiolitis due to RSV peaks around 6 months of age, occurs during the winter months, and is often prevalent in the community; 4) the finding of eosinophilia in the blood or nasal secretions or an elevated serum IgE level (above 20 IU for a child under 1 year of age) is indicative of allergic asthma. In contrast to the older child with asthma, the response to bronchodilators cannot be relied upon to make the diagnosis of reversible obstructive airway disease.

THERAPY

General Principles

Successful management of childhood asthma is contingent upon the patient (depending on age) and his or her parents fully understanding the disease and upon the physician's ability to ultimately prevent physical and psychologic disability. In addition to providing the initial information and detailed instructions, it is frequently necessary to have an ongoing educational process to achieve these goals. The family (and the child if old enough) must not only have some knowledge of how the disease develops, but also must be informed as to how future attacks can be prevented and treated with appropriate pharmacologic agents. The treatment prescribed will vary depending on the severity of the asthma, causes of the child's wheezing, age of the patient, family's psychologic needs, social circumstances, and family resources. Compliance by the patient and family is the essential ingredient of any successful therapy. In treatment regimens provided for patients, special emphasis is placed on the necessity of maintaining physical fitness and for the children to set goals that will allow them to lead as normal a life as possible. They are encouraged to regularly attend school, physical education classes, and participate in sports and other forms of recreation. Obviously, in a few instances some restrictions on activities and career selection may be necessary, such as foregoing becoming a veterinarian.

Specific Therapy

The specific management of asthma consists of three major treatment approaches: avoidance of known precipitating factors (environmental control), specific immunotherapy (hyposensitization), and pharmacologic therapy.

Environmental Control

All children with asthma have some degree of bronchial hyperreactivity. It is therefore essential that those allergens or irritants identified by the history and confirmed when applicable by skin tests be eliminated or avoided to the extent possible within the framework of normal physical and psychologic growth and development. Acute wheezing after exposure to a pet is usually easily recognized, but recommending that the pet be removed from the home is often an unwelcome suggestion. If the asthma is severe and there is a positive skin test, usually parents can be persuaded to remove the animal. On the other hand, although removal of important allergens and irritants is a requisite for good management of asthma, the physician must remain flexible and reasonable, always weighing the potential benefit against any adverse psychologic consequences of his or her recommendations.

Since many patients are allergic to house dust, its elimination is important. Creation of a dust-free bedroom, where the child spends a lot of time, can be accomplished by frequent dusting; encasing pillows, mattresses, box springs, and similar furnishings in airtight plastic covers; and removing bookcases, toys, and unnecessary furnishings. The avoidance of other allergens, however, such as molds and pollens may not be possible, and other therapeutic measures may be necessary.

Immunotherapy

Immunotherapy is indicated for patients who are allergic to specific allergens that cannot be avoided or eliminated and who have failed to

Table 2-3 *Differential Diagnosis of Asthma*

Causes of wheezing under 1 year of age

  Bronchiolitis
  Congenital malformations

   Vascular rings
   Congenital heart disease
   Gastrointestinal anomalies

  Cystic fibrosis
  Bronchopulmonary dysplasia
  Immunodeficiency disorders
  Pulmonary hemosiderosis

Causes of wheezing in toddlers
  and older children

  Aspirated foreign body
  Cystic fibrosis
  Laryngotracheobronchitis
  Gastroesophageal reflux
  Hypersensitivity pneumonitis
  Allergic bronchopulmonary aspergillosis
  Habit cough
  Immotile cilia syndrome
  Parasitic pneumonitis
  α-1-Antitrypsin deficiency
  Collagen diseases

respond to adequate pharmacologic therapy. Although there is substantial evidence that this form of therapy is efficacious for allergic rhinitis, its use for the treatment of asthma has been the subject of considerable controversy. Despite its widespread usage for the treatment of asthma, there has been limited evidence demonstrating its efficacy for this disease. Recently, immunologic changes after immunotherapy, which may relate to clinical improvement, have been documented by a number of investigators. [19] These changes include 1) increases in serum IgG-blocking antibody titers, 2) a decrease in sensitivity of in vitro leukocytes to antigen-induced histamine release, 3) a decline in serum IgE level directed to a specific antigen, and 4) an increased number of specific suppressor T-lymphocytes.

Immunotherapy essentially involves repeated injections of increasing amounts of allergenic extracts until the patient reaches an optimal maintenance dose. (Details of this procedure can be found in all standard allergy texts.) Although the dose considered optimal is somewhat arbitrary and variable, there is considerable evidence to indicate that patients receiving the maximally tolerated doses of antigen achieve the greatest benefit. Recently efforts are being made to modify pollen extracts to reduce their allergenicity without affecting their immunogenecity. Preliminary studies with these antigens, formalin treated (allergoids) and polymerized, produced significant clinical responses with fewer injections and reactions.

Since multiple factors, many of which are nonimmunologic, may influence the course of asthma, it is unlikely that immunotherapy ever "cures" all symptoms. Furthermore, it should be emphasized that this procedure has no place in the therapy of idiopathic (intrinsic) asthma. There is also no evidence for the use of bacterial vaccines or food antigens in the management of asthma.

Pharmacologic Management

The mainstay of treating asthma is the appropriate use of drugs to prevent or relieve airway obstruction. (See Chapters 3 and 16.) In addition, the author and co-workers have published two reviews of pharmacologic management of pediatric allergic disorders.[20,21] Accordingly, despite its importance, only a brief overview of the author's approach to the treatment of acute episodes of wheezing and to the management of chronic asthma will be presented.

Treatment of Acute Attacks

Treatment of acute attacks of asthma depends on the severity and duration of the attack, medications previously taken, and those available. Fortunately most attacks, especially in the early stages, will respond to oral bronchodilators. As soon as wheezing is noted, the child is given orally a short-acting theophylline preparation in the dose of 5–7.5 mg/kg as a solution, chewable tablet, or plain tablet or an oral β-adrenergic agent (metaproterenol, terbutaline, or albuterol). The β-adrenergic agents may be used as a primary bronchodilator or in conjunction with theophylline. Metaproterenol is the only adrenergic agent approved for pediatric use. For children over 6 years of age the dosage is 10–20 mg every 6 hours. For younger children a dosage of 2 mg/kg every 24 hours administered in three doses is usually well tolerated and effective in relieving bronchospasm. Terbutaline and albuterol are available in tablet form; the dosage of the former is 2.5–5 mg every 6 hours, and for albuterol it is 2–4 mg, three to four times a day. Neither of these drugs is approved for patients under 12 years of age. Nevertheless, studies by the author and others have found albuterol to be a very effective bronchodilating drug for children over 2 years of age in dosages of 2 mg three times a day for children under 20 kg and 4 mg three times a day for those weighing more.[22, 23]

For the child who is vomiting, theophylline or aminophylline (85 percent theophylline) administered by rectal solution, 4–6 mg/kg, is reliably absorbed. On the other hand, because of erratic absorption and the potential for overdosage, aminophylline suppositories are contraindicated. Cromolyn sodium may be helpful if used before exposure to a known allergen or before exercise, but it should be discontinued during an acute attack.

In older cooperative children the inhalation of a β-adrenergic aerosol preparation can be used to halt a mild to moderate attack promptly, especially those associated with exercise or occurring at night. Special precautions should always be taken, however, to avoid overdosage and addiction to the nebulizer.

If these measures fail or the patient has severe wheezing, the drug of choice is epinephrine by injection in doses of 0.01 mg/kg or aerosolized adrenergic agents. Although not approved for children, terbutaline (1 mg/ml) in doses of 0.01 mg/kg (up to 0.25 mg) may be substituted in adolescents and young adults. The dose of epinephrine may be repeated twice more at 15- to 20-minute intervals; terbutaline should not be administered more than twice, and the total dose should not exceed 0.5 mg. The unpleasant side effects of epinephrine (pallor, tremor, palpitations, and headache) can be minimized if doses of no more than 0.2–0.3 ml are given at any age. If the patient responds to the initial epinephrine or aerosol therapy, an injection of Sus-Phrine® in the dose of 0.005 ml/kg, with a maximal dose of 0.15 ml may maintain bronchodilation until the oral medication becomes effective.

In children old enough to use them effectively, the use of nebulized brochodilators (metaproterenol, isoetharine, racemic epinephrine, or isoproterenol) are rapidly effective in reversing severe bronchospasm, provided the patient has not been overusing an adrenergic aerosol and become refractory to its effect. Aerosol preparations have the advantage that substantially less drug is required, and accordingly there are fewer associated side effects. A compressor device is the method of choice for delivery of aerosols.

Table 2-4 *Treatment of Acute Attacks*

Drug	Route of Administration	Dosage	Frequency
Epinephrine (1:1000 solution)	Subcutaneous	0.01 mg/kg (maximal 0.3 ml)	15–20 min (three times)
Terbutaline	Subcutaneous	0.01 mg/kg (maximal 0.25 ml)	15–20 min (two times)
Isoproterenol hydrochloride (0.5%)	Aerosol	0.25–0.5 ml in 3-ml saline	q4h
Isoetharine hydrochloride (1%)	Aerosol	0.25–0.5 ml	q4h
metaproterenol	Aerosol	0.1 ml, 2–6 yr 0.2 ml, 6–12 yr 0.3 ml, >12 yr in 3-ml saline	q4h
Racemic epinephrine (2.25%)	Aerosol	0.25–0.5 ml in 3-ml saline	q4h
Epinephrine suspension (1:200) (Sus-Phrine)	Subcutaneous	0.005 ml/kg (maximal 0.15 ml)	Single dose

Intermittent positive pressure breathing devices are no more effective and occasionally may be hazardous because of their potential to induce or worsen a pneumomediastinum or pneumothorax. The dosages of subcutaneous and aerosolized β-adrenergics for the treatment of acute attacks are shown in Table 2–4.

If there is persistent significant wheezing, further therapy should be instituted in an emergency room or hospital setting. A therapeutic serum concentration (10–20 μg/ml) should be obtained rapidly with an intravenous loading dose of aminophylline of 5–7.5 mg/kg diluted in 20–50 ml of saline administered over a period of about 20 minutes. If an intial serum theophylline level cannot be obtained, the loading dose should be modified based on the history of previous theophylline therapy.

When the patient's wheezing is refractory to bronchodilators, intravenous corticosteroids should be promptly administered in large doses in the form of hydrocortisone (Solu-Cortef) or methylprednisolone (Solu-Medrol) or other intravenous preparations in equivalent pharmacologic doses to 2 mg/kg followed by the same dosage over the 24 hours. Tapering the dosage for the sake of minimizing adrenal suppression is unnecessary if steroid therapy has been administered for 5 or less days. Since small airway bronchospasm often persists for more than 1 week, it may be necessary to continue the steroid orally. The dosage usually used by the author is 1–2 mg/kg of prednisone administered as a single morning dose. Once symptoms are adequately controlled, the dosage is tapered by 5 mg/per day.

Management of Chronic Asthma

The goals of the long-term drug management of chronic asthma are to prevent recurrent acute or persistent symptoms and to achieve normal pulmonary function. This may not be feasible in all cases. Care must always be exercised in attempting to create a "symptom-free" patient with normal pulmonary function not to administer agents such as corticosteroids that may produce more serious side effects than asthma.

For children who require "round-the-clock" bronchodilation, theophylline has become the drug of choice. In appropriate doses it reduces the frequency and severity of acute symptoms and minimizes exercise-induced bronchospasm. A close relationship exists between serum theophylline levels and improvement in lung function. Optimal improvement usually occurs with serum levels between 10 and 20 μu/ml, although some asthmatic patients have a maximal response between 7 and 10 μg/ml. Side effects become more frequent as blood levels approach 15–20 μg/ml; however, adverse gastronintestinal symptoms, headaches, behavior and learning dysfunction, and disturbances in sleep may occur with lower levels. Since several methods are now available to measure serum theophylline levels, the dose of each patient can be adjusted to achieve therapeutic effectiveness while avoiding toxicity. Theophylline preparations are available as quick-release tablets and liquid and sustained-release tablets and capsules. The latter are preferable, since they decrease fluctuations in serum concentrations and allow 8- to 12-hour dosing intervals. The bead-filled capsules allow some flexibility in individualizing the dose for infants and children, since they can be opened and the beads sprinkled over a spoonful of soft food such as applesauce without any apparent effect on absorption.

Cromolyn sodium is an alternative agent for the management of chronic asthma. It is a particularly useful drug for patients who are doing poorly with or having significant side effects from theophylline or β-adrenergic agents. Unlike other drugs used to treat asthma, it has no bronchodilator, antimediator, or anti-inflammatory activity. Accordingly, it must be administered prophylactically to exert its beneficial effects. Although children and atopic asthmatic patients appear to respond better than adults and patients with nonallergic asthma, there is increasing evidence that the drug is also beneficial in nonimmunologically mediated asthma. The dosage for children is the same as adults; the contents of one capsule (20 mg) is inhaled four times a day. After a favorable response, the dosage should be reduced to the lowest amount that will control symptoms, usually two or three doses each day. Although a favorable response may be noted within a day or two, occasionally it will take 3–4 weeks before the desired effect becomes apparent. Few side effects have been noted with cromolyn sodium. The most common are local irritant effects on the throat and trachea from inhalation of the powder. This is rarely severe enough to prevents its continued use. To date no long-term adverse effects on the lung have been observed.

If the asthma is not controlled by theophylline or cromolyn sodium, β-adrenergic agents are added. Outside of the United States, the β-adrenergic agents are often used as a primary bronchodilator. Presently the only oral, relatively selective, B_2-adrenergic preparation approved by the Food and Drug Administration (FDA) for children under 12 years of age is metaproterenol. Terbutaline and albuterol have been approved for children over 12 years of age. The dosages of these drugs are the same as that administered for an acute attack. In comparing theophylline administration to oral metaproterenol, it was found that the two drugs were equally effective in controlling chronic asthma. [24] Theophylline caused more side effects, however. Inhaled metaproterenol, albuterol, or isoetharine, one or two inhalations every 4–6 hours, may offer more bronchodilation and avoid systemic side effects, such as tremor and nervousness. They are particularly effective in blocking exercise-induced asthma. Although some tolerance to these agents may develop, it is usually of a degree that does not negate their effectiveness as bronchodilators. As with their use for the control of acute attacks, patients and parents must be warned about potential abuse.

Despite the optimal usage of theophylline, cromolyn sodium, β-adrenergics, a small number of patients who contine to suffer with periodic episodes of severe wheezing or have chronic severe incapacitating asthma will require corticosteroids. Alternate-day prednisone (administered as a single dose in the morning or inhaled beclomethasone dipropionate (Vanceril, Beclovent) are the drugs of choice for long-term use of corticosteroids. A short course of daily prednisone is usually necessary to decrease some of the hyperirritability of the airways and to bring symptoms under control before initiating either of these regimens. Some controversy exists as to which of these methods of administering corticosteroids is preferable. The advantages of alternate-day therapy are its ease of administration, especially to young children, its low cost, and its adverse effects are better known because it has been used since the 1950s. The advantages of beclomethasone aerosol therapy, which the author prefers for older children, are better control of symptoms in most patients, fewer systemic side effects (e.g., cushingoid effects), and less suppressive effects on the pituitary-adrenal axis with the recommended dosage of 400 μg/day. The disadvantages of aerosolized steroids are that their long-term effects remain unknown, although studies to date have not revealed any serious untoward effects. Dosages exceeding 800 μg/day may also lead to supression of the pituitary-adrenal axis. During exacerbations of asthma, daily therapy with corticosteroids should be reinstituted. Once the patient recovers, the previous continuous dosages of alternate-day or aerosol therapy should be resumed. At all times during long-term corticosteroid therapy bronchodilator therapy should be maximized and the dosage or corticosteroids constantly reduced to the minimal amount that will keep the patient's asthma under control.

COMPLICATIONS

The complications of bronchial asthma in children include both the immediate effects arising from an acute attack and the long-term effects of recurrent or persistent asthma. For a more detailed description and information regarding management of these complications the reader is referred to a previous publication by the author and his co-workers.[18] In Table 2-5 various complications are listed. The more common complications encountered in the pediatric age group are infections of one or more parts of the respiratory tract, atelectasis, mediastinal and subcutaneous emphysema, a pneumothorax, growth complications, and status asthmaticus.

PROGNOSIS

Although precise information on the long-term prognosis of asthma is difficult to obtain, a significant number of children with asthma "outgrow" the disease. Nevertheless, recent evidence suggests that despite the lack of clinical manifestations of asthma, there is a persistence of bronchial hyperractivity to methacholene and histamine for 1 to 20 years.[25] In addition, studies from Europe have demonstrated that many patients who seemingly had outgrown their disease experienced symptoms again as they grew older.[26]

The relationship between such factors as the age of onset, presence of atopy, and severity of asthma has been reported to affect the prognosis of childhood asthma. The relationship between age and ultimate outcome is conflicting. It was generally believed that the onset of asthma

Table 2-5 *Complications of Asthma*

- Infection

    Bronchitis
    Pneumonitis
    Sinusitis
    Otitis media

- Atelectasis

- Mediastinal and subcutaneous emphysema

- Pneumothorax

- Growth complications

    Inhibition of linear growth
    Thoracic deformities

- Status asthmaticus

- Chronic irreversible obstructive disease

- Cough syncope

- Bronchiectasis

- Cor pulmonale

- Poliomyelitis-like illness

- Spontaneous fracture of ribs

- Rupture of esophagus

- Myoglobulinuria

- Psychologic problems

- Death

before 2 years, especially under 6 months, entailed a poorer prognosis. Recently, however, the results of a follow-up study of 20 years indicated no correlation between the age of onset and ultimate prognosis. There is a greater consensus that the presence of atopy as demonstrated by positive skin tests, elevated IgE levels, and a family history usually implies a poorer prognosis. Contrarily, there is some suggestion that patients with nonallergic (idiopathic) asthma precipitated mainly by viral respiratory tract infections more likely will become symptom free later in life. Some evidence also has been presented that patients with severe and frequent attacks of wheezing are more likely to have persistent symptoms later in life. Patients who are not symptom free during puberty are unlikely to outgrow their symptoms as young adults. Asthma generallly does not progress to emphysema. In a small proportion of children with severe asthma (especially when complicated by frequent infections), however, it does appear to lead to chronic obstructive airway disease that is irreversible. Despite the fact that relatively few children develop irreversible destructive changes in the lung and a considerable number of children will outgrow asthma, these observations should not be interpreted as a license to withhold therapy. Although certain factors may portend the final outcome, it is difficult to reliably differentiate beforehand those individuals who ultimately do well from those destined to progressive disease.

SUMMARY

Asthma is an extremely common disorder in childhood that is characterized by hyperreactive airways. Multiple immunologic and nonimmunologic factors are known to precipitate acute attacks of wheezing. No unifying theory has been put forth to adequately explain the heterogenous aspects of this disease. Nevertheless, advances in pharmacology, immunology, cellular and membrane biochemistry, and receptor physiology have resulted in a better understanding of the pathophysiologic process of this syndrome. Although no "cure" is presently available, appropriate management will provide significant and adequate control in most children with asthma. Further advances in our knowledge of the basic pathophysiologic process will undoubtedly lead to more effective therapy and ultimately to permanent cures.

References

1. American Thoracic Society, Committee on Diagnostic Standards for Non-Tuberculosis Resiratory Disease: Definition and classification of chronic bronchitis, asthma, and pulmonary emphysema. *Am Rev Respir Dis* 85: 762, 1962.

2. Dodge RR, Burrows B: The prevalence and incidence of asthma-like symptoms in a general population sample. *Am Rev Respir Dis* 12: 567, 1980.

3. Broder I, Higgins MW, Mathews KP, et al: Epidemiology of asthma and allergic rhinitis in a total community, Tecumseh, Michigan: III. Second survey of the community. *J Allergy Clin Immunol* 53: 127, 1974.

4. Wilson JD, Sutherland DC, Thomas AC: Has the change to beta-agonists combined with oral theophylline increased cases of fatal asthma? *Lancet* 1:1235, 1981.

5. Bock SA: The natural history of food sensitivity. *J Allergy Clin Immun Col* 69:177, 1982.

6. Pepys J: Immunopathology of allergic lung disease. *Clin Allergy* 3, 1, 1973.

7. Fink JN, Salvaggio J (eds): N.I.A.I.D. workshop on antigens in hypersensitivity pneumonitides. *J Allerg Clin Immunol* 61:199, 1978.

8. Godfrey S: Childhood asthma, in Clark TJH, Godfrey S (eds): *Asthma.* London, Chapman and Hall Ltd, 1977, p 324.

9. Rachelefsky GS, Coulson A, Siegel SC, et al: Aspirin-intolerance in chronic childhood asthma: detected by oral challenge. *Pediatrics* 56:443, 1975.

10. Vedanthan PK, Menon MM, Bell TD, et al: Aspirin and tartrazine oral challenge: incidence of adverse response in chronic childhood asthma. *J Allerg Clin Immunol* 60:8, 1977.

11. Chand N, Altura BM: Lipoxygenase pathway and hydroperoxy acids: possible relevance to aspirin-induced asthma and hyperirritability of airways in asthmatics. *Prostaglandins Med* 6:249, 1981.

12. Pleskow WW, Stevenson DD, Mathison DA, et al: Aspirin desensitization in aspirin-sensitive patients: clinical characterization of the refractory period. *J Aller Clin Immunol* 69:11, 1983.

13. Middleton E Jr: Antiasthmatic drug therapy and calcium ions: review of pathogenesis and role of calcium. *J Pharm Sci* 69:243, 1980.

14. Frick OL, German DF and Mills J: Development of allergy in children: I. Association with virus infections. *J Allerg Clin Immunol* 63:228, 1979.

15. Cloutier MM, Loughlin GM: Chronic cough in children: a manifestation of airway hyperreactivity. *Pediatrics* 67:6, 1981.

16. Rachelefsky GS, Goldberg M, Katz, et al: Sinus disease in children with respiratory allergy. *J Aller Clin Immunol* 61:310, 1978.

17. Berman BA, MacDonnell KF (eds): *Differential Diagnosis and Treatment of Pediatric Allergy.* Boston, Little Brown & Co, 1981.

18. Siegel SC, Katz RM, Rachelefsky GS: Asthma in infancy and childhood. In Middleton E Jr, Reed CE, Ellis EF (eds): *Allergy: Principles and Practice.* St. Louis, The CV Mosby Co, 1978, p 708.

19. Melam H: Principles of immunologic management of allergic diseases due to extrinsic antigens, in

Patterson R (ed): *Allergic Diseases, Diagnosis and Management.* Philadelphia JB Lippincott Co, 1980, p 326.

20. Siegel SC: Corticosteroids for allergic disorders in children. *Pediatr Ann* 8:57, 1979.

21. Siegel SC, Rachelefsky GS, Katz RM: Pharmacologic management of pediatric disorders. *Curr Probl Pediatr* 9:–., 1979.

22. Rachelefsky GS, Katz RM, Siegel SC: Albuterol syrup in the treatment of the young asthmatic child. *Ann Allergy* 47: 143, 1981.

23. Rachelefsky GS, Katz RM, Siegel SC: Oral albu-terol in the treatment of childhood asthma. *Pediatrics* 69: 397, 1982.

24. Rachelefsky GS, Katz RM, Mickey MR, et al: Metaproterenol and theophylline in asthmatic children. *Ann Allergy* 45:107, 1980.

25. Townley, R.G., Ryo, U.Y., Kolotin, B.M., and Kang, B.: Bronchial sensitivity to methacholine in current and former asthmatic and allergic rhinitis patients and control subjects. *J. Allergy Clin. Immunol.* 5:429, 1975,

26. Blair H: Natural history of childhood asthma. *Arch Dis Child* 52:613, 1977.

3

Exercise-Induced Asthma

Gerd J.A. Cropp

Asthmatic children and adolescents frequently develop wheezing, coughing, and shortness of breath late during and after strenuous exertion. The severity of exercise-induced bronchospasm varies greatly in different patients and even in the same patient at different times. Postexertional asthma usually is most notable 3–5 minutes after the cessation of physical activity. Thereafter the acute airway obstruction tends to resolve gradually and spontaneously. In rare cases, the onset of postexertional bronchospasm is slow but progressive, and the attack may steadily worsen for 30–60 minutes before it resolves. The symptoms associated with exercise-induced airway obstruction are as varied as those seen in other forms of asthma. Once the signs and symptoms of exercise-induced asthma (EIA) are recognized for what they are, appropriate therapy usually prevents their recurrence or terminates them. Since children are more active than adults, this form of asthma is particularly common in the pediatric age group.

During the past few years it has been learned that postexertional bronchospasm is another manifestation of hyperreactivity of the respiratory tree in asthmatic patients. Although acute airway obstruction often follows 6–8 minutes of severe exercise, physical exertion is not necessary to elicit this form of asthma. Any form of hyperpnea will cool the airways, which in turn elicits contraction of bronchial smooth muscles and airway obstruction in patients with active asthma. Since pediatricians are often faced with complaints related to physical exertion, it behooves them to recognize EIA and initiate appropriate preventive or corrective therapy.

INCIDENCE, GRADES OF SEVERITY, AND RELATION BETWEEN EIA AND OTHER BRONCHOPROVOCATION TESTS

Postexertional bronchospasm can be provoked in most active asthmatic patients, provided that sensitive and multiple tests of lung function are used to detect the development of airway obstruction and the environmental conditions are conducive for the development of this type of acute airway obstruction. Asymptomatic asthmatic patients with normal preexercise pulmonary function tests may not develop postexertional bronchospasm. In other patients the airway obstruction may be of such mild degree that they remain unaware of any abnormalities, although pulmonary function tests can detect the presence of airway narrowing. Warm and humid environments lessen the development of EIA, even in highly sensitive patients.

When 60 asthmatic children were tested, it was observed that 85 percent of the boys and 65 percent of the girls developed laboratory and clinical evidence of significant postexertional asthma.[1] There is a good correlation between the incidence of exercise-induced bronchospasm and airway obstruction elicited by the inhalation of methacholine, histamine, or cold dry air.[2] There may be considerable variations in the severity of exercise-induced bronchospasm over the course of a year, with seasonal changes, remissions of asthma with advancing age, or temporary disappearance of symptoms. The temporary or permanent disappearance of EIA usually is associated with a disappearance or lessening of airway hyperreactivity to histamine, methacholine, and cold air.

31

Mild and moderate degrees of exercise-induced bronchospasm occurred with approximately equal frequency in boys and girls. Severe forms of postexertional asthma developed more often in boys than in girls.[1] Most patients experienced the most distressing airway obstruction during the first 5 minutes after exertion, and some even showed detectable and sometimes troublesome wheezing late during exercise. Approximately 5 percent of the children developed gradual increases in airway obstruction that progressed slowly for 30–40 minutes after exercise. Postexertional bronchospasm usually cleared spontaneously without therapy in 15–30 minutes. There were, however, a small but significant number of asthmatic patients who remained quite distressed for 30–60 minutes or longer after exercise, and some required therapy to terminate the acute attacks of bronchospasm.

ENVIRONMENTAL AND OTHER FACTORS

Exercise and hyperpnea-induced asthma is a frequent complaint during the winter months when the absolute humidity and inhaled air temperatures are low. More postexertional airway obstruction also has been observed in hot desertlike climates than in moderate, but humid regions. When patients exercise in an environment with high concentrations of allergens to which they are sensitive, the development of EIA is favored. The presence of a viral respiratory tract infection or a recent vaccination against influenza may increase the severity of postexertional bronchospasm. It appears that any factor which increases the hyperresponsiveness of the respiratory tree will accentuate the response to exercise.

PATHOPHYSIOLOGIC PROCESSES.

During the past few decades numerous theories have been proposed to explain the pathophysiologic mechanisms responsible for EIA. Although some of the previously suggested mechanisms may modulate the development of postexertional airway obstruction, none have adequately explained the frequent and sudden time-limited bronchospasm that develops so often in asthmatic patients after strenuous physical activity. The conditions that were believed to influence the development of EIA included metabolic acidosis, lactate accumulation, abnormalities in free fatty acid utilization, postexertional hypocapnia, excessive α-adrenergic activity, and excessive parasympathetic vagal discharges.[3]

The work of two groups of investigators has now clarified our understanding of the pathophysiologic mechanism of exercise-induced bronchospasm. Strauss et al.[4] and Shturman-Ellstein et al.[5] demonstrated convincingly that postexertional asthma can be prevented by breathing air that is fully saturated with water at body temperature. It also has been shown that exercise-induced bronchospasm can be accentuated by breathing dry and cold air[6] and that voluntary hyperventilation is as effective as exercise in producing acute airway obstruction in sensitive persons. The effects of temperature and humidity in the inhaled air on hyperpnea-induced bronchospasm are illustrated in Figure 3-1.[7] The greatest responses were noted when the inhaled air was dry and very cold; there were no changes in the forced expiratory volume during the first second (FEV_1) when the subjects breathed fully saturated air at body temperature. It may be concluded from these observations that the major trigger of hyperpnea-related asthma is heat loss from the respiratory passages. Deal et al.[8] have shown that there is a remarkably close and predictable relationship between postexertional reductions in expiratory flow rates and heat loss from the respiratory passages (Fig. 3-2).

The way in which heat loss from the respiratory tree causes bronchospasm is not fully understood at this time. It is possible that heat loss stimulates vagal receptors which send afferent discharges to the central nervous system. From there efferent vagal discharges may elicit bronchial smooth muscle constriction and airway obstruction. The existence of such pathways is suggested by the reduction or prevention of EIA in some patients after the inhalation of atropine.[9] Vagal mechanisms are not the only way in which postexertional asthma is brought about. It is likely that mediators contribute to the development of exercise-induced bronchospasm, since cromolyn, a known blocker of mediator release, can prevent or reduce postexertional airway obstruction. It also has been shown that frequent repetitions of strenuous exercise will result in less and less bronchospasm, provided that the activities are separated by less than 1 hour. This observation suggests that the stores of mediators

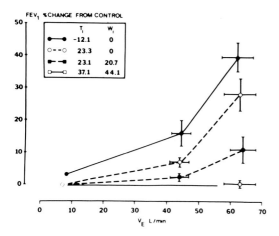

Figure 3-1. Effects of temperature and humidity in inhaled air on development of hyperpnea-induced bronchospasm. (From Deal EC Jr, McFadden ER Jr, Ingram RH Jr, et al: *J Appl Physiol:* 46:476, 1979. With permission.)

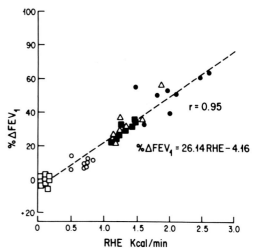

Figure 3-2. Relation between heat loss from respiratory passages and development of EIA. (From Deal EC Jr, McFadden ER Jr, Ingram RH Jr, et al: *J Appl Physiol:* 46:467, 1979. With permission.)

which are responsible for the production of postexertional airway obstruction can be exhausted.

The experimental evidence, clinical observations, and knowledge about the mechanisms of action of various therapeutic agents can be combined in a tentative schema that is shown in Figure 3-3. This illustration demonstrates that exercise and its associated hyperpnea can lead to the stimulation of bronchial smooth muscles by vagal pathways or by the release of chemical mediators. The high sympathetic tone during strenuous exercise or voluntary hyperpnea prevents the development of bronchospasm for as long as the hyperpnea continues. When activity is terminated or the hyperpnea stops, sympathetic transmitters disappear from the circulation within 1 or 2 minutes, but chemical mediators and parasympathetic bronchospastic stimuli remain unopposed and thus produce post-hyperpnea bronchospasm. The magnitude and duration of bronchospasm depend on the amount of mediator released and the duration of the efferent parasympathetic discharges.

DIFFERENTIAL DIAGNOSIS

Exercise-induced asthma should not be confused with the development of dyspnea during exercise in patients with severe, poorly controlled asthma or obstructive lung disease due to

other causes. The patient in whom asthma is not well controlled frequently has limited exercise tolerance, which causes shortness of breath during exertion. This limitation in exercise tolerance can be distinguished from postexertional bronchospasm by noting that it stops as soon as exercise is terminated.

Children and adolescents with other forms of chronic obstructive lung disease may also wheeze and experience shortness of breath during physical activity. This is particularly common in

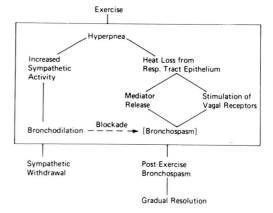

Figure 3-3. Pathophysiologic events responsible for EIA. (From Cropp GJA: *Current Views in Asthma and Immunology.* Atlanta, Ga. With permission.)[14]

patients with cystic fibrosis. Coughing is common in these patients during and after exercise, since physical activity stimulates sputum expectoration. Patients with cystic fibrosis or other forms of nonbronchospastic chronic obstructive lung disease improve when they stop exercise, although it may take several minutes before they return to their preexercise respiratory status. They do not develop postexertional wheezing. The diagnosis of cystic fibrosis usually is obvious from the nutritional state of the patient, chest x-ray examination, findings on clinical examination, and results of a sweat test. Other causes of chronic, nonbronchospastic airway obstruction usually can be identified from a chest x-ray examination, history and physical examination, and appropriate laboratory tests.

A few atopic patients develop serious, prolonged, potentially life-threatening attacks of shortness of breath, wheezing, hives, itching of the skin, stridor, angioedema, choking, gastrointestinal colic, and headaches, and, occasionally hemodynamic collapse shortly after exercise. These attacks are called *exercise-induced anaphylaxis*. They develop rarely in asthmatic patients, but all of these persons are atopic. Exercise-induced anaphylaxis may occur once in a lifetime or can recur repeatedly.[10] There is some evidence that these attacks may be associated with the consumption of foods to which these patients are allergic. The symptoms usually last from 30 minutes to several hours, but the headaches can persist for days. The episodes of exercise-induced anaphylaxis apear to be associated with the release of histamine.[11] Because of the association of exercise-induced anaphylaxis with elevated blood levels of histamine, the attacks are considered to be truly anaphylactic in nature.

DIAGNOSTIC TESTS

Testing Procedures

The occurrence of EIA usually can be determined from the history. When there are doubts about the presence or severity of these attacks, it may be helpful to reproduce them in the laboratory or in the natural setting in which they have been observed. When a child is tested in a natural setting, it is important to remember that a variety of factors can influence the development of postexertional bronchospasm. (See discussion of environmental factors.) In the laboratory exer-

cise can be performed on a treadmill, a cycle ergometer, or other exercise machines which allow sufficient exercise to raise heart rates to 90 percent or more of age-specific maximal levels.[12]

Since they are familiar with bicycles, most youngsters exercise well on a cycle ergometer. Before the test begins, the patients should be familiarized with preexercise and postexercise pulmonary function tests, equipment, and the exercise protocol. Children who are afraid or unable to perform the pulmonary function or exercise tests should be trained until they can do all of the procedures. For the assessment of postexertional bronchospasm it is best to use an 8–10 minute high-load exercise. Once the child has warmed up and started to exercise at a pedal rate of 50–60 rpm, the resistance of the cycle ergometer is rapidly increased until the child exceeds a heart rate of 180 beats/min. This workload is maintained for 6–8 minutes. The child is continually encouraged to perform to the best of his or her ability and is frequently reminded that the test is not of long duration. Most children are able to complete such a test without great difficulties. They breathe from a reservoir that contains dry air at or below room temperature. An electrocardiogram is recorded continuously from two chest electrodes, and the heart rate is computed with a tachometer.

Preexertional and postexertional pulmonary function tests usually include forced vital capacity (FVC) maneuvers, which provide measurements for the FVC, FEV_1 and forced expiratory flow rate between 25 and 75% of FVC ($FEF_{25-75\% VC}$). In many laboratories flow-volume curves can be recorded whenever FVC maneuvers are performed. The equipment and procedures used should satisfy the requirements of the American Thoracic Society guidelines for spirometry.[13] After exercise, only single FVC maneuvers are performed, provided that the patients perform the tests well and the results are within 5 percent of baseline measurements. When there is a deterioration in the test results, at least two measurements are obtained; the FVC and FEV_1 measurements must be within 5 percent of one another to be acceptable. The best test is chosen to represent the patient's pulmonary status.

Before, during, and after exercise the patients should be observed clinically. Careful auscultation of the chest should precede any exercise test, and the attendants should watch for wheezing during and after the exercise test. Careful auscultations and pulmonary function tests are performed 3–5, 10–15, 20–25, and 30–35 minutes after the completion of the exercise test. At the end of the observation period an aerosolized bronchodilator is administered to assure that any residual airway obstruction is eliminated or to test whether preexertional airway obstruction is reversible.

Exercise tests can also be performed with a treadmill. Adolescents and young adults exercise well on these machines. The inhalation of dried and cooled gases is, however, more difficult to arrange. One recommendation is that the grade be set at approximately 10 percent and that the treadmill speed is sufficient to make the person jog at an easy pace, usually 3–5 miles/hr. The duration of exercise testing should be 6–8 minutes at a heart rate of 180 beats/min or above.

The absolute work load needed to elicit bronchospasm varies greatly between persons and depends in part on physical fitness and the type of exercise performed. When muscle groups not commonly used are exercised, the actual amount of work necessary to produce postexertional bronchospasm is less than when well-trained muscle groups are used. This is why arm exercise tends to be more asthmogenic than leg exercise. It is important to realize that exercise lasting less than 2 minutes rarely elicits EIA and quite often produces bronchodilation.[3]

Experienced staff should be in attendance during the performance of exercise tests. The medical and technical personnel need to be certified in cardiopulmonary resuscitation procedures, and use of emergency equipment; appropriate drugs and a defibrillator should be easily accessible. Children should wear clothing that is appropriate for strenuous exercise.

It is useful to score the severity of EIA. Table 3-1 summarizes the deteriorations considered necessary to classify exercise-induced bronchospasm as mild, moderate, or severe. The use of such criteria makes the interpretation of results more uniform and reproducible.

Safety Precautions

When exercise tests are performed in a laboratory, stringent safety precautions must be taken.[12] Patients should be examined carefully before exercise testing is considered. If there is a history suggestive of heart, skeletal or muscular disease, or other significant medical illnesses, it

Table 3-1 *Criteria for Scoring Severity of Exercise-Induced Asthma*

Test	Postexercise Measurements (%)[a]		
	Mild	Moderate	Severe
AES[b]	+1	+2	+3
SGaw[c]	51–70[d]	30–50	<30
(PEFR)[e]	61–75	40–60	<40
FEF$_{25-75\%}$	61–75	40–60	<40
FEV$_1$	66–80	50–65	<50
FVC	81–90	70–80	<70

[a]From Cropp GJA: The exercise bronchoprovocation test: Standardization of procedures and evaluation of response. *J Allergy Clin Immunol* 64:627, 1979. With permission.
[b]AES = Air exchange score; for definition see ref. 1.
[c]Specific airway conductant
[d]Percentage of preexercise values.
[e]Peak expiratory flow rate.

must be assured that the exercise test is safe. When there is evidence of heart disease, it is advisable to have a cardiologist present during the exercise test. There should be a recent 12-lead electrocardiogram available for review and also a recent chest x-ray examination. Blood pressures should be recorded before and during the activity. Exercise should be discontinued when the systolic blood pressure rises over 200 or the diastolic pressure is over 110 mm Hg. Testing should be postponed in asthmatic patients when the baseline pulmonary function tests indicate a moderate degree of airway obstruction. The electrocardiogram should be displayed on a monitor throughout the exercise, and the test should be stopped whenever there are premature ventricular contractions, arrhythmias, or changes in the ST segments.

TREATMENT

EIA can be prevented by the avoidance of strenuous physical activity; however, this is highly undesirable and impossible to achieve in spontaneously active children. Consequently, strategies have to be developed to deal with this common form of reactive airway disease.

Once it has been established that a child develops recurrent EIA during spontaneous play or planned activities, oral bronchodilator therapy can often prevent the occurrence of mild postexertional bronchospasm. When postexertional airway obstruction is marked, oral bronchodilators are usually not sufficient to prevent or reduce EIA to an acceptable level. Under these conditions inhaled β-2-agonists such as albuterol, terbutaline, isoetharine, metaproterenol, or isoproterenol are usually effective in reducing postexertional airway obstruction to a degree so that even strenuous activities can be undertaken. Careful measurements usually show that some degree of postexertional bronchospasm still develops, but it is either of no clinical significance or is mild and of short duration. Cromolyn, which is inhaled before activity, can frequently reduce exercise-induced bronchospasm significantly, although its effectiveness tends to be less than that of inhaled bronchodilators. This is in part due to the absence of any preexertional bronchodilator effect of cromolyn. Patients who have no airway obstruction before exercise usually benefit as much from cromolyn as they do from inhaled bronchodilators. With appropriate therapy before exercise, the majority of asthmatic patients can engage in even strenuous and competitive exercise satisfactorily.

When bronchospasm or hyperinflation develops after exercise, the airway obstruction can be reversed quickly and effectively by the inhalation of a bronchodilator aerosol. Inhaled isoproterenol, metaproterenol, terbutaline, isoetharine, or albuterol are all effective in reversing EIA. Cromolyn has no effect on postexertional bronchospasm. Oral bronchodilators do not act fast enough to terminate an attack of EIA.

When children are known to develop severe postexertional bronchospasm, they should select physical activities which are tolerated relatively well. In general, swimming in indoor pools is better tolerated than running of short or intermediate distances. Football, downhill skiing, and volleyball are better tolerated than soccer, track events, and basketball. Long-lasting endurance exercises such as cross-country skiing and long-distance running are often tolerated surprisingly well; this may be due to the exhaustion of mediator stores during these activities. Environmental conditions, particularly the temperature and relative humidity of the air and the presence of seasonal allergens to which a child may be sensitive, can influence the development of EIA. It is therefore occasionally necessary to select and adjust exercise programs for children so that they can be active during all seasons. This may require participation in indoor sports during the cold winter months or selection of nondemanding physical activites during the allergy season. There is no evidence that inhaled or oral steroids lessen the severity of or prevent EIA.

Physical training will not eliminate EIA. When a child becomes more physically fit, the threshold rises above which exercise-induced bronchospasm will develop. This means that low levels of activities can be performed without distress, and children may require less medication to prevent or control EIA. The reason why training increases the activity threshold is probably due to the lower degree of hyperpnea at any level of oxygen consumption or work load when one is fit than when one is unfit. Since respiratory heat loss is proportional to minute ventilation, any reduction in the ventilatory equivalent ($\dot{V}_E/\dot{V}O_2$) will have a favorable influence on hyperpnea-induced airway obstruction.

CASE PRESENTATION

Figure 3-4 shows the typical exercise-induced pulmonary functional changes in a 12-year-old asthmatic patient with severe postexertional airway obstruction. This patient had a mild degree of preexertional airway obstruction. He was taking slow-release oral bronchodilators for the control of chronic asthma and was unable to tolerate the withdrawal of such medication for more than 12–15 hours. He was steroid dependent, requiring 20 mg. of prednisone every other day. The exercise test was preformed while he was receiving regular bronchodilator therapy. Despite adequate theophylline blood levels, the patient developed mild to moderate wheezing toward the end of strenuous cycle ergometry exercise. His heart rate during the last minute of exercise ranged between 190 and 200 beats/min. When cycling was stopped, severe wheezing, shortness of breath, and hyperinflation developed within 3 minutes. It can be seen in Figure 3-4 that without pretreatment there were notable reductions in vital capacity, forced expiratory flow and specific airway conductance (SGaw), and increases in residual volume. These abnormalities persisted for 30 minutes, but lessened toward the end of the observation period. All abnormalities were eliminated completely by the inhalation of albuterol aerosol. This indicates the pure bronchospastic nature of the airway obstruction associated with EIA. Figure 3-4 also shows that when the patient was treated with inhaled albuterol before exercise, his activity-induced airway obstruction and hyperinflation were greatly reduced.

This patient had perennial asthma. He had no

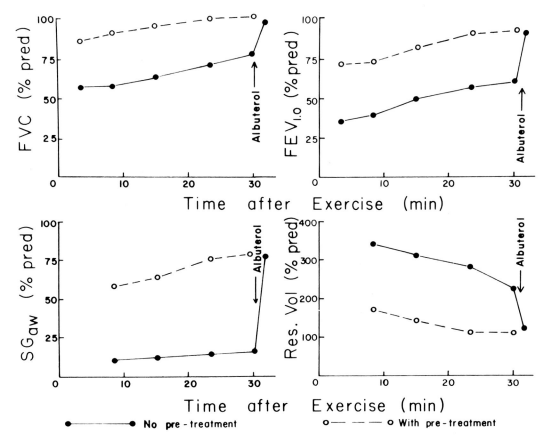

Figure 3-4. Postexertional pulmonary function changes in an asthmatic boy before and after pretreatment with an aerosolized β_2-agonist. Note precipitous falls in the vital capacity, expiratory flow rates, and specific airway conductance and the increase in residual volumes without pretreatment. The functional abnormalities gradually improved over 30 minutes and were completely corrected by the administration of an aerosolized bronchodilator. Pretreatment with albuterol reduced the exercise-induced deteriorations in lung function to such a degree that the child was almost symptom free during the postexercise period.

identifiable sensitivities to environmental antigens. When this boy developed respiratory tract infections, the EIA became more troublesome and exercise tolerance was reduced. The only physical activity he

was unable to perform with appropriate aerosolized bronchodilator therapy was running of intermediate distances (track events). He enjoyed and excelled in swimming and participated in intramural competition.

References

1. Cropp GJA: Grading, time course, and incidence of exercise-induced airway obstruction and hyperinflation in asthmatic children. *Pediatrics* 56: suppl:868, 1975.
2. Chatham M, Bleecker ER, Smith PL et al: A comparison of histamine, methacholine, and exercise airway reactivity in normal and asthmatic subjects. *Am Rev Respir Dis* 126:235, 1982.

3. Cropp GJA: Exercise-induced asthma. *Pediatr Clin North Am* 22:63, 1975.
4. Strauss RH, McFadden ER Jr, Ingram RH Jr, et al: Influence of heat and humidity on the airway obstruction induced by exercise in asthma. *J Clin Invest* 61:433, 1978.
5. Shturman-Ellstein R, Zeballos RJ, Buckley JM et al: The beneficial effect of nasal breathing on

exercise-induced bronchoconstriction. *Am Rev Respir Dis* 118:65, 1978.

6. Strauss RH, McFadden ER Jr, Ingram RH Jr, et al: Enhancement of exercise-induced asthma by cold air. *N Engl J Med* 297:743, 1977.

7. Deal EC Jr, McFadden ER Jr, Ingram RH Jr, et al: Hyperpnea and heat flux: initial reaction sequence in exercise-induced asthma. *J Appl Physiol* 46:476, 1979.

8. Deal EC Jr, McFadden ER Jr, Ingram RH Jr, et al: Role of respiratory heat exchange in production of exercise-induced asthma. *J Appl Physiol* 46:467, 1979.

9. Tinkelman DG, Cavanaugh MJ, Cooper DM: Inhibition of exercise-induced bronchospasm by atropine. *Am Rev Respir Dis* 114:87, 1976.

10. Sheffer AL, Austen KF: Exercise-induced anaphylaxis. *J Allergy Clin Immunol* 1980; 66:106.

11. Soter NA, Sheffer AL, McFadden ER Jr, et al: Exercise-related physical allergy. *J Allergy Clin Immunol* 69:103, 1982.

12. Cropp GJA: The exercise bronchoprovocation test: standarization of procedures and evaluation of response. *J Allergy Clin Immunol* 64:627, 1979.

13. American Thoracic Society Statement. Snowbird Workshop on Standardization of Spirometry. *Am Rev Respir Dis* 119:831, 1979.

14. Cropp GJA: The pathophysiology of airway obstruction in asthma: Basic abnormalities, quantitative assessment and clinical correlates. (Teaching tape and slide presentation.) Published by *Current Views in Asthma and Immunology,* Atlanta, Ga, June 1981.

4

Hypersensitivity Pneumonitis in Children

Zack Haddad
Kumar N. Kulkarni

Diseases due to hypersensitivity reactions in the lung exhibit a diversity that is only partly a function of the different operative mechanisms of hypersensitivity (types I, III, and IV of Gell and Coombs' classification). They are expressed in a variety of frequently similar and occasionally characteristic clinical manifestations.

The route of entry of the culprit antigen is also diverse; antigen may be inhaled, as in farmer's lung (extrinsic allergic alveolitis); ingested, as in drug-induced hypersensitivity pneumonitis (e.g., nitrofurantoin); injected, as in penicillin-induced Löffler's syndrome; or in situ, as occurs in allergic bronchopulmonary aspergillosis (ABPA) due to colonization by fungi.

Both immune and nonimmune mechanisms may be involved in these diseases. If the etiologic agent is undetected and allowed to remain in the patient's environment, irreversible pulmonary damage may ensue. Since signs and symptoms are often nonspecific, diagnosis, management, and ultimately environmental intervention *must* depend on a high index of suspicion; the clinical history must delve deeply into the patient's occupational and recreational activities to provide the clue to the antigen exposure.

DEFINITION

The term *hypersensitivity pneumonitis* comprises a group of diffuse interstitial or alveolar-filling granulomatous pulmonary diseases associated with intense respiratory exposure to finely dispersed organic dust of appropriate particle size.

ETIOLOGY

There are numerous causes of hypersensitivity pneumonitis, and the list continues to expand. The list of causes is summarized in Table 4-1. Antigens such as actinomycetes spores are usually 5 μm or smaller in diameter, so they can enter the alveoli and induce hypersensitivity pneumonitis. The antigens most frequently involved in the etiology of hypersensitivity pneumonitis are the thermophilic actinomycetes, the cause of farmer's lung, which can be isolated from soil, manure, grain, compost, hay, and contaminated forced-air heating and cooling systems. The organisms include *Micropolyspora faeni* and *Thermoactinomyces* species. These microorganisms thrive well at temperature of 40–60°C with approximately 40 percent humidity, thus moldy hay supports their growth well.

Other organisms include fungi such as *Alternaria, Penicillium,* and *Aspergillus* species. Serum proteins also form another important group of antigens. Avian proteins may be inhaled from dried excreta of caged pigeons, chickens, or parakeets. Pituitary snuff, which is made from pituitary glands and used by patients with diabetes insipidus, also can cause hypersensitivity pneumonitis. The proteins involved in this case include bovine and porcine serum and pituitary proteins. Characterization of antigens have been tried by using such procedures as chromatography, gel filtration, and immunochemical and immunoelectrophoretic techniques. Pigeon dropping extracts thus show a heterogeneous mixture of soluble proteins, glycoproteins, and polysaccharides. The major an-

Table 4-1 *Etiology of Hypersensitivity Pneumonitis*

Disease	Exposure	Specific Inhalant
Bagassosis	Moldy sugarcane	*Thermoactinomyces sacchari*
Bat lung	Bat droppings	Bat serum protein
Bird-breeder's lung	Avian dust	Avian serum
Cheese-washer's disease	Cheese mold	*Penicillium casei*
Chicken-handler's disease	Chickens	Feathers serum
Coffee-worker's lung	Coffee dust	Unconfirmed
Coptic disease	Mummies	Mold (not conclusive)
Detergent-worker's lung	Detergent enzymes	*Bacillus subtilis protein*
Duck fever	Duck feathers	Feathers, serum
Farmer's lung	Moldy hay	*Micropolyspora faeni* *Thermoactinomyces vulgaris* *Thermoactinomyces candidus* *Thermoactinomyces viridis*
Furrier's lung	Hair dust	Unconfirmed
Humidifier or forced-air system lung	Fungal spores	*Thermoactinomyces candidus* *Thermoactinomyces vulgaris*
Malt-worker's lung	Malt and barley dust	*Aspergillus clavatus* *Aspergillus fumigatus*
Maple bark disease	Moldy maple bark	*Cryptostroma corticale*
Miller's lung	Contaminated grain	*Acarus siro* (mite) *Sitophilus granarius* (wheat weevil)
Mushroom-worker's disease	Mushroom compost	*Micropolyspora faeni* *Thermoactinomyces vulgaris*
New Guinea lung	Thatched roof dust	*Streptomyces olivaceous*
Paprika-splitter's lung	Moldy pods	*Mucor stolonifer*
Pituitary snuff–taker's disease	Pituitary powder	Bovine and porcine proteins
Rodent-worker's lung	Laboratory animals	Dried rate serum
Sauna-taker's disease	Moldy water and bucket	*Pullularia species*
Sequoiosis	Moldy redwood sawdust	*Aureobasidium pullulans*
Suberosis	Moldy cork dust	*Penicillium frequentans*
Synthetic fiber lung	Orlon, polyester, Bakelite	—unknown
Tobacco-grower's lung	Tobacco plant	Unconfirmed
Turkey-handler's disease	Turkeys	Serum
Urethane foam disease	Urethane foam	Toluene diisocyanate
Wheat weevil disease	Wheat flour	*Sitophilus granarius*
Wood dust disease	Mahogany and oak dust	Unconfirmed
Wood pulp-worker's disease	Moldy logs	*Alternaria tenuis*
Drug-induced pneumonitis		
Nitrofurantoin	Iatrogenic	
Cromolyn sodium	Iatrogenic	
Hydrochlorothiazide	Iatrogenic	

tigens of *Thermoactinomyceces* organisms are acidic glycoproteins, whereas *M. faeni* antigens are polysaccharides.

PATHOLOGIC CONDITION

The basic pathologic condition consists of inflammation of the alveoli and interstitial pulmonary tissue with some bronchiolar involvement. In the acute stage one sees thickening of alveolar septae predominantly with lymphocytes, and plasma cell infiltrates are seen. Foamy macrophages may be present in the alveoli. With chronic disease noncaseating granulomas with epithelioid cells (Langerhan's cells with various degrees of fibrosis) are observed. Pulmonary vasculitis is almost always absent.

INCIDENCE

There are no definitive studies indicating the prevalence of hypersensitivity pneumonitis. The incidence in pigeon breeders is reported to be 6–21 percent, in farmers it is about 7 percent, and in the pediatric age group the incidence is not known.

PATHOGENESIS

The manner by which inhaled organic dusts produce hypersensitivity pneumonitis depends on a complex interrelationship between environmental, genetic, and other host-related factors. Heavy exposure to dust usually is necessary to produce symptoms. It has been calculated that a farmer working with moldy hay can inhale and retain 750,000 spores/min in the lungs, 98 percent of which are actinomycetes. The bulk of evidence is against an infectious etiology.

With regard to host response, the presence of an HLA-associated immune response gene in hypersensitivity pneumonitis has been suggested. For example, in bird-breeder's disease, HLA-1, B8, is frequently associated with active disease.

There is little evidence that IgE-mediated (type I) reactions are involved in the pathogenesis of these diseases. Patients usually have normal IgE levels, and eosinophilia usually is not present. Furthermore, there is no increased incidence of this disease in the atopic population. Immune complex–mediated (type III) tissue

injury has been believed to play an important role. Evidence for this includes the presence of precipitating antibodies against the offending antigen and the detection of specific antigens, immunoglobulins, and complement components in alveolar lesions. On the other hand, precipitating antibodies to organic dusts can be detected in a large percentage of asymptomatic exposed subjects, and pulmonary vasculitis, a manifestation of immune complex injury, usually is *not* seen in the disease process. Furthermore, complement levels are found to decline in asymptomatic, rather than in symptomatic, patients after provocative challenge. The presence of complement components on the surface of alveolar macrophages of patients without the presence of necrotizing vasculitis favors the hypothesis of cytotoxic (type II) allergic tissue injury, rather than type III immune complex–induced disease. A nonimmunologic basis for tissue injury is suggested by direct activation of the alternate complement pathway by organic dust and antigens.

There is increasing evidence, such as granuloma formation, that delayed hypersensitivity (type IV) may be involved in the disease. In vitro tests to detect the presence of delayed hypersensitivity, such as antigen-induced production of migration inhibition factor (MIF) and lymphocyte transformation, can be demonstrated in these patients and these often correlate with activity of the disease process. In animal models for hypersensitivity pneumonitis, classic delayed hypersensitivity reactions at 24–48 hours have been detected by using respiratory tract immunization with thermophilic actinomycete antigens. In summary, it is likely that more than one immunologic, as well as nonimmunologic mechanism may be involved in pathogenesis of hypersensitivity pneumonitis.

DIAGNOSTIC APPROACH

The clinical presentation of patients with hypersensitivity pneumonitis depends on the following factors:

1. The nature of inhaled dust
2. The intensity and frequency of inhalation exposure
3. The intensity and type of immunologic host response

The presence of a concomitant respiratory tract infection can also trigger symptoms. The combination of recurrent symptoms associated with a specific environment should suggest hypersensitivity pneumonitis. The clinical features of illness are similar, regardless of the type and nature of inhaled organic dust. The symptoms can be acute or chronic.

Acute form

Clinical features of the acute form of hypersensitivity pneumonitis are explosive and related to antigenic exposure. The period of sensitization by inhalation of organic dust is variable and may take several months to years.

Symptoms

Symptoms usually occur 4–6 hours after antigen exposure. Systemic symptoms include a temperature as high as 40°C (104°F), chills, myalgia, and malaise. Respiratory symptoms include coughing and dyspnea without wheezing. Symptoms may persist up to 18 hours and spontaneously regress. The attacks recur each time the individual is exposed to large quantities of offending dust. As attacks become more frequent and severe, additional symptoms of anorexia, weight loss, and progressive dyspnea become prominent.

Physical Examination

During the attack the patient is acutely ill and dyspneic. Bibasilar end-inspiratory rales are prominent and may persist for several hours, days, or weeks after the attack subsides.

Laboratory Studies

1. Leukocytosis with a shift to the left may be seen. Although eosinophilia is absent, occasionally up to 10 percent of eosiniphilia may be present.
2. Immunoglobulin levels other than IgE are usually elevated.

Pulmonary Function Studies

Several types of abnormalities may be demonstrated during acute episodes. The most common response occurs 4–6 hours after exposure and consists of a decrease in both the forced vital capacity (FVC) and forced expiratory volume at 1 second (FEV_1) with little alteration in the ratio of these two variables. A decrease in lung compliance and decreased diffusion capacity also occur during the attack. Hypoxemia is detected by arterial blood gas studies. These abnormalities resolve as clinical features subside. With sufficient parenchymal damage, however, changes in pulmonary function in volume and flow rates may be detected even during asymptomatic periods.

A second type of response is seen in patients with pigeon protein or pituitary snuff exposure. This is characterized by an immediate, but transient, decrease in FVC and FEV_1. A late reaction at 4–6 hours with a decrease in these parameters also is seen.

It is important to differentiate the late phase of the dual bronchial obstructive response seen in atopic patients from the late phase of hypersensitivity pneumonitis after antigen challenge. The responses are summarized in Table 4-2. It has been demonstrated that the immediate reaction after antigen challenge in asthma and hypersensitivity pneumonitis is more responsive to bronchodilators, whereas the late response usually is resistant to these drugs. Pretreatment with corticosteroids blocks only the late response, whereas cromolyn sodium can block both responses.

Chest Roentgenography

Chest roentgenography features are variable, ranging from insignificant abnormalities to diffuse fibrosis. The most common findings are diffuse nodular infiltrates and coarse bronchovascular markings. These findings are reversible if the patient avoids further exposure to the offending allergen. During the acute stage soft, patchy, ill-defined parenchymal densities may be seen in both lung fields.

Immunologic Studies

Humoral

1. Serum precipitating antibodies against the specific offending organic dust antigen can be detected by gel filtration or immunoelectrophoresis. With the use of an appropriate antigen, antibodies can be detected in all individuals who are ill. Up to 50 percent of exposed asymptomatic individuals may have precipitating antibodies to the same antigen, however. The presence of antibodies thus is not diagnostic of hypersensitivity pneumonitis. The type of anitbody is usually of the IgG

Table 4-2 *Pulmonary functions after inhalation challenge in dual asthmatic response and in hypersensitivity Pneumonitis*

Tests	Late Phase of Dual Asthmatic Response	Late Phase of Respiratory Response in Hypersensitivity Pneumonitis
FEV_1	↓	↓
FEV_1/FVC ratio	↓	Little or no change
FVC	Usually unchanged	↓
Diffusing capacity	Normal	↓

class, but serum IgM and IgA antibodies have also been detected.

2. The complement level has been noted to be normal or slightly elevated in ill patients. This is not helpful as a diagnostic test.

Cellular studies

Lymphocyte transformation and production of macrophage MIF have been detected in a significant number of patients with bird-breeder's lung. Asymptomatic individuals similarly exposed have negative tests. Symptomatic individuals will have positive precipitin, lymphocyte transformation, and MIF tests, whereas similarly exposed asymptomatic individuals may have precipitating antibodies but are usually negative for lymphocyte transformation and MIF tests.

Histologic examination

In the acute form, there is extensive lymphocytic infiltration in alveolar septae, which are thickened. Alveolar spaces usually contain lymphocytes, plasma cells, and macrophages. The histologic examination will only identify the presence of hypersensitivity pneumonitis, but will not indicate the etiology. Immunoflourescent studies of lung biopsy specimens have detected specific antigens in alveolar septae and the interstitium. Immunoglobulin and complement usually are not demonstrated in such biopsies.

Chronic Form

Patients can develop an insidious form of hypersensitivity pneumonitis, which usually is associated with prolonged exposure to small amounts of antigen.

Symptoms

Symptoms include progressive dyspnea, a cough, malaise, weight loss, and weakness. This form is usually common in individuals who keep several birds in their home.

Clinical Features

Auscultation reveals persistent rales, and pulmonary function testing usually demonstrates restrictive ventilatory impairment, diffusion defects, and hypoxemia. A chest x-ray examination shows diffuse nodulation or fibrosis.

Histologic examination

A lung biopsy may show lymphocytic and plasma cell infiltration of the alveolar walls, which is less prominent than in the acute form of the disease. Extensive fibrosis involving alveolar walls and peribronchial tissue occurs. Granulomas are seen dispersed in interstitial fibrosis. Obstructive bronchiolitis also may be present.

Summary of Diagnostic Features of Hypersensitivity Pneumonitis

1. Hypersensitivity pneumonitis should be considered in the differential diagnosis of every patient with recurrent pulmonary infiltrates or interstitial lung disease. A carefully obtained history may suggest a relationship between an occupation or hobby and symptoms.

2. Patients can present with recurrent "flu-like" episodes, a chronic unexplained cough, dyspnea, or chronic pulmonary impairment. Physical signs are not specific for hypersensitivity pneumonitis. During an

acute attack, fever, bibasilar rales, and leukocytosis with a shift to the left can occur. Spontaneous recovery and subsequent recurrences point to the possibility of hypersensitivity pneumonitis.

3. The most common roentgenographic findings are diffuse nodular infiltrates and coarse bronchovascular markings.

4. Although pulmonary function tests are not diagnostic of hypersensitivity pneumonitis, if a specific environment is suspected, pulmonary function tests can be performed before and for several hours after exposure to an inhalation challenge. If significant changes occur, the environment should be suspected, and immunologic and culture studies should be carried out. Inhalation challenge using potential antigenic materials should be done only in a laboratory or hospital setting, since a severe attack can be precipitated.

5. The most consistent feature of hypersensitivity pneumonitis is the presence of serum precipitating antibodies to the specific antigen source. Antigens from *Thermo actinomyces* and *Aspergillus* species or avian proteins are available to detect precipitins. Additional antigens such as extracts of dusts or fungi cultured from the humidifier or dusts at the place of employment may be needed to demonstrate the presence of precipitating antibodies. Tests for cell-mediated immunity, such as lymphocyte transformation or MIF production, may be even more diagnostic than precipitating antibodies in detecting hypersensitivity pneumonitis from a specific antigen.

6. If other measures fail, a lung biopsy should be carried out. It will indicate the presence of disease and not its source. Immunofluorescent studies for antigens and immunoglobulins in the lung parenchyma may be helpful.

TREATMENT

1. *Avoidance*

   Avoidance of the offending antigen is of utmost importance in the management of hypersensitivity pneumonitis. Once the antigen is identified, various precautions can be taken. Alterations in forced-air heating or cooling systems may be helpful. In some cases a change in occupation may be necessary. Improved ventilation and the use of masks may reduce excessive exposure in bird breeders. Complete avoidance of birds may be necessary at times to prevent the progression of the disease. Individuals with farmer's lung may have to leave the farm, if the diffusing capacity remains abnormal for 2–3 months.

2. *Pharmacologic treatment*

   Pharmacologic treatment is indicated if offending antigens cannot be avoided or if the disease appears to be progressive despite environmental control measures. Corticosteroids are the mainstay of therapy. In acute cases prednisone, 30–60 mg/day for several weeks, may be necessary. Clinical and laboratory responses to steroids may be dramatic. The duration of therapy depends on the clinical response and pulmonary function. Reversal of the disease process depends on how rapidly the diagnosis is made and avoidance carried out. Early identification and avoidance of the offending agent are therefore critical for a good prognosis. Chronic exposure with pulmonary fibrosis is not reversible.

5

Allergic Bronchopulmonary Aspergillosis in Children

Zack Haddad
Kumar N. Kulkarni

Aspergillus organisms are ubiquitous molds found in air, soil, decaying vegetation, swimming pool water, house dust, and bedding. Many species of *Aspergillus* may infect humans, but the most common is *A. fumigatus*. The following are five types of lung disease caused by *Aspergillus* organisms:

1. *Invasive or septicemic aspergillosis* occurs in patients whose immune function has been compromised. There is invasion of the bronchial wall, producing bronchitis, pneumonia, mycotic abscesses, and chronic granulomas.
2. *Aspergilloma* is the most common form of aspergillosis. The organism colonizes preexisting anatomic abnormalities, such as a bronchiectactic or tuberculous cavity. There is superficial invasion of tissue.
3. *Bronchial asthma* IgE–mediated bronchial asthma can be caused by *Aspergillus* organisms.
4. *Extrinsic allergic alveolitis* can be caused by *A. clavus* growing in moldy barley on floors of breweries.
5. *Allergic bronchopulmonary aspergillosis* is characterized by bronchospasm, pulmonary infiltrates, eosinophilia, and immunologic evidence of allergy to the antigens of *Aspergillus* species.

In 1952 Hinson et al. first described allergic bronchopulmonary aspergillosis (ABPA) in three patients with wheezing; recurrent febrile episodes; blood eosinophilia; sputum plugs containing fungi, neutrophils, and eosinophils; and x-ray evidence of pulmonary consolidation.

EPIDEMIOLOGY

The most common species of *Aspergillus* associated with ABPA is *A. fumigatus,* although other species, such as *A. flavus, A. niger,* and *A. nidulans,* have been implicated occasionally. Because of the ubiquitous distribution of the fungus, failure to obtain a definitive history of exposure is common. The incidence is higher in fall and winter months (September to March) when spore counts are higher. Nosocomial outbreaks of ABPA can occur and are linked to increased spore counts in ventilation systems. There is no sex predilection, and the disorder has been described in all age groups. The majority of cases occur in those less than 35 years of age.

INCIDENCE

The incidence of ABPA is reported to be much greater in the United Kingdom than in the United States. It is the most common cause of asthma with pulmonary eosinophilia in the United Kingdom. The first case of ABPA was reported in the United States in 1968. An accurate incidence is difficult to obtain. The incidence is believed to be increased in patients with cystic fibrosis. In a large series of studies on cystic fibrosis, the incidence of ABPA was found to be 11 percent.

PATHOGENESIS

ABPA is believed to be initiated with inhalation and trapping of short-chain spores of *A. fumigatus* in viscid secretions of the respiratory tract of asthmatic patients. *A. fumigatus* spores

45

germinate and form mycelia at body temperature. Tissue invasion by fungus is believed not to occur. The antigen source continues to grow in the bronchial lumen and continuously sheds antigens into the tissues.

The exact mechanisms involved in the pathogenesis are unknown, but evidence suggests that type I (immediate hypersensitivity) and type III (immune-complex) reactions are involved. The immediate hypersensitivity reaction is believed to be IgE mediated and accounts for bronchospastic symptoms that are the hallmark of this disorder. The type III reaction is probably responsible for the roentgenographic features of ABPA, as well as destructive changes in the bronchi.

Both IgE skin-sensitizing and IgG precipitating antibodies are required for expression of the disease and dual skin-test responses present in ABPA. It is believed that IgE immunoglobulins enhance the tissue-damaging effects of IgG precipitating antibodies. Patients with ABPA have small amounts of precipitating antibodies and demonstrate vigorous late skin-test response, as opposed to patients with aspergilloma, who show weak or negative immediate skin reactivity and negative late skin-test reaction despite high titers of precipitating antibodies. The low precipitating titler provides a condition of moderate antigen excess, leading to formation of toxic immune complexes.

The importance of precipitating antibodies in pathogenesis has been demonstrated by passive transfer experiments in monkeys. Transfusion of serum from a patient with ABPA to a monkey, followed by aerosol challenge with *Aspergillus* antigens, resulted in development of pulmonary lesions consistent with ABPA. Transfusion of skin-sensitizing antibodies alone, however, caused no pulmonary lesions. Recently a possible role for cell-mediated hypersensitivity (type IV) reactions has been inferred from demonstration of in vitro lymphocyte transformation to *Aspergillus* antigens in patients with ABPA. Granulomas and mononuclear cell infiltration also are present in histopathologic processes of the lungs. Finally, the complement system may be operative in the pathogenesis. Circulating immune complexes and evidence of activation of the classic complement pathway have been demonstrated during the acute phase of allergic aspergillosis. Using in vitro systems, *Aspergillus* antigens have been shown to directly activate the alternate complement pathway.

HISTOLOGIC AND PATHOLGIC PROCESSES

Bronchial walls are usually not invaded, and fungal hyphae may be identified in the exudate. The parenchyma usually shows extensive consolidation, chronic inflammatory cells, and a large number of granulomas. The alveolar walls may show thickening. Granulomas have central necrosis and multinucleated giant cells with prominent infiltration of eosinophils. Immunofluorescent staining is usually absent, indicating no vascular deposits of immune complex. Chronic sequelae of ABPA include changes such as fibrosis, bronchiectasis, lung contraction, and lobar shrinkage.

DIAGNOSTIC APPROACH

History

Patients with ABPA are almost always atopic and have a history of bronchial asthma for variable lengths of time. Patients with early-onset asthma have the highest incidence of personal and family history of allergy compared to those with late-onset asthma. The interval may vary from 3–5 years to 24 years between the onset of asthma and appearance of ABPA. ABPA is a recurrent disorder with a wide range of clinical presentations. Bronchospasm and dyspnea are the most common symptoms. An intermittent or chronic cough is present in 98 percent of patients. A productive cough is common, and expectoration of sputum plugs is present in about 54 percent of patients. Sputum plugs are usually hard, solid lumps of different sizes, shapes, and color, ranging from brown to dirty green. Hemoptysis, although usually minimal, is present in 34–85 percent of patients. Localized pleuritic chest pain is present in about 50 percent of patients. Generalized constitutional symptoms include fever, usually low-grade, malaise, anorexia, headaches, and loss of energy.

Physical Examination

Wheezing and airway obstruction are usually present. Crepitant rales can be heard over lung segments that are shown to be involved on roentgenography.

Laboratory Tests

Roentgenographic Examination

A variety of roentgenographic abnormalities have been described in patients with ABPA. The most common is a massive homogeneous density, and indicating areas of consolidation. The upper lobes are usually involved, and the radiodensity shadow can be patchy, triangular, or lobar. These opacities may shift from one site to the other rapidly. Another frequently seen abnormality due to edema of the bronchial wall consists of two parallel hairline shadows extending from the hilum in the direction of bronchi and is called a *tramline shadow*. Secretions in dilated bronchi give rise to "toothpaste" shadows that revert to normal once mucous plugs are expectorated. Other findings reported on chest x-ray examination are atelectasis, lobar emphysema, lobar shrinkage, and cavitation. Patients may be relatively free of symptoms but have extensive involvement roentgenographically. Consolidation may resolve but frequently leaves evidence of permanent lung damage in the form of bronchiectasis.

Bronchography

The most common finding on bronchographic examination is proximal saccular bronchiectasis, with normal filling of distal bronchi. This finding is unique to ABPA.

Pulmonary Function Tests

Pulmonary function tests reflect the underlying lung disease and vary from obstructive to restrictive functional abnormalities. All patients have a decrease in the forced expiratory volume in 1 second (FEV_1) and forced vital capacity (FVC). The ratio of FEV_1/FVC usually is less than 70 percent. There is evidence of increased airway resistance. Evidence of reversible bronchospasm with the use of bronchodilators may be minimal. The diffusion capacity is decreased in most of the patients and usually correlates with the duration of the disease.

Eosinophil Count

Peripheral blood eosinophilia is a universal feature of ABPA. An absolute eosinophil count greater than 500/mm^3 is the rule and generally exceeds over 100/mm^3. Values greater than 3000/mm^3 are common. Blood eosinophilia usually parallels the activity of pulmonary involvement.

Sputum Examination

Direct examination of sputum reveals a large number of eosinophils and fungal mycelia. Mycelia usually have good preservation of cytoplasm, which is indicative of active growth. In contrast, patients with aspergilloma usually have mycelia that are devoid of cytoplasm.

Positive cultures are not diagnostic of ABPA because of the ubiquitous distribution of fungus, and negative cultures are not uncommon. Routine sputum cultures from asthmatic patients yield positive growth in about 10 percent of patients.

Serum IgE Levels

Total IgE levels and IgE levels specific for *Aspergillus* organisms are elevated in patients with ABPA. IgE levels are considerably higher than in patients with extrinisic asthma. For example, values greater than 15,000 ng/ml are not unusual in ABPA. The majority of this IgE response results from nonspecific stimulation of IgE-producing plasma cells by the *Aspergillus* organism. It now appears that IgE levels correlate best with disease activity. IgE levels often rise before clinical exacerbation and decrease on remission.

Skin Tests

Intradermal testing with 1 or 10 mg/ml of the protein fraction of *A. fumigatus* results in dual skin-test responses in almost all patients with ABPA. The immediate wheal and flare reaction subsides, and in 4 hours erythema and poorly defined edema appears, reaching peak response at 8 hours and resolving by 24 hours. If the immediate skin-test response is negative, it is unlikely that ABPA is causing the clinical symptoms. Immediate positivity is not diagnostic of ABPA, since it is present in about 25 percent of asthmatic patients. Similarly dual skin responses have been reported in 4 percent of healthy individuals, 36 percent of allergic asthmatic patients, and up to 96 percent of patients with aspergilloma. Standardization of the antigenic extracts used for skin testing has not yet been accomplished. Most commercially available preparations contain mixtures of extracts of different species of *Aspergillus*. Lower potency extracts may give rise to false-negative reactions.

Table 5-1 *Criteria for Diagnosis of Allergic Bronchopulmonary Aspergillosis*

- Primary criteria

    Episodic bronchial obstruction
    Peripheral blood eosinophilia
    Immediate skin reactivity
    to *Aspergillus* antigens
    Serum precipitins to *Aspergillus* antigens
    Elevated serum IgE level
    History of infiltrates
    Central bronchiectasis

- Secondary criteria

    Aspergillus organisms in sputum
    History of mucous plug expectoration
    Late skin-test reactivity to *Aspergillus* antigens

Serum Precipitins

The precipitating antibodies to *A. fumigatus* are generally of the IgG type: Two techniques, double immunodiffusion and counterimmunoelectrophoresis (CIE), are used to detect precipitins. The immunodiffusion technique can be made more sensitive by concentrating the serum threefold to fourfold. Serum precipitins are positive in about 92 percent of patients with ABPA when the serum is concentrated, as opposed to 72 percent in those with unconcentrated serum. The presence of precipitating antibodies to *A. fumigatus* is not diagnostic of ABPA, since it is present in 9 percent of hospitalized patients, 3 percent of healthy office workers, and 27 percent of patients with allergic asthma. In addition, almost all patients with an aspergilloma have positive serum precipitins.

Bronchial Challenge

Bronchial challenge with *Aspergillus* antigen is seldom necessary for diagnosis and can be dangerous. The bronchial response is dual, like the skin test, with an immediate fall in FEV_1 associated with wheezing, which resolves, followed in 4–6 hours by a second fall in FEV_1. Late responses may last for many hours and are difficult to reverse. Patients with atopic bronchial asthma due to *A. fumigatus* show only immediate responses. Patients with aspergilloma have a fever without asthma 6 hours after bronchial challenge.

DIAGNOSTIC CRITERIA

ABPA has few specific, pathologic, or roentgenographic features unique to itself. A high index of suspicion is necessary to arrive at the diagnosis. Criteria for the diagnosis of ABPA are shown in Table 5-1. The diagnosis of ABPA is considered likely if the first six primary criteria are present and certain if all seven are present.

DIFFERENTIAL DIAGNOSIS

Bacterial pneumonia, tuberculosis, and carcinoma need to be differentiated in patients suffering from asthma and pulmonary shadows. Many patients with cystic fibrosis have positive precipitating antibodies and immediate-type skin tests. An elevated sweat chloride test, a positive family history, and lack of eosinophilia or extremely high IgE levels help to differentiate it from ABPA. Eosinophilic pneumonias caused by chemical substances, helminths and various mycotic antigens usually begin with a cough and anorexia. A chest x-ray examination shows transient, migratory infiltrates, and bronchiectasis seldom occurs. Extrinsic allergic alveolitis is usually seen in nonatopic patients and consists of interstitial pulmonary infiltrates with normal levels of IgE and eosinophils.

TREATMENT

Early and vigorous treatment is important, because it is difficult to clear the fungus once bronchial damage had occurred. Corticosteroids are the most effective drugs in the treatment of ABPA. They decrease allergic inflammatory responses, pulmonary infiltration, and the amount of viscid secretions. Prednisone initially is given for 2–3 months in dosages of 1–2 mg/kg/day, ideally until complete clearing of the chest x-ray film occurs. Then a daily dose of 0.5 mg/for each kilogram of body weight is continued for 2 weeks, followed by an alternate-day schedule for another 3 months. Over the next 3 months, the dose is tapered and discontinued. Long-term steroid therapy seems essential to prevent recurrences. This schedule must be flexible to the patient's clinical and laboratory response.

FOLLOW-UP CARE

Since one third of acute exacerbations of ABPA are asymptomatic, patients need to be monitored carefully. IgE levels increase with recurrence and decrease with remission. Serial IgE measurements should be done once a month for 2 years. The chest film should be obtained every 4 months for a 2-year period. Any exacerbation should be treated by corticosteroid therapy. Routine bronchodilator therapy with vigorous postural drainage and chest percussion should be continued indefinitely.

PROGNOSIS

If untreated, ABPA becomes chronic, leading to airway obstruction, pulmonary consolidation, and progressive bronchiectasis. Intelligent management can result in an improved prognosis.

REFERENCES

Fink JN: Hypersensitivity pneumonitis, in Middleton E Jr, Reed CE, Ellis EF (eds); *Allergy: Principles and Practice.* St Louis, The CV Mosby Co., 1978, p 855.

Fink JN: Immunologic lung diseases. *Hospital Practice* 16:53, 1981.

Glimp RA, Bayer AS: Fungal pneumonias: Allergic bronchopulmonary aspergillosis. *Chest* 80(pt 3):85, 1980.

Henderson AH: Allergic aspergillosis: review of 32 cases. *Thorax* 23:501, 1968.

Hinson KFW, Moon AJ, Plummer NS: Bronchopulmonary aspergillosis: a review and a report of eight new cases. *Thorax* 73:317, 1952.

Lopez M, Salvaggio J: Hypersensitivity pneumonitis: current concepts of etiology and pathogenesis. *Annu Rev Med* 27:453, 1976.

Pepys J: Hypersensitivity diseases of the lungs due to fungi and organic dusts, in *Monographs in Allergy.* Vol. 5 Munich, Basel S Karger, 1969.

Rosenberg M, Patterson R, Roberts M, et al: The assessment of immunologic and clinical changes occurring during corticosteroid therapy for allergic bronchopulmonary aspergillosis. *Am J Med* 64:599, 1978.

Slavin RG: Allergic bronchopulmonary aspergillosis, in Middleton E Jr, Reed CE, Ellis EF (eds): *Allergy: Principles and Practice.* St Louis, The CV Mosby Co, 1978, p 843.

Wang JLF, Patterson R, Mintzer R, et al: Allergic bronchopulmonary aspergillosis in pediatric practice. *J Pediatr* 94:376, 1979.

Wang JLF, Patterson R, Roberts M, et al: The management of allergic bronchopulmonary aspergillosis. *Am Rev Respir Dis* 120:87, 1979.

6

Deficiency in Host Defense Mechanisms of the Lung

Stanley P. Galant

The nonrespiratory activity of purifying inspired air and keeping lung tissue free of infection is collectively referred to as *lung host defense mechanisms*.[1,2] Elements of the defense system are spaced along the entire respiratory tract from air entry at the nares to the level of oxygen uptake in the alveolar surface. Different mechanisms operate along the conducting airways compared to the air exchange units (Table 6-1). The conducting airways extend from the nares to the terminal bronchioles. Factors important at this level include anatomic barriers, branching of the respiratory tree, mucus entrapment, mucociliary clearance, cough response, bronchoconstriction, and locally produced secretory IgA (SIgA). Distal to the terminal bronchioles in air exchange units other elements become more important, such as the lining material of the alveoli (surfactant), iron-containing proteins (transferrin), IgG, properdin and factor B (important in the alternative complement pathway), and the pulmonary alveolar macrohpage (PAM), which is the principal phagocytic cell of the airways and scavenger of the alveolar surface. Many of these resistance factors are mechanical or nonspecific interactions that form the first line of defense. Although these factors frequently are effective, it is the inflammatory amplification capability of the lung working throught the immune system that provides the greatest protection for the lung particularly when the first line of defense is breached. The immune system is the major focus of this discussion.

Several excellent papers[1,2] review the nonspecific defense mechanisms and will not be discussed further. In this chapter the most important immune mechanisms in the lung will be explored, followed by a description of clinical entities that have been associated with several types of deficiency in host defense mechanisms. Finally, a therapeutic approach to these deficiencies will be briefly presented.

THE LUNG AS AN IMMUNOLOGICAL ORGAN

It is not commonly appreciated that the lung is an important lymphoid organ. In the late 1950s Humphrey and co-workers showed that after intravenous hyperimmunization of a rabbit with killed pneumococcal organisms, the lung tissue exceeded the bone marrow, the spleen, and lymphoid glands in antibody synthesis.[3] The lung can respond with antibody synthesis after local antigen inoculation without the participation of extrapulmonary lymphoid tissue. Morphologically, the tremendous distribution of lymphoid tissue within the lung would support the impression of an active immunologic organ. Lymphoid aggregates are present in bronchial mucosa, nodules are seen in the walls of large- and medium-sized bronchi, lymph nodes are present in the hilar area, and lymphoid cells are seen in the small airways and among the bronchoalveolar cell population. Perhaps the most fascinating organization of pulmonary lymphoid tissue consists of lymphoid nodules referred to as *bronchial-associated lymphoid tissue* (BALT)[4] These nodules, located at bifurcations of the bronchial tree,

Table 6-1 *Host Defenses of Lung*

Level of Lung	Nonspecific Factors	Specific Immunologically Stimulated Factors
Upper airways	Anatomic barriers	Secretory IgA
	Branching of tracheobronchial tree	T-lymphocytes
	Mucous entrapment	Bronchus-associated lymphoid
	Mucociliary clearance	Tissue (BALT)
	Cough response	
	Bronchoconstriction	
Lower airways	Surfactant	IgG
	Transferrin	T-lymphocytes
	Complement	Complement
	Pulmonary alveolar macrophage (PAM)	Pulmonary alveolar macrophage (PAM) (activated)
	Polymorphonuclear cell	Polymorphonuclear cell

are covered by a specialized flat lymphoepithelium lining and are devoid of glandular goblet cells, which facilitates antigen uptake. The BALT cell population consists of 20 percent thymus-derived T-lymphocytes, 50 percent bursal-derived B-lymphocytes that have only surface-staining immunoglobulin markers (showing immaturity), and 30 percent null cells. Unlike lymph nodes, BALT contains no true germinal centers or plasma cells and a lower percentage of T-lymphocytes. B-lymphocytes in BALT are believed to be precursors of SIgA plasma cells. Several studies suggest a common network between BALT and similar cells in lymphoid tissue in the gastrointestinal tract (e.g., Peyer's patches). Cells leaving BALT are believed to undergo maturation into IgA-secreting cells, which then relocate in the lamina propria and submucosa of the respiratory and gastrointestinal tracts.[5]

SIgA is believed to provide major mucosal protection in the upper respiratory tract, including the tracheobronchial tree. Several studies have validated this concept by showing better correlation between the presence of specific SIgA antibodies to respiratory microbes and the prevention of clinical manifestations than correlation with serum antibodies.[6] In contrast to serum in which IgG predominates, IgA exceeds IgG in bronchial and nasal secretions.[7] SIgA is a dimer consisting of two IgA molecules (IgA$_2$ subclass predominantly) bound together by two additional nonimmunoglobulin moieties known as *secretory piece* and J chain, respectively. This configuration apparently stabilizes the molecule

in secretions, thus increasing its resistance to proteolysis. The antimicrobial action of SIgA apparently is related to its ability to specifically block adsorption of macromolecules to the mucosal surface.[8] This facilitates normal degradative processes, resulting in the clearance of potentially harmful substances. IgE plasma cells are located in similar sites to those of IgA. Although viral antibody activity has been shown for IgE, its role in host defenses remains undefined.[9] Furthermore, stimulation of these cells can result in hypersensitivity phenomena in the lung.

Protection of the lower respiratory tract is associated with a different set of immunologic factors. It is believed that the predominant immunologic response at the alveolar level is not IgA, but IgG. Secretions from the upper and lower portions of the respiratory tract thus differ in their content of immunoglobulins. IgA-secreting cells predominate in the upper and middle levels of the tract, but rarely are found as far down as the bronchioles, even in the presence of infection. When alveolar space washings are tested, they resemble serum in terms of IgG/IgA ratios (Table 6-1).

Cells from the distal air spaces obtained by bronchial lavage consist of the PAMs, T- and B-lymphocytes, plasma cells, neutrophils, and eosinophils. The similarity of T- and B-lymphocyte proportions in serum and the alveolar space suggests interchange between these two compartments. Although local cell-mediated immunity has been shown after aerosolization of bacillus Calmette Guerin (BCG) organisms, similar protection from virulent *Mycobacterium tuberculosis* was seen after parenteral immunization. The PAM is the resident mononuclear phagocyte of the lung and functions as the primary defense mechanism against particulate matter.[10] Developing from the precursor bone marrow monocyte, it functions in such tasks as antigen processing and scavenging the alveolar surface. Particles ingested by the macrophage are either cleared in the mucociliary escalator or in the lung interstitium through the pulmonary lymphatics. The PAM kills microbes after their attachment to the cell surface and phagocytosis. This process is facilitated by IgG and complement opsonization of the microbe, which then binds to cell-surface Fc fragment and complement C3b receptor sites. PAMs which can be activated directly by microbes or T-lymphocytes through the release of lymphokines, have increased numbers of these important receptors and are more effective in their antimicrobial function. Microbicidal mechanisms are poorly understood, but are believed to involve oxidative metabolism, including the production of superoxide anion and hydrogen peroxide in conjunction with a halide anion. Several factors have been shown to modify PAM performance. For example, surfactants enhance PAM killing, whereas tobacco smoke and viral infections inhibit phagocytosis and killing. The latter is consistent with the observation that respiratory tract viral infections frequently precede bacterial infections in the lung. PAMs are most important when the route of inoculation is inhalation and the microbes are primarily intracellular. These include viruses, fungi, and several bacteria (e.g., *Mycobacteria* organisms). *Staphylococcus* organisms are also handled by PAMs. The neutrophil is the other important phagocytic cell in lung defenses, particularly at the alveolar level. It may be more effective in clearing pneumococci than staphylicocci, although it is important for both microbes.

In summary, pulmonary defenses can be viewed as a two-layered system. First, there are nonspecific factors such as anatomic barriers, clearance mechanisms, inhibitory substances such as transferrin and surfactants, complement components, and nonactivated macrophages. This system is reasonably adequate to protect against the usual microbial inoculum. With an unusually large or virulent inoculum, however, the amplification system is initiated in the immune host, which generates an appropriate inflammatory response to combat the infection.

This second line of defense includes the activated PAMs, sensitized T-lymphocytes, opsonic antibodies, complement, and neutrophils.

CONSEQUENCES OF HOST DEFENSE DEFICIENCIES

In this discussion deficiencies of immunologic and inflammatory factors will be correlated with their clinical pulmonary manifestation. The examples given are not intended to be comprehensive nor inclusive of extrapulmonary involvement.

Antibody Deficiency States

As seen in Table 6-2, antibody deficiency, particularly of the IgG class, results in pyogenic parenchymal lung infections with highly virulent bacteria such as pneumococci, *Haemophilus influenzae*, streptococci, and *Pseudomonas aeruginosa*.[11] This would be expected, since IgG protects the lung parenchyma by forming opsonic antibodies against these microbes. Serious chronic lung infections associated with broncheictasis have been reported in such antibody deficiency states as X-linked agammaglobulinemia and the common variable type of hypogammaglobulinemia primarily due to the lack of IgG. Recently, Beck and Heiner described four patients with severe recurrent sinopulmonary infections associated with an isolated absence of IgG_4 subclass.[12] Patients with IgA deficiency are known to have an increased prevalance of respiratory tract infections and respiratory allergies such as allergic rhinitis and bronchial asthma.[13] IgA deficiency is not necessarily associated with clinical manifestations, however, perhaps because the function IgA can be replaced by IgM in these cases.

Deficiencies in Cell-mediated Immunity

Patients who lack T-lymphocyte function suffer from severe chronic pulmonary infections with organisms that are usually of low pathogenicity in the normal host.[14] These opportunistic infections include viruses such as cytomegalovirus and herpes simplex; intracellular bacteria, including *Mycobacterium avium intracellulare,* and *Klebsiella pneumoniae;* fungi, including *Candida albicans;* and protozoa such as *Pneumocystis carinii* and *Toxoplasma gondii.* In children with

Table 6-2 *Immunologic Defense Mechanisms*

Host Factor Deficiency	Type of Infection	Clinical Example
Antibodies	Pyogenic bacteria	X-linked agammaglobulinemia Common-variable hypogamma- globulinemia
Cell-mediated immunity	Intracellular microbes, viruses, fungi, bacteria	Thymic aplasia
Combined deficiency	Any type, *Pneumocystis* *carinii*	Severe combined immune deficiency Wiskott-Aldrich syndrome Ataxia telangiectasia

primary congenital immunodeficiencies, however, pure B-lymphocyte defects have also been associated with *Pneumocystis* disease. Patients with combined T- and B-lymphocyte deficiencies, however, appear to be most predisposed to infection with this organism. An example of T-lymphocyte immunodeficiency is thymic aplasia (DiGeorge syndrome).

Combined T- and B-lymphocyte Deficiencies

Patients with a spectrum of primary T- and B-lymphocyte deficiencies have been reported.[15] Infections include those previously mentioned with *Pneumocystis carinii* and cytomegalovirus being particularly prominent. These agents should be suspected in the compromised host whenever there is roentgenographic evidence of interstitial or alveolar pneumonia. Fever is uncommon, but respiratory distress associated with hypoxemia and few auscultatory findings is characteristic. In patients with severe combined immunodeficiency, these infections tend to be severe and occur in early childhood. Examples of less severe combined T- and B-lymphocyte immunodeficiencies include Wiskott-Aldrich syndrome, immunodeficiency with thymoma, and ataxia telangiectasia.

Abnormalities of the Phagocyte

Although the immune deficiencies just described are well recognized, less appreciated until recently have been defects in the factors that create the inflammatory response. These abnormalities may also result in chronic recurrent pulmonary infections (Table 6-3). These entities include the abnormal number and function of phagocytic cells (monocyte-macrophage and neutrophil) and abnormalities in complement.

Deficiency of phagocytic cell number or defective cellular function have best been studied for the neutrophil because it is a more accessible cell than the monocyte-macrophage. Both cell types protect the surface of the respiratory tract as major scavengers of microbes and other particulate matter in the lung parenchyma. Since there is less known about monocyte abnormalities and they commonly occur in conjunction with neutrophil defects, the latter will be discussed more fully. Neutropenia of either a persistent or cyclic variety can be associated with pyogenic pulmonary infections. In addition these patients may encounter such opportunistic bacteria as *Serratia* and *Pseudomonas* organisms, *Staphylococcus epidermidis,* and several fungi. Patients with defects in neutrophil movement (chemotaxis) have severe skin and pulmonary infections with *Staphylococcus aureus* and *Candida albicans.* Buckley (1977) has described several patients with similar clinical and laboratory findings characterized by an unusual facies, impaired neutrophil chemotaxis, and extremely elevated serum IgE levels.[16] The mechanism responsible for increased susceptibility to infection is complex, since the chemotactic defect is not constant, and other abnormalities such as T-lymphocyte dysfunction may also be present. Patients with chronic granulomatous disease (CGD) who have neutrophils that can phagocytize, but cannot kill catalase-positive organisms, have serious infections with *Staphylococcus aureus, pseudomonas* organisms, *Serratia marcescens,* and several fungi. Recently a child was reported to have disseminated atypical mycobacteria infection

Table 6-3 *Inflammatory Factor Deficiency*

Host Factor Deficiency	Type of Infection	Clinical Example
Phagocytic cell (monocyte or neutrophil)		
Leukocytopenia	Pyogenic bacteria	Cyclic neutropenia
Chemotaxis	*Staphylococcus aureus, Candida* organisms	Hyper-IgE syndrome
Killing	Catalase-positive bacteria	Chronic granulomatous disease
	Both catalase-positive and catalase-negative microbes	Chédiak-Higashi syndrome
Complement	Pyogenic bacteria	Hypercatabolism of C3
C3 Hypocomplementation		

who possibly had a defective monocyte-killing capability.[17] Isolated monocyte-macrophage abnormalities have also been reported in malacoplakia and pulmonary alveolar proteinosis.[18] Patients with Chédiak-Higashi syndrome have similar symptoms to those with CGD, but in addition have difficulty with catalase-negative organisms.

Complement Abnormalities

Deficiencies of nearly all of the complement components have been associated with clinical manifestations of infection or autoimmune phenomena.[19] Probably the most profound pulmonary infections arise from deficiency of C3, which can occur either as a result of absent synthesis or increased degradation. Infections with pyogenic organisms similar to that seen with IgG hypogammaglobulinemia occur.

DIAGNOSTIC CONSIDERATIONS

A brief overview of clinical and laboratory findings that should point to the correct diagnosis will be presented here.

Clinical Clues

Perhaps the most important consideration in suggesting a deficiency in host defenses is the presence of chronic, recurrent, severe sinopulmonary infections with organisms of high virulence such as staphylococci or pneumococci or, on the other hand, infections with opportunistic microbes such as *Serratia marcescens*. It is thus incumbent on the physician to identify the organism. Tracheal aspiration and at times an open or closed lung biopsy may be warranted. This helps in suggesting the presence of immune deficiency and provides a good rationale in specific therapy.

Laboratory Tests

Antibody Deficiency States

The key points in assessing antibody deficiency states include first, adequate quantitation of IgG, IgM, and IgA by techniques such as radial immunodiffusion followed by correct interpretation using age- and sex-matched controls. Second, assessment of antibody-producing capacity using antibody formation to tetanus, diphtheria, rubella, streptococci for IgG, and isohemagglutinins A and B for IgM synthesis. Suspicion should be raised when immunoglobulin levels are less than 2 standard deviations (SD) from the mean, and antibody synthesis is inadequate for age and exposure. Once a deficiency state has been diagnosed, more sophisticated investigation can be carried out, such as identification of B-lymphocyte surface markers and assessment of in vitro antibody synthesis.

Deficiencies in Cell-mediated Immunity

Helpful screening tests for deficiencies in cell-mediated immunity include the search for lymphocytopenia (less than 1500 lymphocytes/mm^3), absence of a thymic shadow on chest films, and lack of delayed hypersensitivity reactions to several microbial antigens such as tetanus toxoid, *Candida albicans*, and streptokinase-streptodornase. More definitive assessment includes in vitro responses of the T-lymphocyte to antigen and mitogen stimulation, as well as subpopulation characterization with monoclonal antibodies.

Abnormalities of the Phagocyte

After determining the neutrophil number, one can screen for killing and phagocytic capability with the qualitative nitroblue tetrazolium (NBT) test. Chemotaxis is usually assessed using a Boyden chamber and a variety of chemoattractants.

Complement Abnormalities

A search for abnormalities in complement is measured in two ways: functional assays based on hemolytic activity and radial immunodiffusion which can quantitate individual complement proteins.

THERAPEUTIC STRATEGY

A complete discussion of therapy in patients with host deficiencies is beyond the scope of this paper. Furthermore, only the principles of replacement therapy will be given, and description of therapies aimed at specific microbes will not be covered. Interested readers are referred to the literature for a more comprehensive discussion on the subject.[20]

Antibody Deficiency States

The major immunoglobulins involved in protection of the respiratory tract are IgA (upper) and IgG (lower). Deficiencies that warrant replacement therapy demostrate serum levels less than 2 SD below the mean for age and sex, inability to adequately synthesize antibodies, and significant clinical expression such as pyogenic sinopulmonary infections.

Currently there are no effective and practical means of replacing IgA. Commercial γ-globulin contains insufficient amounts of IgA for replacement therapy, but sufficient amounts to sensitize the patient to IgA. This could lead to the development of anti-IgA antibodies and anaphylaxis after subsequent exposure. It is therefore contraindicated. Improvement was reported in a single patient after infusions of fresh frozen plasma, which resulted in normal IgA levels.

Additional therapy to be considered is the use of bovine and human colostrum, which are both rich sources of IgA. Most recommend, however, directing therapy toward the specific disease entity associated with an IgA deficiency.

Patients with a significant IgG deficiency (as defined above) should receive 100 mg/kg/month (0.6 ml/kg) of commercially available Cohn fractioned γ-globulin *intramuscularly* after administering double this amount as a loading dose. Since no specific serum levels of γ-globulin are known to ensure antimicrobial protection, serial determinations are not recommended. Plasma infusions are effective in delivering substantial quantities of IgG, IgA, and IgM and are useful when large volumes of γ-globulin are necessary. Since this procedure carries the potential risk of serum hepatitis, however, there usually is a need for a relative as a donor. Intravenous preparations of γ-globulin treated with sulfhydryl agents and iodoacetamide have been under clinical trial in the United States and appear to be safe and effective. This form of γ-globulin therapy has recently become commercially available.[21]

Deficiencies in Cell-mediated Immunity

Several preparations have been used for replacement therapy in patients with either T- or combined T- and B-lymphocyte deficiency. The results have been mixed, depending on the agent used and the particular deficiency state. The fetal thymus works dramatically in patients with thymic aplasia (DiGeorge syndrome) injected parenterally or within a millipore chamber, suggesting that clinical efficacy may be at least in part due to a thymus humoral factor. Its effect in combined immune deficiency and syndromes such as Nezelof syndrome or ataxia telangiectasia has been extremely variable. Cultured thymus epithelium and the thymus hormone thymosin also have resulted in adequate replacement therapy in some patients with T-lymphocyte or combined deficiency states. Transfer factor has generally proven disappointing when used to improve general T-lymphocyte function, although some patients with the Wiskott-Aldrich syndrome appear to show temporary remissions. Patients with severe combined immunodeficiency benefit most from bone marrow transplantation from a histocompatible sibling, matched at the HLA loci, particularly HLA-D. In the absence of a suitable bone marrow donor several other approaches have been taken, including transplantation of fetal liver, fetal thymus, and the combination of the two with some measure of success.

Amplification System

Replacement or correctional therapy related to neutrophil disorders remains experimental at this time. Patients with complement deficiencies generally benefit from replacement with fresh human plasma. Replacement with specific factors is currently being studied.

Case Report

The following case report illustrates several of the concepts in the diagnosis and therapy of immune deficiency previously discussed.

An 18-year-old man came to the office because of recurrent pneumonia. He had frequent upper respiratory tract infections and bilateral otitis media during his preschool years and at least five episodes of pneumococcal or *Haemophilus influenzae* pneumonia documented by sputum culture and chest films from ages 5 to 15 years. He had the usual childhood diseases, including rubeola and varicella, without unusual complications. A tonsillectomy and adenoidectomy were performed at age 15 years, and chronic bronchitis with sputum production and occasional hemoptysis was noted at 16 years. After a diagnosis of bronchiectasis of the left lower lobe of the lung was made, a partial lobectomy was performed. In the last 2 years he has had recurrent sneezing, wheezing, and headaches. Sinus films showed air-fluid levels of the maxillary sinuses. The history and allergy skin tests revealed sensitivity to several inhalant allergens. Treatment consisted of theophylline, antihistamines, and injection therapy. Since starting this program, however, he has continued to have otitis media and pneumonia. The family history reveals that both parents have allergic rhinitis, and a sister has asthma. No history was noted of early death or immune deficiency in the family.

Physical examination revealed a thin, tall, chronically ill man in no distress. The nasal mucosa was hyperemic and swollen, and a purulent discharge also was noted in the nasal cavity. No adenopathy was palpable. Examination of the chest revealed decreased breath sounds on the right, with bilateral rhonchi, rales, and wheezes. No clubbing or cyanosis was present.

Laboratory tests included the following data. The complete blood count was unremarkable with white blood cells of 7000/mm^3, 45 percent lymphocytes and 1 percent eosinophils. The IgG level was 10 mg/100ml, the IgA and IgM levels were 0, and the IgE level was 33 IU/ml. Antibody function was poor to tetanus toxoid immunization, and anti-A (his blood type is B) isohemagglutinins were less than 1:2. T-lymphocyte function assessed by skin tests and in vitro stimulation with antigen and mitogen was normal. B lymphocyte number, determined by polyvalen flourescent antisera, was normal.

Because of these clinical and laboratory findings the patient was given an intramuscular injection of γ-globulin. After several injections the patient developed flushing of the face, tightness in the chest, dyspnea, and hypotension several minutes after an injection.

Discussion

This patient has the common variable type of hypogammaglobulinemia and IgE-induced bronchial asthma. Allergen-induced asthma is suggested by the history and positive skin tests to several common allergens. Findings suggestive of common variable hypogammaglobulinemia include the onset of defective antibody synthesis starting after infancy and the presence of normal numbers of B-lymphocytes (indicated by surface immunoglobulin receptors) that are unable to normally differentiate into antibody-secreting plasma cells. Despite considerable humoral deficiency, however, the patient was still capable of synthesizing and secreting IgE antibodies. T-lymphocyte function, which can also be abnormal in this syndrome, was normal.

This patient demonstrates the necessary criteria for life-long intramuscular γ-globulin therapy. These criteria include a serum IgG level greater than two standard deviations below age and sex corrected mean values, the inability to make antibodies, and serious pyogenic infections. Intravenous plasma therapy, assuming an appropriate donor, and a new intravenous gamma globulin preparation[21] would be other options.

The anaphylactic-type reaction described after γ-globulin injection is most often due to complement activation by γ-globulin aggregates even when the injection is intramuscular. Long-term management of this problem is difficult. If the reaction is due to aggregates, the use of a supernatant preparation after ultracentrifugation of the γ-globulin may be helpful.

Finally, although not common, asthma has been well documented with a variety of immune deficiency states. In addition, several types of immunologic aberrations occur in the atopic asthmatic individual. Partial T-lymphocyte deficiency, particularly of the T-suppressor subpopulation, abnormal IgA responses, and impaired non-IgE antibody synthesis have been noted.

REFERENCES

1. Reynolds HY: Lung host defenses: a status report. *Chest* 75(suppl):239, 1979.
2. Newhouse M, Sanchis J, and Bienenstock J: Lung defense mechanisms. N Engl J Med 295:990, 1976.
3. Humphrey JH, Sulitzeanu BD: The use of (^{14}C) amino acids to study sites and rates of antibody synthesis in living hyperimmune rabbits. Biochem J 68:146, 1958.
4. Bienenstock J, Clancy RL, Perey DYE: Bronchus associated lymphoid tissue (BALT): its relationship to mucosal immunity, in Kirkpatrick CH, Reynolds HY (eds): *Immunologic and Infectious Reactions in the Lung.* New York, Marcel Dekker, Inc., 1976, p 29.
5. Craig SW, Cebra JJ: Peyers patches: an enriched source of precursors for IgA producing immunocytes in the rabbit. *J Exp Med* 134:188, 1971.
6. Rossen RD, Kasel JA, Corich RB: The secretory immune system: its relation to respiratory viral infection. *Prog Med Virol* 13:194, 1971.
7. Kaltreider HB, Chan M: Immunoglobulin composition of fluid obtained from various levels of the canine respiratory tract. Read before the International Congress on Lung Diseases, Montreal, Quebec, May 18–21, 1975.
8. Williams RC, Gibbons RJ: Inhibition of bacterial adherence by secretary immunoglobulin A: a mechanism of antigen dosposal. *Science* 177:697, 1972.
9. Welliver RC, Kaul TN, Ogra PL: The appearance of cell bound IgE in respiratory-tract epithelium after respiratory-syncytial virus infection. *N Engl J Med* 303:1198, 1980.
10. Hocking WG, Golde OW: The pulmonary-alveolar macrophage. *N Engl J Med* 301: 580, 639, 1979.
11. Ochs HD, Wedgewood RJ: Disorders of the B-cell system, in Stiehm ER, Fulginiti VA (eds): *Immunologic Disorders in Infants and Children.* Philadelphia, WB Saunders Co, 1980, p 239.
12. Beck CS, Heiner DC: Selective immunoglobulin G4 deficiency and recurrent infections of the respiratory tract. *Am Rev Respir Dis.* 124:94, 1981.
13. Ammann AJ, Hong R: Selective IgA deficiency: presentation of 30 cases and a review of the literature. Medicine 50:223, 1971.
14. Hughes WT: *Pneumocystis carinii* pneumonia. *N Engl J Med* 297:1381, 1977.
15. Ammann AJ: T cell and T-B cell immunodeficiency disorders. *Pediatr Clin North Am* 24:293, 1977.
16. Buckley RH: Disorders of the IgE system, in Stiehm ER, Fulginiti VA (eds): *Immunologic Disorders in Infants and Children.* Philadelphia, WB Saunders Co, 1980, p 274.
17. Uchiyama N, Greene GR, Warren BJ, et al: Possible monocyte killing defect in familial atypical mycobacteriosis. *J Pediatr* 98:785, 1981.
18. Poplack DG, Blaese RM: Disorders of the mononuclear phagocytic system, in Stiehm ER, Fulginiti VA (eds): *Immunologic Disorders in Infants and Children.* Philadelphia, WB Saunders Co, 1980, p 367.
19. Johnston LB, Stroud RM: Complement and host defense against infection. *J Pediatr* 1977; 90:169.
20. Stiehm ER: Immunodeficiency disorders—general consideration, in Stiehm ER, Fulginiti VA (eds): *Immunologic Disorders in Infants and Children.* Philadelphia, WB Saunders Co, 1980, p 183.
21. Ochs HD: Intravenous immunoglobulin therapy of patients with primary immunodeficiency syndromes: Efficacy and safety of a new modified immune globulin preparation, in Alving BM (ed) *Immunoglobulins: characteristics and uses of intravenous preparations.* Washington, D.C., U.S. Government Printing Office 1980, p. 9.

7

Pulmonary Hemosiderosis

Thomas F. Boat

INTRODUCTION

Pulmonary hemosiderosis results from bleeding into the airways of the lung and conversion of hemoglobin into hemosiderin by alveolar macrophages that ingest the extravasated red blood cells. Hemosiderosis transiently follows acute blood loss into the lungs, for example, from an arteriovenous malformation or hemangioma, erosion of a blood vessel due to bronchiectasis, or aspiration of blood in the pharynx. In this case, hemosiderin is formed and cleared with 1–2 weeks. Few symptoms appear unless acute bleeding has been massive or is repetitive. Pulmonary hemosiderosis usually occurs as a result of persistent, low-grade, diffuse alveolar bleeding, often with superimposed episodes of more brisk diffuse hemorrhage. The alveioli fill with phagocytic cells and cell debris. Interstitial inflammation and, ultimately, fibrosis appear. Gas exchange is compromised. Hemosiderosis may be secondary to nonpulmonary processes, such as left ventricular failure with increased pulmonary venous and capillary pressure, or collagen-vascular diseases with vasculitis-related disruption of pulmonary vascular endothelial barriers. More commonly in children pulmonary hemosderosis is a primary disease of the lung, albeit with multiple pathogenic mechanisms.

Pulmonary hemosiderosis of any etiology in children is uncommon. Because of its extensive morbidity and not infrequent mortality in children, prompt recognition and appropriate therapy are imperative.

BASIC MECHANISMS

Pathogenesis

Diffuse primary pulmonary hemorrhage can be classified on the basis of immunopathologic mechanisms into (1) Goodpasture's syndrome, (2) diffuse pulmonary hemorrhage accompanied by immune complex–mediated glomerulonephritis, (3) idiopathic pulmonary hemosiderosis, and (4) cow's milk–related pulmonary hemosiderosis.

In *Goodpasture's syndrome* antibasement membrane antibodies are detected in serum, and linear IgG deposits are seen along glomerular and alveolar basement membranes. These antibodies probably damage the alveolar-capillary barrier and allow movement of red blood cells into alveoli. Pulmonary hemorrhage may precede clinical evidence for renal dysfunction so that a kidney biopsy is required to make or definitively exclude this diagnosis in cases of isolated pulmonary hemosiderosis.

In diffuse pulmonary hemorrhage accompanied by immune complex–mediated glomerulonephritis granular deposits of immunoglobulins and complement are seen by immunofluorescence in basement membranes and the mesagium of the kidney, but not necessarily in the lung. These renal lesions also are characteristic of nephritis in systemic lupus erythematosus, but the two conditions can be differentiated by the presence or absence of circulating antinuclear antibodies.

In idiopathic pulmonary hemosiderisis no known immune mechanism is demonstrable. In some cases thickening and breaks in the continuity of alveolar-capillary basement membranes have been noted by electron microscopy, but the relationship of these ultrastructural lesions to diffuse hemorrhage has not been firmly established. Familial occurrence has been reported, suggesting a genetic basis for this condition. It is unlikely, however, that this condition represents a homogeneous disease process.

Especially in young children, *pulmonary hemosiderosis can be associated with the presence of precipitating antibodies to cow's milk proteins and milk-related symptoms.* These symptoms can include vomiting and diarrhea, chronic blood loss in the stool, and chronic rhinitis. Although the precipitins are IgG antibodies and immune complex–mediated reactions have been postulated, no single immunologic mechanism has been found to explain the development of hemosiderosis in milk-sensitive patients. These children may be subject in early life to repeat aspiration of milk or have IgA deficiency, both of which are known to promote the generation of milk precipitins in high titers.

Pulmonary hemosiderosis also may occur in conditions causing pulmonary vasculitis (systemic lupus erythematosus, Wegener's granulomatosis, rheumatoid arthritis, anaphylactoid purpura) or pulmonary venous hypertension (mitral stenosis, chronic left ventricular failure). In the former situation, vascular inflammation appears to disrupt the integrity of the pulmonary vessel endothelium, whereas in the latter, a chronic increase in capillary pressure favors diapedesis of red blood cells into alveolar spaces.

Pathologic Mechanisms

Acute hemorrhage is seen in both alveolar and interstitial regions. Hemosiderin-laden macrophages also appear in both locations within 72–96 hours after hemorrhage. Alveoli often are filled with phaygocytic cells, and alveolar septae are thickened by an influx of inflammatory cells and ultimately by fibrosis. Both mechanisms produce a restrictive lung condition. In larger airways, blood is an irritant, causing bronchial wall edema, bronchospasm, and increased secretion of mucus, leading to obstruction of airflow. Severe, long-term hemosiderosis may be accompanied by diffuse interstitial fibrosis and pulmonary hypertension, characterized by hypertrophy of arteriolar walls.

CLINICAL MANIFESTATIONS

Pulmonary manifestations common to all forms of pulmonary hemosiderosis are those to be expected in alveolar filling diseases, such as tachypnea, tachycardia, shortness of breath with exertion, easy fatigability, dyspnea, and cyanosis. A hacking or productive cough may accompany these symptoms and signs, and wheezing is not infrequent. Brisk, diffuse bleeding may result in frank hemoptysis. Growth failure is seen in longstanding cases. In all chronic cases iron deficiency anemia accompanies these pulmonary manifestations and is attended by pallor and fatigue. This finding always is suggestive of hemosiderosis.

Physical findings may include pallor, a repetitive cough, sputum production, rales and rhonchi, digital clubbing, and cyanosis. Chest roentgenograms show variable changes, including evanescent small infiltrates in mild disease, soft diffuse perihilar infiltrates in some cases, and extensive stippling and fine linear densities in severe disease. (Fig. 7-1) Pulmonary function testing generally demonstrates restrictive lung changes, occasionally with a superimposed obstructive component.

Idiopathic Pulmonary Hemosiderosis

Idiopathic pulmonary hemosiderosis appears most often in 1- to 7-year-old children and is frequently carried into adolescence or adulthood. It tends to be more episodic than other types of hemosiderosis, and exacerbations can be severe, even life threatening. These exacerbations are more frequent at times of viral illnesses and often are attended by fever and shaking chills. Because the manifestations are sufficiently variable, this condition cannot be distinguished on clinical grounds from the immunologically based types of hemosiderosis.

Goodpasture's Syndrome

This unusual condition occurs most often in young adult men. Only six children under 16 years of age have been described. Pulmonary bleeding may be relentless and severe. In the past, however, death has usually occurred because of renal failure. When pulmonary hemorrhage precedes evidence of nephritis, this condition may be indistinguishable clinically from idiopathic pulmonary hemosiderosis.

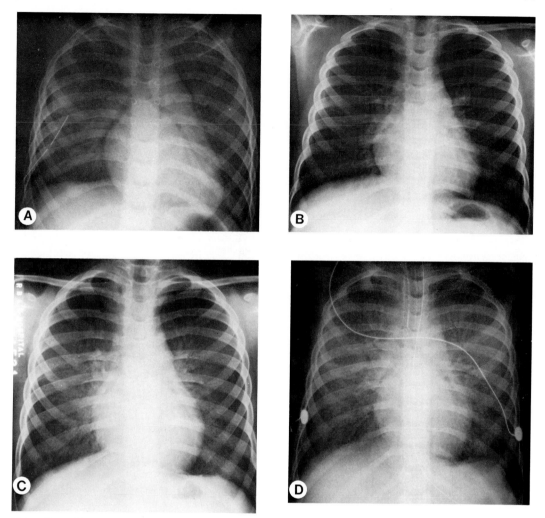

Figure 7-1. Chest roentgenograms of an 8-year-old boy with idiopathic pulmonary hemosiderosis, showing the episodic nature of this disease. (A) Diffuse interstitial and alveolar filling densities produce a hazy shadowing of both lung fields. Aeration is better in the apices than in the lower lobes. Air bronchograms are prominent. The chest tube was inserted at the time of the lung biopsy, 1 day earlier. (B) Considerable clearing of both lung fields after 6 weeks of corticosteroid therapy (2 mg/kg/day tapered to 1 mg/kg/day on week four). A few faint nodular densities persist bilaterally. (C) Exacerbation of linear and finely nodular densities, most prominent in a perihilar distribution, 5 months after diagnosis. Patient was receiving 10 mg of prednisone daily at this time. Symptoms included shortness of breath and increased coughing. (D) Severe exacerbation of acute pulmonary hemorrhage with bilateral diffuse infiltrates and poor aeration of both lungs. The patient was intubated, but despite high-dose corticosteroid therapy, did not recover.

Pulmonary Hemosiderosis with Immune Complex Nephritis

The two children reported (Loughlin et al, 1978) displayed pulmonary manifestations similar to those of idiopathic pulmonary hemosiderosis. Both developed frank hemoptysis and anemia.

Pulmonary Hemosiderosis with Cow's Milk Precipitins

Children with cow's milk precipitins develop pulmonary hemosiderosis early in life, frequently in infancy. Black children who are not breast fed appear to be especially susceptible. Manifestations include transient pulmonary infiltrates or atelectasis, intermittent wheezing, eosinophilia, mild to moderately severe iron deficiency anemia, hepatosplenomegaly, failure to thrive, and striking elevations of serum IgE levels. Frequent extrapulmonary manifestations include gastrointestinal effects (vomiting, diarrhea, occult blood in the stool) and chronic rhinorrhea with nasal obstruction, occasionally accompanied by striking hypertrophy of pharyngeal lymphoid tissue and obstructive alveolar hypoventilation with cor pulmonale (Fig. 7-2).

Recurrent Pulmonary Hemorrhage in Infants.

Massive, acute, but diffuse, pulmonary hemorrhage recently has been noted in three previously healthy infants beyond the newborn period; in one case it was recurrent and fatal. In these children hemosiderin-laden macrophages appeared 2–5 days after onset of bleeding and disappeared after 2 weeks. Although no definite etiology for the hemorrhage was discovered, exposure to marijuana smoke preceded bleeding episodes in two infants. This form of hemorrhage appears to be different from that seen in newborns with respiratory distress syndrome or other serious illness during the first month of life.

DIFFERENTIAL DIAGNOSIS

Pulmonary hemosiderosis can mimic nearly every chronic pulmonary condition of infants and children, including asthma, cystic fibrosis, and alveolar filling diseases such as pulmonary alveolar proteinosis and desquamative interstitial pneumonia. The chief differentiating feature is hypochromic, microcytic anemia, which can be profound. Hemoptysis also strongly points toward the diagnosis of pulmonary hemosiderosis in children who do not have bronchiectasis or pulmonary tuberculosis. Recurrent or persistent lung disease with anemia also may occur in sickle cell disease and chronic severe lung infection, but these can be easily distinguished from pulmonary hemosiderosis with appropriate testing.

KEY DIAGNOSTIC TESTS

The diagnosis of pulmonary hemosiderosis is established by the detection of hemosiderin-laden pulmonary macrophages. These cells can

be seen in smears of sputum or bronchial aspirates stained with potassium ferrocyanide. If bronchial secretions cannot be obtained, diagnostic efforts may have to include open lung biopsy. Some physicians have looked for hemosiderin-containing alveolar macrophages in early morning gastric aspirates. These samples do not always contain intact, easily identified macrophages, however. Hemosiderin-laden macrophages appear within 48–72 hours after bleeding in the lung and may disappear almost completely from the lung within 2–4 weeks after an acute bleeding episode. This information is helpful in differentiating a single bleeding episode from persistent lung hemorrhage. Documentation of iron deficiency anemia may require assessment of hemoglobin and hematocrit levels, red cell indices, serum iron and iron-binding capacity, or serum ferritin or erythrocyte protoporphyrin levels.

Children potentially having idiopathic or immunopathologic pulmonary hemosiderosis should be tested for antibasement membrane antibodies, antinuclear antibodies, and precipitins to cow's milk proteins in serum. Careful studies of renal function are indicated. Immunofluorescence and electron microscopy of lung or kidney biopsy specimens may be helpful in differentiating idiopathic pulmonary hemosiderosis from Goodpasture's syndrome and pulmonary hemosiderosis associated with immune complex–mediated nephritis. Secretory or blood eosinophilia and high IgE levels suggest milk-related pulmonary bleeding. The identification of multiple serum precipitins to defatted cow's milk by double gel diffusion (Ouchterlony) analysis confirms the diagnosis. Precipitins most often are directed against bovine γ-globulins. If milk-related hemosiderosis is strongly suspected, a trial cow's milk–free diet is warranted. If clinical and laboratory manifestations disappear, rechallenge and documentation of original manifestations on two separate occasions is strong supporting evidence for this diagnosis. Tests to rule out contributing factors such as congenital heart disease and collagen vascular diseases should be used as indicated.

THERAPY

The therapy selected for hemosiderosis in children depends largely on the identification of pathogenic factors. A number of general thera-

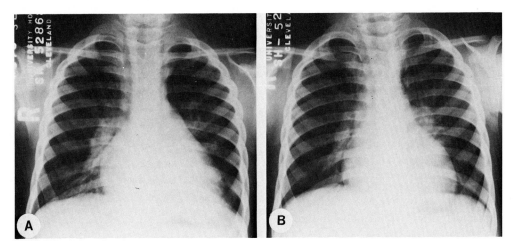

Figure 7-2. (A) Chest roentgenogram of a 3-year-old with cow's milk–induced pulmonary hemosiderosis and upper airway obstruction. Right lower lobe infiltrate, prominence of pulmonary arteries, and enlargement of the heart are evident. (B) Chest roentgenogram of the same child, 3 months after removal of cow's milk from the diet and an adenoidectomy. In addition to clearing of infiltrates, the heart diameter decreased dramatically, and the pulmonary artery segments are less prominent.

peutic principles should be recognized, however. Children with pulmonary hemosiderosis frequently present with considerable respiratory distress and hypoxemia. Supplementary oxygen is often required, and assisted ventilation occasionally may be necessary. Blood transfusions are indicated to treat profound anemia. Superimposed hypersecretion, bronchospasm, or bronchial infection should be recognized and treated appropriately with brochodilators or antimicrobials.

Idiopathic Pulmonary Hemosiderosis

Most authorities agree that high-dose corticosteroids are beneficial at the time of acute exacerbations. Dosages should range from 10 to 20 mg/kg/day of hydrocortisone or an equivalent dose of another glucocorticoid. These doses should be continued for 5–7 days after brisk, diffuse bleeding appears to have stopped, then tapered slowly over 2 or more weeks. There is little direct evidence that long-term steriod therapy is beneficial for prevention of recurrent exacerbations, although some children seem to have fewer relapses if steroids are continued. In these cases, alternate-day regimens using minimal effective doses are preferable. Recurrent severe exacerbations have been successfully treated with other immunosuppressants, most notably azathioprine (Imuran), 2–3 kg/day. If the child has been

symptom free after receiving these drugs for 1–2 yers, the drug should be withdrawn and the child carefully observed. Reinstitution of maintenance immunotherapy may be required. Chronic severe pulmonary symptoms due to continued blood loss and deposition of iron in interstitial areas of the lung may respond in part to iron-chelation therapy with desferrioxamine. There is no evidence that milk restriction is helpful for this form of pulmonary hemosiderosis.

Goodpasture's Syndrome

This condition is perhaps the most refractory to medical therapy of the pulmonary hemosiderosis syndromes. Improvement of pulmonary hemorrhage can be attributed to corticosteroid or azathioprine therapy in less than one third of trials. A bilateral nephrectomy has resulted in remission of pulmonary disease in 40 percent of patients in whom it was performed. This observation suggests that the antibasement membrane antibody in some cases is produced to kidney antigen and that lung basement membranes are secondarily involved.

Pulmonary Hemosiderosis with Immune Complex Nephritis

Both children described with this condition have reponsed satisfactorily to corticosteroids.

Pulmonary Hemosiderosis with Cow's Milk Precipitins

In well-documented cases, pulmonary hemo-siderosis disappears within a few weeks when cow's milk and its products are removed from the diet. In at least one documented case, pulmonary hemosiderosis and upper airway obstruction with cor pulmonale resolved and then returned and resulted in unexpected death after unsupervised ingestion of milk. Milk and its products usually can be safely reintroduced after a 2- to 3-year, symptom-free interval. A reaction to soy-base formula, mimicking that to cow's milk formula, has been observed by the author in one child. Failure of children to respond when switched to soy milk may be due to this situation or to another etiology for pulmonary symptoms. An adenoidectomy with or without tonsillectomy may be indicated if the hemosiderosis is accom-paned by upper airway obstruction and evidence of alveolar hypoventilation.

Secondary Pulmonary Hemosiderosis

In general, precipitating factors such as left ventricular failure, mitral stenosis, or underlying systemic disease with vasculitis should be treated vigorously. As in primary pulmonary hemosid-erosis, symptomatic pulmonary therapy and treatment of superimposed factors such as bron-chospasm or infection may also be indicated.

FOLLOW-UP AND PROGNOSIS

Because pulmonary hemosiderosis is a life-threatening condition in many children, close medical supervision by a knowledgeable physi-cian is required. Activity of disease can be monitored by obtaining serial hematocrit levels and reticulocyte counts and performing cytologic examinations of sputum for hemosiderin-laden macrophages. Iron metabolism and hemoglobin production also should be monitored and iron supplements administered for well-documented hypochromic, microcytic anemia accompanied by evidence of iron deficiency. Ventilatory status can be monitored by chest roentgenograms every 6–12 months and by serial pulmonary function tests, including arterial oxygen tensions.

Milk-related and secondary pulmonary hemo-siderosis rarely cause irreversible chronic lung disease and disappear if the offending condition is controlled or removed. Idiopathic pulmonary hemosiderosis often is attended by alterations of pulmonary function that cannot be reversed and may be fatal. Bleeding may be massive and life threatening. One 8-year-old child with idiopathic pulmonary hemosiderosis who was observed closely at Rainbow Babies and Children's Hospi-tal, Cleveland, and treated with alternate-day steroids therapy, experienced massive lung bleeding and had a cardiopulmonary arrest, apparently due to profound hypoxemia. He could not be resuscitated in the emergency room 1 hour after bleeding was noted. The prognosis for Goodpasture's syndrome is bleak; about one half of all patients die of asphyxia after pulmon-ary hemorrhage.

Case Report # 1:

Idiopathic pulmonary hemosiderosis fre-quently appears early in childhood, may be life-threatening, and has an unpredictable course. This report documents an apparent re-sponse to immounosuppressive therapy and a favorable outcome.

S.A., a 1600-g. twin, had no neonatal respiratory problems and was well for the first 6 months of life. At that age she developed respiratory distress with cough-ing and wheezing. Chest roentgenograms were "clear." Symptoms abated with supportive therapy for bron-chiolitis. A cough reappeared intermittently, there-after, and chest roentgenograms demonstrated patchy infiltrates in the right lower and middle lobes and the lingula at 8 months of age. The hemacrit level was 17 percent, and the reticulocyte count was 8 percent. The red blood cells were microcytic and hypochromic, and iron saturation was 3 percent. Little hemosiderin was present in bone marrow aspirate. The hematocrit level promptly rose to 35 percent after oral administration of ferrous sulfate and an iron dextran injection (Imferon). Initial infiltrates cleared, but new infiltrates and epi-sodes of coughing and fever associated with anemia were documented repeatedly over the next 4 months. At 12 months of age, her height and weight were below the third percentile. Further evaluation revealed a sweat chloride test result of 7 mEq/L and normal serum immunoglobulins. Results of stool guaiac examinations were repeatedly negative. Milk precipitins were not found in serum. An open lung biopsy showed diffuse hemorrhage, numerous hemosiderin-laden macroph-ages within alveoli and the interstitium, and thickened alveolar septae with evidence of early fibrosis. No immunoglobulin or complement deposits were seen in lung tissue by immunofluorescence. Prednisone was adminstered at a dosage of 2 mg/kg/day initially and then tapered to 10–15 mg every other day. During the second year of life, two additional episodes of coughing, respiratory distress, fever, infiltrative lung disease, and falling hematocrit levels necessitated hospitalization and larger doses of corticosteroids. Each time the symptoms resolved quickly, but chest roentgenograms retained linear densities bilaterally. Her height and weight remained between the third and tenth percentile. After a third episode of brisk pulmonary hemorrhage at 32 months of age, azathioprine in a dosage of 25–50 g/day was added to low-dose alternate-day corticosteroid therapy. Thereafter, no more pulmonary hemorrhage episodes were documented. S.A. grew well, attaining the twentieth to fiftieth percentile for height and weight. Chest roentgenograms continued to show diffuse nodular densities until 50 months of age; thereafter, only prominent interstitial markings were noted. Good health was maintained through the eighth year of life and for the last 12 months S.A. was not receiving immunosuppressive therapy.

Case Report # 2:

A number of children with pulmonary hemosiderosis also show evidence for immunologic reaction to cow's milk proteins. While the relationship of these 2 findings is not understood, the child presented here displays the typical features of this syndrome.

J.C. suffered birth asphyxia, resulting in cortical blindness and delayed speech and motor development, but no spasticity. Occasional choking episodes occured during feeding in the first year of life. He required medical attention repeatedly in infancy for episodes of respiratory distress with wheezing, coughing, and fever. Persistent right upper lobe atelectasis and transient patchy bilateral infiltrates were documented

by chest roentgenography during the first 3 years of life. Purulent rhinitis and noisy breathing were also chronic problems. At 1 year of age an esophogram demonstrated reflux but no evidence of aspiration, and sweat chloride test results were 15 mEq/L. Intermediate-strength purified protein derivatives were negatives. The hematocrit level was 25 percent, the reticulocyte count was 3 percent and iron saturation was 3 percent with a total iron-binding capacity of 465 mg/dL. The hematocrit level responded to iron therapy, but subsequently fell to previous levels. An electrocardiogram suggested right ventricular hypertrophy, but cardiac catheterization failed to demonstrate a congenital abnormality of the heart.

At 3 years of age, clinical manifestation persisted. Growth was greatly retarded. Large tonsils and adenoids were noted, and obstructive hypoventilation due to lymphoid hyperplasia was believed to be responsible for continuing evidence of right ventricular hypertrophy. In addition, precipitins (at least three) to cow's milk proteins were detected in his serum. Greater than 1 cm induration was noted at 15 minutes and again at 4 hours after subcutaneous injection of filtered cow's milk. The stool guaiac examination results were trace to 1+. Serum IgE levels were greater than 1500 units. A tonsillectony and an adenoidectomy were performed to relieve ventilatory obstruction. Aspiration of airways through an endotracheal tube at surgery revealed large numbers of hemosiderin-laden macrophages.

Because of a suspected relationship between nasopharyngeal obstruction, pulmonary hemosiderosis, and hyperreactivity to cow's milk proteins, all cow's milk and milk products were removed from the diet. No subsequent episodes of pneumonia were documented, and anemia did not recur. An electrocardiogram was normal, and chronic rhinitis disappeared. Growth resumed at an anticipated rate for the child's age. J.C. was fed a soy-based milk for two years, after which he tolerated cow's milk without further problems.

REFERENCES

Beckerman RC, Taussig LM, Pinnas JL: Familial idiopathic pulmonary hemosiderosis. *AM J Dis Child* 133:609, 1979.

Boat TF, Polmar SH, Whitman V, et al: Hyperreactivity to cow milk in young children with pulmonary hemosiderosis and cor pulmonale secondary to nasopharyngeal obstruction. *J Pediatr* 87:23, 1975.

Heiner DC, Sears JW, Kniker WT: Multiple precipitins to cow's milk in chronic respiratory disease. *Am J Dis Child.* 103:40, 1962.

Loughlin GM, Taussig LM, Murphy SA, et al: Immune-complex-mediated glomerulonephritis and pulmonary hemorrhage simulating Goodpasture syndrome. *J Pediatr.* 93:181, 1978.

Proskey AJ, Weatherbee L, Easterling RE, et al: Goodpasture's syndrome: a report of five cases and review of the literature. *Am J Med* 48:162, 1970.

Soergel KH, Sommers SC: Idiopathic pulmonary hemosiderosis and related syndromes. *Am J Med* 32:499, 1962.

Stafford HA, Polmar SH, Boat TF: Immunologic studies in cow's milk-induced pulmonary hemosiderosis. *Pediatr Res* 11:898, 1977.

Thomas HM, Irwin RS: Classification of diffuse intrapulmonary hemorrhage. *Chest* 68:483, 1975.

8

Gastroesophageal Reflux

Gary S. Rachelefsky
William E. Berquist

The most acceptable general definition of gastro-esophageal reflux (GER) is the presence of gastric contents in the esophagus. Such an event may produce a variety of disorders yet may also be a physiologic event. As a result, controversy remains about the mechanisms producing GER and diagnostic criteria for implicating GER as an etiologic agent. Since the early observations in the 1950s by Berenberg and Neuhauser, however, great strides have been made in characterizing GER and its contribution to various pathologic disorders. In this chapter the physiology, manifestations, diagnostic tests, management, and role of pathologic GER will be discussed, with particular emphasis on the relationship of GER to pulmonary disease.

HISTORY

The association of GER with a variety of disorders has been recognized and recorded as early as 1887. Subsequently, several reports have suggested that GER has been etiologic in the development of pulmonary disorders, including such diverse entities as chronic coughing, asthma, bronchitis, sudden infant death syn-

Supported by CRC Grant No.#RR-00865, Allergy Research Foundation, Inc., University of California, Los Angeles, Department of Pediatrics.
We wish to thank Susan August for secretarial assistance.
The figures in this chapter are from Berquist WE: Gastroesophageal reflux in children: a clinical review. *Pediatr Ann* 1982; 11:135. With permission.

drome, recurrent pneumonias, and pulmonary fibrosis.

Early reports of GER and associated pulmonary disease were confined mostly to literature on adults. Reports that are responsible for leading to the association of GER and pulmonary disease first appear in reviews on the complications of achalasia. Although Plummer and Vinson[1] emphasize that patients with achalasia of the cardia are likely to develop pulmonary complication, the relationship between bronchopulmonary disease and esophageal dysfunction was not widely recognized until Vinson[2] explained the cause and effect in a case of achalasia complicated by lung abscess.

In 1949 Belcher[3] reviewed a series of 48 patients with esophageal disorders who had developed such pulmonary complications as abscess, bronchiectasis, pneumonitis, and even lung collapse. He found that 18 had little or no esophageal symptoms despite serious underlying esophageal disease. More recently, Kennedy[4] has discussed 25 patients who entered the hospital with pulmonary complaints and were then found to have GER either secondary to hiatal hernia or achalasia. Fifteen had surgical treatment of the abnormal esophageal gastric junction and subsequent amelioration of the lung complaints. The course of 28 asthmatic patients with long-term coughing and wheezing and associated hiatal hernias have been described by Overholt and Ashraf.[5] After surgical correction of the hernias, 24 had moderate to complete relief of the chronic pulmonary symptoms.

Mays[6] reported on 28 adults who have severe

asthma without an allergic component. Eighteen (64 percent) were found to have hiatal hernias and 13 (46 percent) were found to have demonstrable GER. His data suggests aspiration of gastric acid as a "trigger" of severe asthma and that it should be routinely sought in the treatment of patients that are difficult to control.

Overholt and Voorhees[7] reported the finding of hiatal hernia and reflux in 30 percent of their patients with intractable asthma. Cure of asthma symptoms was accomplished in a high proportion of their patients by surgical restoration of effective esophagel sphincter function. A helpful diagnostic clue to esophageal-respiratory association was sudden development of asthma in late life with no other evident cause except massive high GER. Urshel and Paulson[8] and Davis[9] reported that a majority of their patients with severe asthma were cured of symptoms after successful surgical repair of GER.

It is important to realize, however, that studies which have selected patients with GER and looked for pulmonary disease have demonstrated that usually reflux does not lead to chronic airway disease. Vraney and Pokorny[10] report that there is no statistically significant difference in pulmonary function studies between patients with or without GER. Another recent study[11] found that patients with reflux esophagitis undergoing antireflux operations actually had a lower incidence of obstructive lung disease (38 percent) than other general surgical patients (52 percent). Pellegrini, DeMeester, and Johnson[12] have recently reported the results of 24-hour pH monitoring of the esophagus in 100 consecutive patients, 48 of whom were suspected of having episodes of pulmonary aspiration based on a history of nocturnal coughing or pulmonary symptoms associated with heartburn. In 13 of these patients who developed pulmonary symptoms during the monitoring period, 8 aspirated reflux gastric contents. In the remaining 5 patients, an episode of coughing or wheezing was preceded by a reflux episode. Of the 8 patients who have aspirated refluxed gastric contents, 4 had no history of heartburn. Five of the 8 had an antireflux operation, and, when evaluated 4 months later, they had relief of pulmonary symptoms and normal 24-hour pH studies.

Abnormal reflux of gastric contents into the esophagus as a cause of gastroesophageal and respiratory signs and symptoms in adults is thus amply documented. Early studies reported figures for GER in children with chronic pulmonary disese varying from 16 to 75 percent. These studies involved prior population selection and reliance on the less sensitive esophagram as the only diagnostic test. More recent reports in children will be detailed later in the chapter.

PATHOPHYSIOLOGIC MECHANISM

The esophagus is a collapsed hollow tube that carries food from the mouth to the stomach.[13,14] It is lined by squamous epithelium, with the upper third containing striated muscle and the lower third containing smooth muscle. Food entering the esophagus is propelled downward by progressive waves of contractions induced by a swallow (primary peristalsis). Secondary waves of peristalsis may be induced by the presence of substances in the esophageal lumen. Uncoordinated contraction (tertiary waves) can occur, especially in individuals with esophagitis. The distal end of the esophagus acts as a sphincter; the junction of stomach and esophagus has a zone of elevated pressure, the lower esophageal sphincter (LES). The LES is 3–5 cm in length and normally maintains a pressure between 15 and 30 mm. Hg, which is generated by the intrinsic musculature of the sphincter. It is not anatomically a distinct sphincter. Displacement of the sphincter into the thorax (hiatal hernia) does not diminish its pressure or competence. The esophagus enters the stomach at an angle that probably contributes to the formation of a flop valve, aiding in sphincter competence. The gastroesophageal sphincter is connected to the diaphragm by ligaments that also help to maintain sphincter function. This sphincter pressure, the mucosal choke mechanism, a flop valve mechanism, intraabdominal position, and the anchoring by phrenoesophagel ligaments all contribute to the competence of the junction between the esophagus and stomach.

The sphincter mechanism is the major barrier to GER in humans. Some abnormality in LES muscular function allows the sphincter to become weaker and then incompetent, leading to retrograde flow into the esophagus. Three abnormalities in LES function have been described: a decrease in LES pressure, a reduction in adaptive response of the sphincter to increases in intraabdominal pressure, and defect in release of gastrin during eating. A decrease in LES pressure (less than 10 mm HG) has been demonstrated in most patients with GER. An individual with normal LES function who increases intraabdominal pressure (i.e., Valsalva's maneuver, tight clothing) will increase LES pressure to prevent reflux. Persons with GER do not have this adaptive mechanism. Gastrin release from the antrum and duodenum will stimulate the LES and raise its intrinsic pressure. Individuals with symptomatic GER appear to release less gastrin in response to food, thus leading to less increase in the LES pressure compared to normal persons. The exact role of gastrin in the pathophysiologic process of GER, however, has not been fully worked out. Other gastric hormones—motilin, substance P, and pancreatin polypeptide—also have been shown to have an effect similar to gastrin. On the other hand, secretin, cholecystokinin, glucagon, vasoactive intestinal polypeptides, and gastric inhibitory polypeptide all decrease LES pressure. At the present time, it is not clear what the physiologic role of these peptides is in esophageal function.

Multiple other factors are involved in control of the LES. Stimulation of the vagus leads to relaxation of the LES. Tetrodotoxin, an agent that blocks nerve conduction, however, does not affect LES tone in the opossum.

Recent studies of smooth muscle strips of the opossum LES suggest that LES tension requires prostaglandin synthetase. Indomethacin, a prostaglandin synthetase inhibitor, decreases LES tension in vitro. Other studies suggest that LES tone depends on nonneural factors besides a hormonal substance. They suggest the presence of an autoregulatory mechanism intrinsic to the smooth muscle cells of the LES. Animal studies have shown that certain antiasthmatic medication, isoproterenol and theophylline, will decrease the LES pressure. The authors[15] and others[16] have demonstrated that theophylline (given orally and intravenously) will lower the LES pressure and also cause GER. The authors could not demonstrate such an effect with orally administered metaproterenol (Alupent, a relatively selective 2_2 adrenergic agent), however. In fact, this agent appears to lessen the degree of GER in normal persons and asthmatic patients.

What then accounts for the pathogenesis of GER? In the past it was believed that a sliding hiatal hernia played a major role; however, this appears not to be a prerequisite. The predominant factor in the pathogenesis of GER is incompetence of the LES. The exact cause for sphincter incompetence is unknown.

MANIFESTATIONS

Many symptoms and signs have been attributed to GER. With continuous intraesophageal pH monitoring it is now clear that episodes of GER occur frequently without symptoms or sequelae in normal individuals. When symptoms occur that are considered to result from GER, it is imperative to ascertain if the pattern of GER is "physiologic" with symptoms arising primarily from abnormalities in controlling the reflux material in the esophagus. Second, attempts should be made to link the event of GER with its effects which may result either from excessive GER or inabilities in controlling GER in the esophagus. This organization will aid in the comprehension of the manifestations of GER, since in some patients the event of reflux will be silent and its effects more prominent. (Table 8-1).

The primary symptom of an event of GER is chronic vomiting. This symptom is an objective event and may appear in some patients as regurgitation or rumination.

Secondary effects of the event of GER depend on the organ or tissue affected by gastric contents. These symptoms may be divided into nonpulmonary symptoms, such as heartburn, abdominal pain, water brash or taste, and pulmonary symptoms, such as coughing, aspiration pneumonias, or chronic bronchitis.

The most typical presentation of GER is postprandial, nonbilious vomiting or regurgitation. It is usually not forceful, but is easily induced with abdominal compression or recumbency. Before clinicians begin to diagnose GER in a vomiting patient, a prerequisite consideration is the chronicity of the symptoms. Acute vomiting due to infections and metabolic, toxic, and neurologic etiologies should be excluded in all age groups. Subsequently, it is critical to determine the frequency, consistency, volume, timing, and nature of the emesis with careful consideration as to circumstances about the onset of the vomiting.

With continuous intraesophageal pH monitoring the pattern of overt vomiting may vary considerably despite the clinical ease of documentation of the GER episode. Some patients with frequent emesis have only brief episodes of

Table 8-1 *Clinical Manifestations of Gastroesophageal Reflux*

- *Primary Manifestations*

  Vomiting

  Regurgitation

  Rumination

- *Secondary Manifestations*

  Nonpulmonary symptoms

  Hematemesis
  Dysphagia (odynophagia)
  Heartburn
  Irritability
  Abdominal pain
  Heme-positive stools
  Iron deficiency anemia
  Sandifer syndrome (head locking)

  Pulmonary symptoms

  Coughing
  Cyanosis
  Apnea
  Recurrent pneumonias (aspiration pattern)
  Chronic asthma
  Bronchitis
  Diffuse pulmonary fibrosis
  Bronchiectasis
  Sinusitis, otitis
  Fibrosis
  Hemoptysis

reflux, whereas others may have prolonged clearance of gastric acid in the esophagus. This pattern of reflux may be indicative of the underlying etiology, such as an incompetent lower esophageal or a distal gastric outlet obstruction. Another easily documented event of GER includes rumination, which is a pleasurable self-stimulative return of ingested food to the mouth. This commonly is seen in sensory-deprived infants with damage of the central nervous system. Regurgitation or nonforceful emesis frequently is seen in infancy and resolves with maturity or introduction of solid foods.

Symptoms Resulting from Gastroesophageal Reflux

Nonpulmonary manifestations center around the presence of esophageal irritation with gradual damage to the mucosa. Early symptoms include heartburn (midline retrosternal burning sensa-

tion or discomfort without radiation). In infants such pain may be manifested by irritability, crying, and twisting of the neck. Older children may not be able to localize pain or describe it well but may complain of abdominal or chest pain. Water brash, bad breath, or a bitter taste from gastric acid in the mouth may occur without emesis. Children may have an odor of gastric acid and undigested food. Positive results from guaiac stool tests, iron deficiency anemia, or hematemesis may result from reflux-induced esophagitis. Dysphagia, or odynolphagia (pain with swallowing), and stricture formation occur with severe esophagitis.

Neurologic symptoms such as seizures, neck twisting, or head locking (torticollis) (Sandifer syndrome) have been noted to improve after antireflux treatment. GER symptoms of regurgitation, emesis, and rumination are often prominent in children with severe mental retardation or central nervous system damage. Failure to thrive as a result of excessive emesis, strictures, or pulmonary disease related to GER has been noted and may be the only manifestation.

Pulmonary Manifestations

In patients with or without emesis, pulmonary symptoms may result from massive, mild, or infrequent aspiration (Table 8-1). Choking after meals, with cyanosis or apnea spells (near sudden infant death syndrome included), are frequent presentations. Recurrent pneumonia in the upper lobes and right middle lobe may suggest recurrent aspiration, particularly in supine patients. The event of reflux may induce bronchospasm and chronic asthmatic symptoms through reflex vagal mechanisms or recurrent aspiration. Chronic bronchitis may also result from continued exposure to aspirated gastric contents.[3,4,12] Patients with esophageal disorders (achalasia, tracheoesophageal fistulas, or esophageal strictures) are particularly prone to such symptoms, which resolve after antireflux measures are taken. Nocturnal coughing is relatively nonspecific in pulmonary disorders but has been noted in patients with GER.

DIAGNOSTIC EVALUATION

If a history is compatible with GER, the clinician must decide how extensive an evaluation is warranted. The evaluation may be divided according to three purposes: (1) to evaluate the extent and relationship of reflux to the patient's clinical symptoms, (2) to evaluate the potential causes or contributing factors that produce GER, and (3) to determine the presence and severity of pathologic sequelae. Table 8-2 summarizes these tests.

Roentgenographic Studies

The routine chest film may give evidence of recurrent aspiration-like pneumonias (Figs. 8-1 and 8-2), whereas a routine abdominal series may reveal evidence of an obstructed duodenum. A barium esophagram with upper gastrointetinal series will evaluate the stomach for pyloric stenosis, duodenal or pyloric channel ulcers, antral web, duodenal atresia or stenosis, and antral dysmotility. A videoesophagram or cine-esophagram should be done to evaluate esophageal peristalsis and the extent of reflux.[17,18] If there is dysphagia, the patient also should be fluoroscopically monitored during swallowing. The effectiveness of antral movements and gastric emptying are evaluated, and malrotation should be excluded. Various techniques to improve the roentgenographic evaluation have been advocated, such as the water siphon test, in which the stomach is filled with barium, and the patient is given small swallows of water.[19] Unfortunately, large numbers of normal persons will reflux with the water siphon test, particularly since the LES relaxes normally with swallows.

Scintigraphic Studies

Scintigraphic studies have been advocated and used to evaluate the extent and severity of GER. These tests are performed by mixing technetium-99m (^{99}mTc) with food or liquid.[20–24] Scanning is done over the esophagus, stomach, and small intestine. The quantitation of gastric emptying may be assessed in cases in which outlet obstruction is questioned, and reflux is assessed by scanning over the esophagus. The degree of radiation exposure is equivalent to one chest film. This test is convenient and easily performed on patients of all ages on an outpatient basis. Scintigraphy is more physiologic in evaluating emptying disorders of both the esophagus and stomach, since it is quantitative and may be used in monitoring response to therapy. The scinti-

Table 8-2 *Diagnostic Evaluation for Gastroesophageal Reflux*

- *History, physical*

- *Video esophagram, upper gastrointestinal tract series*

    Anatomic defects
    Grade reflux
    Assess swallowing mechanism
    Assess esophageal peristalsis, obstruction
    Diagnose aspiration
    Evaluate gastric outlet and emptying

- *Chest x-ray examination*

- *Esophageal manometry*

- *Gastric emptying (scintigraphic) study*

- *Tuttle test (standard acid reflux test)*

- *Continuous intraesophageal pH monitoring*

    On-and-off medication, evaluation of lung pulmonary function tests
    After antireflux therapy

- *Esophagastroduodenoscopy*

- *Esophageal biopsies*

- *Technetium-99 reflux and gastric emptying scintiscan*

graphic studies have been used to assess aspiration[25] but have not proven successful in minor episodes of aspiration.

Esophageal Manometry

A continuously perfused multilumen catheter assembly is used to locate the LES area and assess peristalsis in the body of the esophagus and resting LES pressure.[26–28] Ineffective peristalsis of low amplitude may result from esophagitis and either primarily or secondarily may contribute to prolonged stasis of acid in the esophagus with poor clearance. This may induce further injury to the esophageal mucosa. The amplitude, sequence, and duration of peristalsis in the esophageal body may be assessed by the use of manometry. If the LES pressure is below 10 mm Hg, there is a high correlation with a continuously incompetent sphincter mechanism, permitting frequent massive reflux. When the LES pressure is greater than 20 mm Hg, it may be intermittently incompetent or competent with other causes for GER.

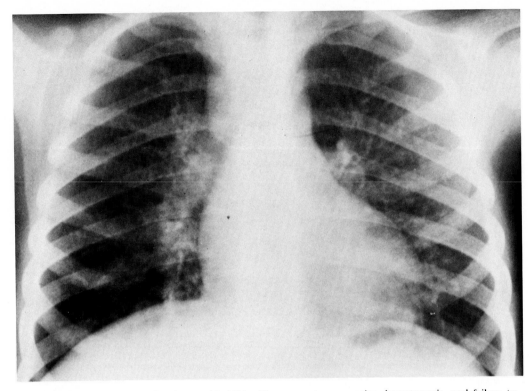

Figure 8-1. Chest x-ray film of a 4-year-old child with recurrent pneumonias, hematemesis, and failure to thrive. GER with esophagitis was demonstrated. From Krantman JH, Rachelefsky GS, Lipson M, et al: Recurrent pulmonary infiltrates, digital clubbing and failure to thrive in a 4-year-old boy. *J Allergy Clin Immunol* 61:403, 1978. With permission.

Intraesophageal pH Monitoring

There are many versions of pH monitoring. The initial evaluation was described by Tuttle and Grossman,[29] and subsequently a standard acid reflux test was derived for both adults and children. This test proved useful in assessing gross degrees of reflux. The standard acid reflux test (Tuttle test)[30,31] is performed by instilling 300 ml of 0.1N hydrochloric acid for each 1.73 m² of body surface area into the stomach through a nasogastric tube. The tube is removed, and a pH probe is positioned 5cm above the LES in adults or at a level of 13 percent of the distance from the nares to the LES in children. In most infants, the pH probe tip is placed approximately 2–3 cm above the LES. With the pH probe in place (once the patient has swallowed and cleared the acid from the esophagus), the patient is monitored for episodes of reflux (an intraesophagal pH less

than 4) and graded on a scale as to the number of episodes that occur within 1 hour. Ninety percent of normal individuals will have reflux less than two times in an hour. The test is extremely sensitive, and patients with severe reflux usually have a positive test. Because of the need to improve and quantitate correlation between symptoms and episodes of GER, 24-hour monitoring of the intraesophageal pH has been developed.[32–34] This test (Fig. 8-3) has been useful for diagnosing GER and assessing the effectiveness of various therapies. The probe is placed in the same manner as for the standard acid reflux test. It is critical to place the probe accurately and check it during the period monitored to be certain that it has not moved into the stomach or upward into the esophagus during the procedure. The probe is calibrated against two buffers of pH levels 4 and 7 and remains taped to the nares for the duration of the study. Probes

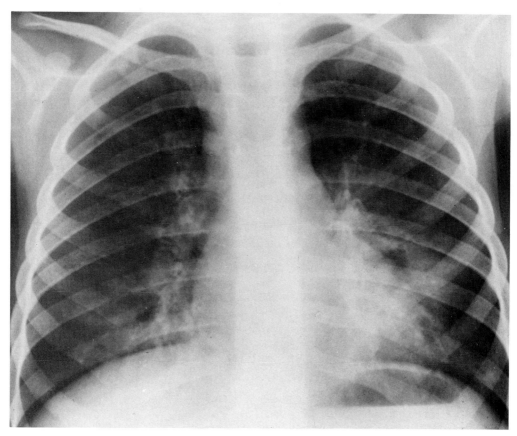

Figure 8-2. Chest x-ray film of the same child before fundoplication with changing pulmonary infiltrates. From Krantman HJ, Rachelefsky GS, Lipson M, et al: Recurrent pulmonary infiltrates, digital clubbing and failure to thrive in a 4-year-old boy. *J Allergy Clin Immunol* 61:403, 1978. With permission.

are available for infants and children and are the size of an 8 French feeding tube. With a probe and a reference electrode connected to a bioisolator or directly to a portable pH meter, the pH level is continuously recorded on a recording device. Asymptomatic individuals (Fig. 8-4) have approximately one episode of reflux every hour and no reflux during sleep. Individuals with severe esophagitis (Fig. 8-5) frequently have the most severe and prolonged reflux and have poor acid clearance from the esophagus. Some individuals have reflux 50 percent of the time monitored. In patients who have respiratory complaints or apneic episodes, there may be a correlation between the apneic episode or respiratory symptoms and episodes of reflux. Recently the authors evaluated an infant with episodes of severe cyanosis (Fig. 8-6) who re-

quired resuscitation and paramedic transport to a hospital. On monitoring in the hospital, the infant was noted to have an episode of cyanosis after a feeding and good correlation with reflux at the time of cyanosis. One year after fundoplication (Fig. 8-7) this infant has had no further apneic or cyanotic spells.

Any episode of reflux may be considered pathologic if it correlates with symptoms or sequelae such as cyanosis or severe apnea (Fig. 8-8). Monitoring the pH level is a direct physiologic measurement of GER and esophageal clearance, but does not pinpoint the pathologic abnormality that is causing the reflux. It quantitatively assesses the frequency and duration of reflux episodes and correlates these episodes with the clinical symptoms. It is also useful for evaluating therapy of GER.

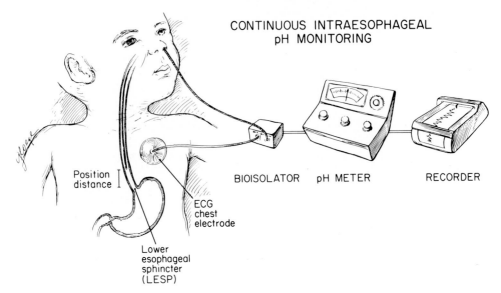

Figure 8-3. Schematic representation of intraesophageal pH monitoring in a child. The probe is placed in the esophagus 2–5 cm above the LES. The probe and a reference electrode are connected to a bioisolator and then to a pH meter. The pH level is continuously recorded.

Endoscopy and Esophageal Biopsies

Esophagoscopy in children with the use of flexible fiberoptic endoscopes may be safely performed routinely in children without the use of general anesthesia. The purpose of endoscopy is to evaluate abnormalities noted in the roentgenographic study and to assess with greater sensitivity the presence of esophagitis, which may be the major sequelae of significant GER, leading to stricture formation or Barret's esophagus. The esophageal lumen is assessed for evidence of gross erythema, easily induced friability, loss of the normal vascular pattern, erosions, webs, ulcerations, and strictures. Biopsies may be performed through the endoscope with the use of grasp forceps to confirm esophagitis, and the specimen may be submitted for culture. The esophageal biopsy specimens are assessed for the presence of polymorphonuclear cells infiltrating the mucosa, basal cell hyperplasia, and a change in the ratio of the rete pegs to the esophageal epithelial layer, which are sensitive indicators of esophagitis. It is important that the specimens be obtained at least 3 cm orad from the LES. The stomach, antrum, pylorus, duodenal bulb, and duodenum may be assessed for evidence of webs, ulcers, inflammation, stenosis, or any outlet obstruction.

GASTROESOPHAGEAL REFLUX–INDUCED PULMONARY DISEASE IN CHILDREN

In the infant or child, the gastrointestinal manifestations of GER (vomiting, dysphagia, failure to thrive, esophagitis, and esophageal stricture) are the most commonly reported. The serious pulmonary complications resulting from GER are being recognized with increased frequency. Pearson and Wilson[35] described the association of esophageal hiatal hernia as a cause of benign, pulmonary fibrosis. Davis and Fiuzat[36] discussed regurgitation and aspiration as one of the causes of recurrent pulmonary infection in infants and children. Of 55 infants and children surgically treated for GER by Johnson et al.,[37] recurrent aspiration pneumonia was the indication for operation in 13.

Darling, Fischer, and Gellis[38] reviewed barium esophagrams on 507 children with the presence of GER or hiatal hernia and found 79 cases with coexisting pulmonary disease. Danus et al.[39] evaluated 44 children with recurrent

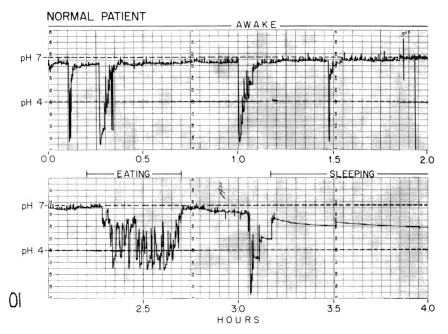

Figure 8-4. Intraesophageal pH monitoring in an asymptomatic adult. A pH level of 4 is used as a standard measure of GER. Note that episodes are of brief duration, usually less than 2 minutes. The eating interval is excluded from calculations, since the patient is given fluid with a pH level of 4.

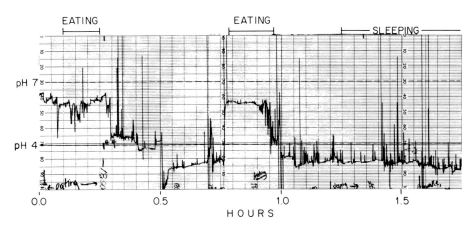

Figure 8-5. Intraesophageal pH monitoring in a 2-year-old with hematemesis and gross esophagitis. LES pressure was low (5 mm Hg). This tracing shows prolonged GER with poor acid clearance.

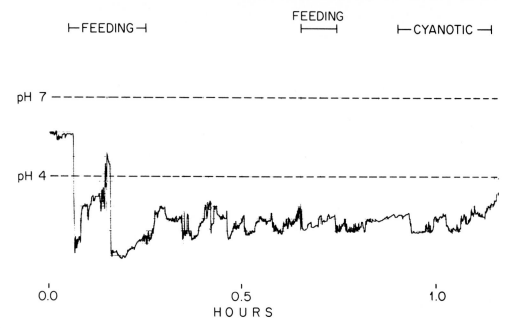

Figure 8-6. Intraesophageal pH monitoring in an infant with episodes of cyanosis. The patient required resuscitation several times by nurses and paramedics. The tracing demonstrates prolonged reflux accompanied by a cyanotic episode. No further episodes have occurred up to 1 year after fundoplication.

bronchitis using both roentgenographic and manometric techniques. Of the 44, 26 (59 percent) had GER. Shapiro and Christie[40] studied 19 steroid-dependent asthmatic children, some with a history of pneumonia. Using esophagrams, manometry, and Tuttle tests, they diagnosed GER in 9 children (43 percent). The authors[41] prospectively evaluated 30 children (1–18 years of age) with recurrent pulmonary disease—

chronic asthma or two or more documented pneumonias. The tests employed included esophagrams, the Tuttle test, manometry, and esophagoscopy with esophageal biopsy. Nineteen (63 percent) had GER based on two or more positive tests. Of those with GER, 17 had a history of nocturnal coughing and 8 vomited during infancy.

The authors[42] evaluated GER in 82 other

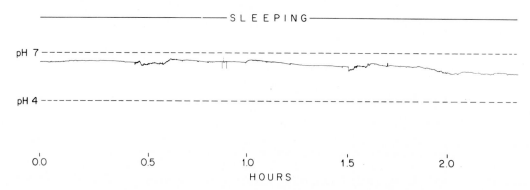

Figure 8-7. Normal intraesophageal pH tracing after fundoplication in a child with GER and an episode of cyanosis.

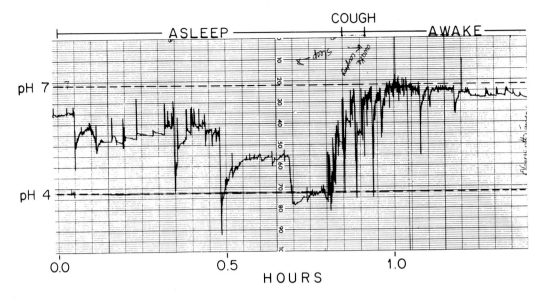

Figure 8-8. Intraesophageal pH monitoring in an 8-month-old child with chronic coughing and recurrent pneumonias. Note that the patient is asleep and awakes only after a reflux episode of approximately 8 minutes. There were no further episodes of coughing or recurrent pneumonia after fundoplication.

children with chronic asthma or recurrent pneumonias using five standardized tests for GER. Children with chronic asthma and gastroesophageal symptoms had the highest incidence of GER. Chronic asthmatic children had a 51 percent incidence of GER, whereas 43 percent of patients with recurrent pneumonia had a diagnosis of GER for a combined incidence of 49 percent. These findings were similar to the previously reported 47–63 percent incidence of GER in patients with chronic pulmonary disease.[39,40]

The respiratory symptoms improved in most of the authors' patients with GER who had antireflux management. Fundoplication proved to be a more successful treatment, with six patients becoming entirely asymptomatic. Although most asthmatic children had favorable improvement, reflected by less need for steroid therapy, only two (17 percent) became asymptomatic in comparison to four of seven (57 percent) patients with recurrent pneumonias only who underwent fundoplication. The authors know that failure of medical antireflux management did not preclude a favorable response of subsequent surgical antireflux management. Similarly, Shapiro and Christie[40] observed . that medical management had little effect on improving symptoms in

steroid-dependent asthmatic children after a careful 3-week trial.

The successful resolution of pulmonary disease with fundoplication in 25 percent of the authors' patients and improvement of symptoms in another 67 percent is similar to the recent success reported by others.

Jolley et al.[43] attempted to correlate respiratory symptoms caused by GER in 27 children less than 6 months of age with documented reflux and associated respiratory disease. Their study was controlled by 14 children with reflux without respiratory symptoms; continuous pH monitoring was employed. The mean duration of reflux during sleep was greater than 4 minutes, with a majority being greater than 6 minutes. The authors also noted in an 8-month-old infant with recurrent pneumonias, coughing and reflux during sleep (Fig. 8-6).

In a recently completed study, the authors[44] observed that asthmatic children have a greater frequency and more prolonged GER (using continuous pH monitoring) during sleep compared to normal adults. Those who treat patients having asthma are familiar with the repeated complaints that the asthmatic attacks are more severe at night than in the daytime and that the attacks are often preceded by severe bouts of coughing that suddenly awaken the patient from sleep. One of the possible causes of nocturnal asthma is GER in the presence of a hyper-reactive airway. Patients with hiatal hernia or reflux frequently reflux the stomach contents into the esophagus when they are prone. Whether nocturnal asthma in the presence of GER is a result of aspiration of stomach contents or vagal stimulation has not been established.

Although evidence exists for an association between bronchial asthma and esophageal reflux, the exact mechanism is unclear. Is it aspiration or a reflex action? A majority of investigators suggest the aspiration of gastric contents, with two recent studies demonstrating the presence of aspiration in asthmatic patients with esophageal disease. Pelligrini, DeMeester, and Johnson[12] showed an association between wheezing and a drop in the esophageal pH level. Larrain et al.[45] demonstrated that a majority of patients with asthma and GER had the same type of lesions on the posterior larynx as had patients seeking medical care for reflux. Scintigraphic techniques would be ideal for demonstrating aspiration in asthmatic patients with GER; the few studies to date have not done so.

The reflex mechanism for bronchial asthma in patients with GER was first prognosed by Bray[46] in 1934. Friedland, Yamate, and Marinkovich[47] proposed that a vagal reflex from an area of damaged esophageal mucose could lead to bronchospasm. Mansfield and Stein[48] placed acid in the esophagus of asthmatic patients with GER and performed a variety of pulmonary function tests. Only airflow resistance changed with such a challenge. In their study of acid provocation in 15 asthmatic patients with GER, Kjellen[49] observed a significant decrease in vital capacity and an increase in the slope of alveolar plateau. The former was reversed with antacids.

GER in infants frequently is not diagnosed, either clinically or roentgenographically. If respiratory complications are present, then pneumonia, cystic fibrosis, or congenital heart disease may be suspected. If apneic spells intervene, then sepsis, aspiration or neurologic disorders may be suspected. Frequently the diagnosis of GER is not considered, or, if it is, demonstrated reflux is believed to be unrelated. Respiratory arrests and death resulting from GER rarely have been reported. One report[50] describes children under the age of 6 months who had respiratory arrests secondary to GER. Those patients had no evidence of gross aspiration. They postulated that a small quantity of refluxed gastric contents is aspirated, thereby producing apnea secondary to laryngospasm. Do some of these patients represent possibly aborted crib deaths? The recognition that GER may cause respiratory arrests in term infants after the neonatal period raises the question of whether occult GER may be one cause of sudden infant death syndrome. Certain epidemiologic aspects of sudden infant death syndrome are consistent with GER as a causal mechanism. The peak age incidence is the same as in infants 1–6 months of age. Most occur during sleep when the patient is in a horizontal position. There were respiratory symptoms in 48 hours preceding death in 25–45 percent of babies with sudden infant death syndrome; the symptoms may have been secondary to unrecognized minor episodes of aspiration. Some pathologic evidence strongly suggests that crib deaths are respiratory in origin. Changes observed in the larynx at autopsies support the hypothesis that laryngospasm is the final, fatal event in some patients with sudden infant death syndrome.

Most infants with esophageal atresia and tracheoesophageal fistulas now survive. Many have recurrent or chronic respiratory tract infections.[51] It has been shown that recurrent episodes of pneumonitis in these patients, after the repair, are often due to an incompetent LES with GER and aspiration.[52] Distorted peristalsis in the body of the esophagus or the degree of stricture at the site of anastamosis have been held accountable for continuing aspiration in these children.

The literature, along with the authors' experiences, link GER in children with a variety of pulmonary disorders. One needs to consider this association in any child with unexplained or difficult to treat pulmonary disease, and, if GER is diagnosed, then appropriate medical and possibly surgical treatment should be instituted.

TREATMENT OF GASTROESOPHAGEAL REFLUX

Before treatment of GER is instituted, a concerted effort must be made to elucidate the cause and identify the sequelae. In the first 6 months of life, evaluation of GER must be carefully undertaken only when significant sequelae occur such as listed in Table 8-1. Once the diagnosis of GER has been confirmed by two or more positive tests, therapy must be initiated. Upright positioning and thickened feedings will not change the physiologic abnormalities. They may, however, diminish the overt amount of reflux and, in cases of less severe reflux, may permit postponement of further therapy; the patient may outgrow the degree of vomiting. This treatment may be used empirically when the only complaint is frequent vomiting, and evaluation reveals the sequelae of GER. The upright position must be maintained for at least 2 hours after each meal and may be necessary nearly continuously. Bethanechol at a dose of 9 mg/mm^2 may be useful in some infants and may allow a sufficient period for maturity.[53–55]

If any patient has significant sequelae, particularly severe failure to thrive, gross esophagitis, recurrent apnea, cyanosis, or pneumonia, surgical intervention is warranted. Fundoplication is preferred by many institutions. In this procedure, the gastric fundus is wrapped around the distal esophagus. With continuous pH monitoring, surgical therapy has been demonstrated to result in even less reflux than in controls.[56] If the infant under 6 months of age is having no significant sequelae but continues to vomit, the surgical decision may be postponed; careful monitoring for any developing sequelae should continue, however. Success of therapy or improvement of GER also may be evaluated by repeat intraesophageal pH monitoring.

Another modality of treatment for GER is antacids. They are taken when symptoms occur. Alginic acid (Gaviscon), a substance that coats the esophagus and promotes salivation to neutralize acid reflux, is also useful to relieve heartburn.[57] In addition, cimetidine has been used,[58] although not approved for children with GER. It may be taken at a dosage of 20–40 mg/kg/day, in a maximum of four divided doses for continuous coverage, or once at bedtime to ensure adequate antacid protection during recumbency. Cimetidine and antacids may relieve the pain of heartburn; however, they may not prevent continued injury to the body of the esophagus.

Numerous surgical operations are available to prevent GER. One of the more popular is fundoplication as just described. Additional procedures include the Belsey repair and Hill operation, which provide lesser degrees of fundoplication and gastropexy. In all of the techniques, fixation of the LES below the diaphragm and creation of a longer narrowing of the distal esophagus are mechanisms that may contribute to improved LES competence.

Attention to the correction of antral dysmotility in infants should be mentioned. As discussed, occasionally a funnel-shaped antrum and delayed gastric emptying are found on both barium study and gastric-emptying studies;[59] the LES remains normal. Surgery of choice in this instance is a long myotomy similar to the Ramstedt operation, with extension of the myotomy over the antrum. This may relieve the obstruction in some children, resulting in resolution of vomiting and significant GER.

SUMMARY

There is no doubt that a causal effect exists between the reflux of gastric contents into the esophagus and a variety of respiratory complaints and disorders. An extensive review of this association has been presented along with the diagnostic approach and treatment regimens available. Hopefully this chapter will stimulate further interest and investigation into the mechanisms involved.

REFERENCES

1. Plummer HS, Vinson PP: Cardiospasm: a report of 301 cases. *Med Clin North Am* 5:355, 1921
2. Vinson PP: Cardiospasm complicated by pulmonary abscess: a case report. *Am J Surg* 2:359, 1927
3. Belcher JR: The pulmonary complications of dysphagia. *Thorax* 4:4, 1949.
4. Kennedy JH: "Silent" gastroesophageal reflux: an important but little known cause of pulmonary complications. *Dis Chest* 42:42, 1962.
5. Overholt RH, Ashraf MM: Esophageal reflux as a trigger in asthma. NY *Med* 66:3030, 1966
6. Mays EE: Intrinsic Asthma in adults: association with gastroesophageal reflux. *JAMA* 236:2626, 1976.
7. Overholt RH, Vooorhees JR: Esophageal reflux as a trigger in asthma. *Dis Chest* 49:464–466, 1966.
8. Urshel HC, Paulson DL: Gastroesophageal reflux

and hiatal hernia: complications and therapy. *J Thorac Cardiovasc Surg* 58:21, 1967.

9. Davis MV: Evolving concepts regarding hiatus hernia and gastroesophageal reflux. *Ann Thorac Surg* 7: 120, 1969.

10. Vraney GA, Pokorny C: Pulmonary function in patients with gastroesophageal reflux. *Chest* 76:678, 1979.

11. Skinner DB, DeMeester TR: Gastroesophageal reflux. *Curr Probl Surg* 13:2–62, 1976.

12. Pellegrini CA, DeMeester TR, Johnson LF: Relationship between pulmonary aspiration and gastroesophageal reflux. Read before the fortieth annual meeting of the Society of University Surgeons, Salt Lake City, Feb 15–17, 1979.

13. Cohen S, Snape WJ: The pathophysiology and treatment of gastroesophageal reflux disease. *Arch Intern Med* 138:1398, 1978.

14. Herbst JJ: Gastroesophageal reflux. *J Peditr* 98:859–870, 1981.

15. Berquist WE, Rachelefsky GS, Kadden M, et al: The effect of theophylline on gastroesophageal reflux in normal adults. *J Allergy Clin Immunol* 67:407, 1981.

16. Stein MR, Weber RW, Towner TG: The effect of theophylline on the lower esophageal sphincter pressure (LESP). *Ann Allergy* 45:239, 1980.

17. Berenberg W, Neuhauser EBD: Cardioesophageal relaxation (chalasia) as a cause of vomiting in infants. *Pediatrics* 5:414–420, 1950.

18. McCauley RGK, Darling DB, Leonidas JC, et al: Gastroesophageal reflux in infants and children: a useful classification and reliable physiologic technique for its demonstration. *Am J Roentgenol* 130: 47–50, 1978.

19. Linsman JF: Gastroesophageal reflux elicited while drinking water (water siphonage test)—its clinical correlation with pyrosis. *AJR* 94:325–332, 1965.

20. Fisher RS, Malamud LS, Roberts GS, et al: Gastroesophageal (GE) scintiscanning to detect and quantitate GE reflux. *Gastroenterology* 70:301–308, 1976.

21. Chaudhuri TK, Greenwald AJ, Heading RC: A new radioscopic technic for the measurement of gastric emptying of a solid meal. *Am J Gastroenterol* 65:46–51, 1976.

22. Tolin, RD, Malamud LS, Reilley J, et al: Esophageal scintography to quantitate esophageal transit (quantitation of esophageal transit). *Gastroenterology* 76:1402–1408, 1979.

23. Rudd TG, Christie DSL: Demonstration of gastroesophageal reflux in children by radionuclide gastroesophagraphy. *Radiology* 131:483–486, 1979.

24. Heyman S, Kirkpatrick JA, Winter HS, et al: An improved radionuclide method for diagnosis of gastroesophageal reflux and aspirations in children (milk scan). *Radiology* 131:479–482, 1979.

25. Reich SB, Earley WC, Ravin TH, et al: Evaluation of gastropulmonary aspiration by a radioactive technique: Concise communication. *J Nucl Med* 18:1079–1081, 1977.

26. Cohen S: Developmental characteristics of lower esophageal sphincter function: a possible mechanism for infantile achalasia. *Gastroenterology* 67:252–258, 1974.

27. Euler AR, Ament ME: Value of esophageal manometric studies in the gastroesophageal reflux in infancy. *Pediatrics* 59:58–61, 1977.

28. Dodds WJ: Instrumentation and methods of intraluminal esophageal manometry. *Arch Intern Med* 136:515–523, 1976.

29. Tuttle SG, Grossman MI: Detection of gastroesophageal reflux by simultaneous measurement of intraluminal pressure and pH. *Proc Soc Exp Biol Med* 98:225–227, 1958.

30. Venkatachalam B, DaCosta LR, Ip SKL, et al: What is a normal esophagogastric junction? *Gastroenterology* 62:521–527, 1972.

31. Euler AR, Ament ME: Detection of gastroesophageal reflux in the pediatric age patient by esophageal intraluminal pH probe measurement (Tuttle test). *Pediatrics* 60: 65–68, 1972.

32. Johnson LF, DeMeester TR: Twenty-four hour pH monitoring of the distal esophagus. *Am J Gastroenterol* 62: 325–332, 1974.

33. Sondheimer JM: Continuous monitoring of distal esophageal pH: a diagnostic test for gastroesophageal reflux in infants. *J Pediatr* 96:804–807, 1980.

34. Jolley SG, Johnson DG, Herbst JJ, et al: An assessment of gastroesophageal reflux in children by extended pH monitoring of the distal esophagus. *Surgery* 84:16–24, 1978.

35. Pearson JE, Wilson RS: Diffuse pulmonary fibrosis and hiatus hernia. *Thorax* 26:300, 1971.

36. Davis MV, Fuizat J: Application of the Belsey hiatal hernia repair to infants and children with recurrent bronchitis, bronchiolitis and pneumonitis due to regurgitation and aspiration. *Ann Thorac Surg* 3:99, 1967.

37. Johnson DG, Herbst JJ, Oliveros MA, et al: Evaluation of gastroesophageal reflux surgery in children. *Pediatrics* 59:62, 1977.

38. Darling DB, Fisher JH, Gellis SS: Hiatal hernia and gastroesophageal reflux in infants and children: analysis of the incidence in North American children. *Pediatrics* 54:450, 1974.

39. Danus O, Casar C, Larrain A, et al: Esophageal reflux—an unrecognized cause of recurrent obstructive bronchitis in children. *J Pediatr* 89:220, 1976.

40. Shapiro GG, Christie DL: Gastroesophageal reflux in steroid-dependent asthmatic youths. *Pediatrics* 63: 207–212, 1979.

41. Euler AR, Byrne WJ, Ament ME, et al: Recurrent pulmonary disease in children: a complication of gastroesophageal reflux. *Pediatrics* 63:47, 1979.

42. Berquist WE, Rachelefsky GS, Kadden M, et al: Gastroesophageal reflux associated with recurrent pneumonia and chronic asthma in children. *Pediatrics* 68:29, 1981.

43. Jolley SG, Herbst JJ, Johnson DG, et al: Esophageal pH monitoring during sleep identifies children with respiratory symptoms from gastroesophageal reflux. *Gastroenterology* 80:1501, 1981.

44. Rachelefsky GS, Berquist WE, Rowshan N, et al: Gastroesophageal reflux (GER) in asthmatic children compared to normals. *J Allergy Clin Immunol* 69:143, 1982.

45. Larrain A, Lira E, Otero M, et al: Posterior laryngitis—a useful marker of esophageal reflux, in Kjellen G: *Oesophageal Dysfunction and Bronchial Asthma*. Linköping University Medical Dissertations No. 111, Linköping, Sweden, 1981.

46. Bray GW: Recent advances in the treatment of asthma and hay fever. *Practitioner* 34:368, 1934.

47. Friedland GW, Yamate M, Marinkovich VA: Hiatal hernia and chronic unremitting asthma. *Pediatr Radiol* 1:156, 1973.

48. Mansfield LE, Stein MR: Gastroesophageal reflux and asthma: a possible reflex mechanism. *Ann Allergy* 41:224, 1978.

49. Kjellen G: *Oesophageal dysfunction and bronchial asthma*. Linköping University Medical Dissertations No. 111, Linköping, Sweden, 1981.

50. Herbst JJ, Book LS, Bray PF: Gastroesophageal reflux in the "near miss" sudden infant death syndrome. *J Pediatr* 92:73, 1978.

51. Milligan DWA, Levinson H: Lung function in children following repair of tracheoesophageal fistula. *J Pediatr* 95:24, 1979.

52. Whitington PF, Shermeta DW, Seto DS, et al: Rose of lower esophageal sphincter incompetence in recurrent pneumonia after repair of esophageal atresia. *J Pediatr* 91:550, 1977.

53. Farrell RL, Roling GT, Castell DO: Cholinergic therapy of chronic heartburn. *Ann Intern Med* 80:573, 1974.

54. Thanik KD, Chey WY, Shah AN, et al: Reflux esophagitis: effect of oral bethanechol on symptoms and endoscopic findings. *Ann Intern Med* 93:805, 1980.

55. Euler AR: Use of bethanechol for the treatment of gastroesophageal reflux. *J Pediatr* 96:321, 1980.

56. Berquist WE, Fonkalsrud EW, Ament ME: Effectiveness of Nissen fundoplication on gastroesophageal reflux in children measured by 24-hour intraesophageal pH monitoring. *J Pediatr Surg* 16:872, 1981.

57. McHardy G: A multicenter randomized clinical trial of Gaviscon in reflux esophagitis. *South Med J* 71:16, 1978.

58. Behar J, Brand DL, Brown FC: Cimetidine in the treatment of symptomatic gastroesophageal reflux: a double-blind controlled trial. *Gastroenterology* 74:441, 1978.

59. Byrne WJ, Kangarloo H, Ament ME, et al: Antral dysmotility: an unrecognized cause of chronic vomiting during infancy. *Ann Surg.* (In press.)

9

Bronchopulmonary Dysplasia

Kathy E. Wedig
Margaret C. Bruce
Richard J. Martin
Avroy A. Fanaroff

In newborns bronchopulmonary dysplasia (BPD) is a clinicopathologic symptom complex associated with prolonged oxygen and ventilator therapy. It is a frustrating entity that continues to raise many perplexing questions. Intellectual controversy reigns regarding the individual contributions of oxygen, endotracheal tubes, ventilatory pressure, and infection to this clinicopathologic process. The incidence, 5 percent of neonatal intensive care admissions, can only be estimated because diagnostic criteria are not clearly defined. Infants who develop BPD have complicated clinical courses exacerbated by infection, atelectasis, and congestive heart failure in addition to compromised nutritional status and a delicate fluid balance.

This chapter will address the persistently perplexing problems of BPD. New beliefs regarding the pathophysiologic process of oxygen toxicity, as well as a discussion of current therapy, will be presented.

PATHOPHYSIOLOGIC PROCESS

Bronchopulmonary dysplasia (BPD), first described by Northway in 1967,[1] is now a well-recognized sequela of prolonged oxygen and ventilator therapy for neonatal respiratory distress. Northway observed that this chronic lung disease was most likely to occur in infants exposed to an inspired oxygen concentration (F_{IO_2}) in excess of 0.80 and high ventilator pressures for greater than 150 hours. Since Northway's original description, BPD also has been reported after exposure to an F_{IO_2} greater

than 0.40 over a relatively prolonged period, as well as in infants whose exposure to an F_{IO_2} greater than 0.80 was less than 24 hours. The precise combination of oxygen exposure, ventilator settings, and time that results in the development of BPD in an individual infant is clearly a complex question that remains unanswered.

Northway, Rosan, and Porter[1] described in detail the pathologic features of four stages leading to the development of BPD. In the earliest stage, occurring on days 2 and 3, the lungs are hyperemic and atelectatic with hyaline membranes. They also observed occasional loss of ciliated epithelial cells along with necrosis and metaplasia of the bronchiolar mucosa. Stage II, observed in infants 4–10 days old, was characterized by persisting hyaline membranes, necrosis, and repair of alveolar epithelial cells. They also found emphysematous coalescence of alveoli, thickening of capillary basement membranes, bronchiolar necrosis, and squamous metaplasia. Stage III, described as the period of transition to chronic disease, occurred in infants 10–20 days old. In this stage hyaline membranes were absent, and there was widespread bronchial and bronchiolar mucosal metaplasia and hyperplasia. Alveolar macrophages and histiocytes, as well as abundant mucus, were observed in the airways. Progressive alveolar coalescence resulted in groups of emphysematous alveoli surrounded by atelectatic areas. Thickening of basement membranes was more apparent than in stage II. In stage IV (infants older than 1 month), there was widespread bronchiolar smooth muscle. The emphysematous alveoli were circumscribed by increased reticulum, collagen, and irregularly formed elastin. Pulmonary arterioles were involved and showed intimal thickening with medial hypertrophy.

Roentgenographic staging of BPD frequently underestimates the severity of the pathologic changes that have occurred. Edwards, Colby, and Northway[2] compared roentgenographic and pathologic stages in 142 infants. In 63 percent, the pathologic stage of BPD was more advanced than the stage indicated roentgenographically. Roentgenographic and pathologic stages were the same in 34 percent of the infants, and in 3 percent the roentgenographic stage exceeded the pathologic stage. The authors reported a significan correlation between roentgenographic and pathologic staging with the caveat that x-ray films underestimate more frequently than they overestimate the severity of BPD.

Cytologic examination of tracheobronchial aspirates has also been explored as an alternative method for determining the severity of BPD. Merrit et al.[3] found that changes in the cytologic examination of tracheobronchial aspirates were closely correlated with duration and intensity of oxygen and ventilation therapy. These authors reported that a characteristic pattern of cellular changes occurred after 10 days of life, primarily in those infants who ultimately developed BPD. This pattern, consisting of squamous metaplasia, chronic inflammation, regenerating epithelial cells, and multinucleated histiocytes, enabled a diagnosis of BPD to be made earlier than by roentgenographic changes alone in 70 percent of the cases.

The relative contribution of each form of therapy, particularly oxygen concentration versus ventilator pressure, toward the development of BPD is difficult to delineate. Historically, the introduction of intermittent positive pressure ventilation (IPPV) resulted in an increased incidence of BPD. With the use of negative pressure ventilation, BPD was apparently not observed, possibly secondary to the absence of IPPV or the accompanying endotracheal tube. Unfortunately, the technical difficulties inherent in negative pressure ventilation around the infant's thorax prevented the widespread acceptance of this mode of therapy. Meanwhile, Berg et al.[4] reported in 1975 that the supplementation of IPPV with positive end expiratory pressure (PEEP) reduced the incidence of BPD, possibly because of a concomitant reduction in F_{IO_2}.

In 1976 Taghizadeh and Reynolds[5] described certain pulmonary changes in BPD that appeared to be primarily the result of mechanical ventilation with high positive inspiratory pressures. Only those infants receiving positive inspiratory pressures greater than 35 cm H_2O showed narrowing and obstruction of bronchial lumina by epithelial hyperplasia and fibroblastic proliferation. Severe parenchymal damage with centrilobular peribronchiolar fibrosis was also found. The authors suggested that the main factor initiating the process of BPD is distortion and disruption of terminal airways with resultant obliteration of the lumina associated with obstructive or compensatory emphysema. When ventilator pressures were decreased to 25 cm H_2O the incidence of BPD appeared to decrease despite inspired oxygen concentrations of greater than 80 percent during IPPV. Apart from the high peak inspiratory pressures that may be needed during IPPV, the presence of an endotracheal tube may act as a foreign body, affecting both the volume of secretions and mucociliary transport in general. In addition, Watts, Ariagno, and Brady,[6] documented a significantly higher incidence of pulmonary intersitital emphysema in infants who developed BPD.

BIOCHEMISTRY OF OXYGEN TOXICITY

Despite the implications that IPPV is a major etiologic factor in the development of BPD, there is much indirect evidence that oxygen toxicity also plays a key role. The pathologic changes in the lung observed in both humans and animals exposed to high concentrations of oxygen are essentially identical to the pathologic changes observed in the lungs of infants with BPD.[7] Studies with experimental animals have demonstrated that the initial lesion is in the capillary endothelial cells, resulting in a serous and cellular exudate in the air spaces. This initial exudative stage of oxygen toxicity is characterized by edema, alveolar hemorrhage, hyaline membranes, and inflammation. As the exposure to high concentrations of oxygen continues, the type I alveolar epithelial cells are damaged, as are bronchiolar and tracheal ciliated cells. The proliferative stage occurs approximately 5 days after the onset of oxygen exposure and may overlap to some extent with the exudative stage. The proliferative stage is characterized by proliferation of alveolar type II epithelial cells, nonciliated secretory (Clara) cells, and fibroblasts.

The cell damage resulting from exposure to high concentrations of oxygen is believed to be caused by the oxygen radicals and other chemically reactive oxygen metabolites formed during the in vivo reduction of inhaled oxygen. Although most inhaled oxygen is reduced to water, a small fraction is reduced to hydrogen peroxide, which decomposes to form the highly reactive hydroxyl and superoxide radicals. When these radicals are produced in concentrations that overwhelm their respective defense mechanisms (i.e., superoxide dismutase, catalase, and peroxidase), they alter the structural integrity of cells by peroxidizing membrane lipids, oxidizing protein sulfydryls, depolymerizing mucopolysaccharides, and damaging nucleic acids.

Boat[8] used human neonatal tracheal explants to study the effect of oxygen on ciliary movement, mucociliary transport, and secretory activity. He observed that exposure to 80 percent oxygen for 48–96 hours resulted in abnormal ciliary activity with failure of mucociliary function as evidence by carbon particle transport coincident with evidence of squamous mataplasia histologically. Whereas initial exposure to high concentrations of oxygen resulted in increased glandular activity and increased lysozyme and mucin production and secretion, continued exposure produced diminished surface secretions related temporarily to loss of goblet cells from the surface epithelium and failure to discharge secretions from submucous glands that became distended. Exposure of the same explants to 21 percent oxygen in the same medium was associated with normal mucociliary transport and glandular activity throughout the 168-hour study period. He concluded that the abnormal mucociliary transport and glandular function after oxygen therapy may play a significant role in the pathogenesis of BPD.

PROTEOLYTIC ENZYMES IN BRONCHOPULMONARY DYSPLASIA

Recent evidence suggests that proteolytic enzymes also may contribute to the pathologic changes associated with both oxygen toxicity and BPD. Many of the observed pathologic changes in infants with BPD, such as focal emphysema, damage to ciliated cells, and squamous metapla-

sia of the bronchiolar epithelium, may be initiated or exacerbated by proteolytic enzymes. The presence in lung tissue of polymorphonuclear cells (PMNs) containing proteolytic enzymes has been well documented in infants with BPD. The authors, too, have observed that PMNs are the predominant cell type in endotracheal tube secretions obtained from 30 infants receiving ventilation therapy who were exposed to F_{IO_2} greater than 0.4. Animal studies have also shown that exposure to oxygen greater than 95 percent for 66 hours causes a sevenfold increase in the number of PMNs lavaged from rat lungs,[9] which suggests that oxygen therapy alone may evoke an inflammatory response in these infants. In addition, infants with severe respiratory distress syndrome frequently develop pulmonary infections and the attendant inflammatory response would further increase proteinase challenge to the lungs. Proteolytic enzymes contained in PMNs (elastase, cathepsin G, collagenase) are capable of destroying the three general types of structural proteins (elastin, collagen, structual glycoconjugates) of the lungs. Insoluble (crosslinked) elastin is solubilized by elastase, collagen is digested by collagenase and elastase and the soluble form of elastin (the uncrosslinked precursors to insoluble elastin) and proteoglycans are digested by elastase and cathepsin G.

Susceptibility of α_1 proteinase inhibitor (α_1PI) to oxidative inactivation has been demonstrated by in vivo and in vitro exposure to oxidants such as ozone, chloramine T, and N-chlorosuccinimide, as well as cigarette smoke. Dimished activity of α_1PI obtained from the lung lavage of cigarette smokers compared with α_1PI obtained from nonsmoking control subjects has been attributed to oxidation of the active site methionine of α_1PI by oxidants of cigarette smoke.[10] (This impaired proteinase activity could result in the development of pulmonary emphysema in chronic smokers.)

Infants who develop respiratory distress frequently require prolonged exposure to high F_{IO_2} and ventilatory assistance. Bruce[11] studied airway secretions from infants treated with high concentrations of oxygen to determine whether chronic exposure to high F_{IO_2} results in oxidative inactivation of α_1PI. She demonstrated that exposure to greater than 60 percent inspired oxygen for 6 or more days resulted in notable impairment of the elastase inhibitory capacity of α_1PI. Restoration of some activity after treatment with a reducing agent, DL-dithiothreitol, suggests that loss of activity of α_1PI is due, in part, to oxidative inactivation. Furthermore, as detailed previously, exposure to high FIO_2 results in an increase in polymorphonuclear leukocytes containing proteolytic enzymes in the lungs. This, coupled with inactivation of α_1PI, supports the hypothesis that proteolytic destruction of lung tissue could occur in infants chronically exposed to high FIO_2.

CLINICAL FEATURES

BPD is a disease of varying severity that encompasses a relatively broad spectrum of pulmonary complications. Epidemiologic studies vary widely in defining precise diagnostic criteria and appropriate neonatal population denominators for comparative studies.[12] As a result, the incidence of BPD can only be approximated at 5 percent of all infants admitted for neonatal intensive care and requiring IPPV. At one end of the spectrum of severity are the mildest cases that typically consist of premature infants recovering from respiratory distress syndrome who may demonstrate a plateau in both ventilator settings or inspired oxygen requirements during weaning, associated with nonspecific roentgenographic findings of mild pulmonary infiltrates. Some clinicians would classify these babies as having a prolonged course of respiratory distress syndrome, whereas others would call it early or mild BPD. At the other end of the spectrum BPD is characterized by severe cystic emphysema. As noted earlier, BPD is not confined to infants with a history of respiratory distress syndrome, but may develop in term or postterm infants after meconium aspiration syndrome, persistent fetal circulation, neonatal pneumonia, or a surgical problem such as congenital diaphragmatic hernia. These babies usually require higher ventilator settings or more prolonged inspired oxygen exposure to develop the disease than do premature infants. The development of BPD often is first suspected when substantial ventilator and oxygen dependence extends beyond 7 days. Nonetheless, definitive roentgenographic features may not typically develop until later in the course, usually around the third week of life.

The roentgenographic sequence of four stages of BPD initially described by Northway[1] is no longer commonly seen. The initial picture is essentially indistinguishable from that of uncomplicated respiratory distress syndrome. The subsequent development of parenchymal opacification may simulate another process, such as congestive heart failure from a patent ductus arteriosus, pulmonary hemorrhage, or infection (Fig. 9-1). The typical lacy or bubbly pattern is not necessarily seen, and, when it does appear, it may not follow a period of parenchymal opacity. Finally, the characteristic picture of chronic lung disease ultimately appears at 3–4 weeks. The typical hyperinflation interspersed with areas of patchy opacification or atelectasis must be differentiated from a wide range of disorders at this age, giving a comparable roentgenographic picture (Table 9-1).[13]

Clinical and roentgenographic recovery run a variably protracted course, interrupted by acute exacerbations of cardiorespiratory symptoms. The latter are typically precipitated by either infections, atelectasis, or episodes of congestive heart failure, and their clinical differentiation is often a diagnostic dilemma. Cardiomegaly infrequently is seen on roentgenographic examination because of pulmonary hyperexpansion, and changes in the pulmonary vasculature may be obscured by the parenchymal disease. Pulmonary infections are usually nonspecific in appearance and location and frequently related to the aspiration of feedings. Recurrent atelectasis with segmental collapse is a frequent problem in patients with BPD and may occur anywhere in the lungs, although the left lower lobe frequently is involved.

MANAGEMENT

The successful treatment of BPD is a long-term process that requires a major commitment from the medical, nursing, and respiratory therapy staff, not to mention the role of other ancillary personnel and, most important, the parents.

Cardiorespiratory Care

Long-term mechanical ventilation requires dedicated staff who are well versed in all aspects of respiratory therapy. During the prolonged process of weaning from IPPV, intermittent mandatory ventilation (IMV) is a form of assisted ventilation that allows the infant to breathe

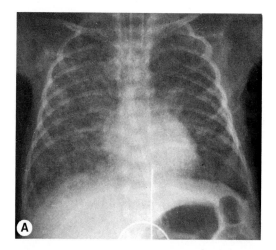

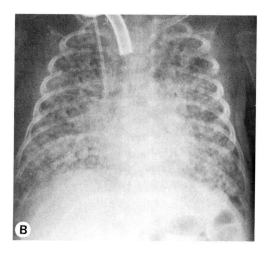

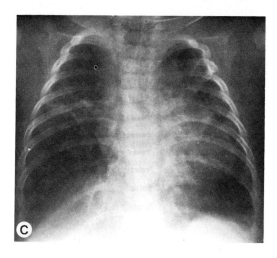

Fig. 9-1. Typical roentgenographic progression of BPD from early BPD (**A**) through stage III (**B**) and later stage IV disease (**C**). From Fox WW, Morray JP, Martin RJ: Chronic pulmonary diseases of the neonate, in Fanaroff AA, Martin RJ (eds): *Behrman's Neonatal-Perinatal Medicine*, ed 3. St Louis, The CV Mosby Co, 1983.

spontaneously between a set number of mechanical breaths for each minute. A low PEEP is maintained in order to stabilize lung volume. An IMV rate is selected that allows Pa_{AO_2} in the 50–70 mm Hg range. Adequacy of gas exchange should be monitored by arterial blood gases at intervals dictated by the child's clinical condition. During times of stability, transcutaneous po_2 measurements are useful. Long-term mechanical ventilation requires the presence of a secure airway that may be provided by a well-fitting endotracheal tube of an appropriate size. If prolonged mechanical ventilation is required, tracheostomy may be a more appropriate form of airway control. Precise timing for this therapy is unknown at this time. Prolonged use of oversized endotracheal tubes may result in a high incidence

of subglottic stenosis, as well as lesser forms of tracheal damage.

Weaning from IMV may be a long, slow process, taking many months in extreme cases. After IMV has been discontinued, the infant may benefit from endotracheal constant positive airway pressure for 1–2 weeks. Weaning from oxygen should progress concurrently and with even greater caution. Reduction in inspired oxygen of as little as 2 percent may result in a profound change in the infant's clinical condition and requires constant reassessment.[14] Chest physiotherapy is performed at variable intervals (depending on secretions) in an attempt to prevent atelectasis and pooling of secretions. Infants with both subacute and chronic forms of BPD may exhibit clinical elements of bronchospasm, and a trial of bronchodilators may be indicated.

Infants with BPD are particularly susceptible to pulmonary edema, perhaps because of abnormal lymphatic drainage or the deleterious effects of right-sided heart failure on left ventricular function. Fluids are restricted as much as possible while still considering the need for a high caloric intake. Chronic diuretic therapy is instituted with a thiazide or a loop diuretic such as furosemide. Parameters that need frequent monitoring in-

Table 9-1 *Radiographic Differential Diagnosis of Bronchopulmonary Dysplasia*

1. Wilson-Mikity syndrome
2. Meconium aspiration syndrome
3. Pulmonary interstital emphysema
4. Overhydration
5. Viral pneumonia (especially cytomegalovirus)
6. Total anomalous pulmonary venous return (type III)
7. Pulmonary lymphangiectasia
8. Recurrent pneumonitis or aspiration (immune deficiency, gastroesophageal reflux, H-type tracheoesophageal fistula, etc.)
9. Cystic fibrosis
10. Idiopathic pulmonary fibrosis (Hamman-Rich syndrome)

From Edwards DK: Radiographic aspects of bronchopulmonary dysplasia. *J Pediatr* 95:823, 1979. With permission.

clude intake and output, electrolytes, urine specific gravity, body weight, rales, peripheral edema, and liver enlargement.

General Supportive Care

Maintaining an adequate nutritional status is a key component of the care of infants with BPD. Malnutrition will result in a delay in the development of new alveoli, making weaning from mechanical ventilation almost impossible. An aggressive approach should thus be taken toward supplying a parenteral or oral caloric intake that is adequate for growth. High-calorie formulas and supplements may be used to maximize the intake of calories while restricting fluid intake to prevent congestive heart failure. Adequacy of nutrition should be closely monitored, and growth charts for height, weight, and head circumference need to be kept. Rib fractures noted on routine chest roentgenograms together with generalized bone demineralization are not frequently observed in BPD but are usually a manifestation of rickets and may require additional calcium or vitamin D supplementation.

Vitamin E supplementation has recently been suggested in the therapy of BPD. Vitamin E is a naturally occurring antioxidant that was first identified in 1922. Since the premature infant is

deficient in vitamin E, containing only 6 percent of the adult stores, much research has focused on the use of vitamin E in premature infants specifically to prevent retrolental fibroplasia and, more recently, in the amelioration of BPD. Investigation with vitamin E in retrolental fibroplasia actually commenced as early as 1949 when Owens and Owens gave alternate low birth–weight infants vitamin E 150 mg/day as soon as they could commence feeding. They noticed that 4 percent of the vitamin E–treated infants developed retrolental fibroplasia compared with 22 percent of the controls. Furthermore, they noted that progression of the lesions was arrested in a number of cases when vitamin E was commenced. At that time the etiology of retrolental fibroplasia was still unknown, and this work was largely forgotten. Research efforts were revived in the 1970s when it was theorized that oxygen toxicity may be mediated through radical production and could therefore be counteracted by antioxidants and other free radical scavengers such as vitamin E.

The use of vitamin E as a potential therapy for BPD was based on animal experiments in which vitamin E reduced the pulmonary damage from oxygen exposure. Ehrenkrantz[15] in 1978 used large doses of vitamin E to prevent BPD in humans. He documented that infants treated with vitamin E had shorter exposure to oxygen and mechanical ventilation but the results did not reach statistical significance. Critical evaluation of the study pointed out the lack of randomization of subjects, the absence of a placebo group, and imprecise roentgenographic categorization and diagnosis of BPD, and the study design made it difficult to separate the severity of disease and effects of therapy. Ehrenkrantz therefore redesigned his study in 1979 as a randomized, double-blind control study using 20 mg/kg/day of vitamin E. To date all the infants have survived, and there has been no significant difference in the number of hours of oxygen or mechanical ventilation.

In a number of other studies relating the use of vitamin E to prevention or amelioration of BPD, conflicting data have been obtained. In some animal experiments investigators showed a positive effect of vitamin E, whereas in two clinical studies no significant difference has been noted between the control and the treated group.

In view of the fact that there appear to be few harmful side effects and in view of the beneficial effects of vitamin E in the prevention of severe RLF, it appears prudent to initiate its use for low birth–weight infants requiring assisted ventilation.

The infant with severe BPD may be ventilator dependent for many months and thus deprived of normal levels of environmental stimulation. To minimize the risk of developmental delays, a well-organized program of infant stimulation may help the infant achieve maximal potential. Such a program will instruct the caretakers in helping the infant with various social, language, cognitive, and motor skills. Parental participation in many aspects of the child's care is critical for the child's normal development and for establishment of normal relationships. Therefore parents are encouraged to visit as frequently as possible and are educated about relevant medical equipment and procedures. In time many are able to assume complete responsibility for procedures such as chest physiotherapy and tracheal suctioning, in addition to holding and playing with their child. During prolonged hospitalization every effort must be made to assign a consistent physician and nursing team to oversee the child's care and be available for continuing parental support.

PROGNOSIS

The initial mortality of infants with severe BPD before discharge remains quite high due to a combination of respiratory failure, infection, and congestive heart failure. Nonetheless, with adequate nutrition, somatic growth, and control of infection and heart failure, pulmonary function may gradually improve and roentgenographic healing occur. Nonspecific infections of the upper and lower respiratory tract are common during the first year of life, whereas episodes of wheezing suggestive of asthma or bronchiolitis have an increased incidence in the first 2 years. Although the incidence of severe handicaps in pulmonary function or neurologic performance may be as high as 35 percent, prognosis for future development compares favorably to that of ventilated infants who required IPPV but did not develop BPD.[16] Smyth[17] observed a high incidence of obstructive airway disease at 8 years in a small group of BPD survivors. Other data also indicate that pulmonary function may be impaired beyond infancy even though many of the infants may be asymptomatic. Data on longer term follow-up studies of pulmonary function in infants with BPD will be eagerly awaited in the future.

REFERENCES

1. Northway WH Jr, Rosan RC, Porter DY: Pulmonary disease following respirator therapy of hyaline membrane disease. *N Engl J Med* 276:357, 1967.
2. Edwards DK, Colby TV, Northway WH: Radiographic-pathologic correlation in bronchopulmonary dysplasia. *J Pediatr* 95:834, 1979.
3. Merritt A, Stuard ID, Puccia J, et al: Newborn tracheal aspirate cytology: classification during respiratory distress syndrome and bronchopulmonary dysplasia. *J Pediatr* 98:949, 1981.
4. Berg TJ, Pagtakhan RK, Reed MH, et al: Bronchopulmonary dysplasia and lung rupture in hyaline membrane disease: influence of continuous distending pressure. *Pediatrics* 55:51, 1975.
5. Taghizadeh A, Reynolds EOR: Pathogenesis of bronchopulmonary dysplasia following hyaline membrane disease. *Am J Pathol* 82:241, 1976.
6. Watts JL, Ariagno RL, Brady JP: Chronic pulmonary disease in neonates after artificial ventilation: distribution of ventilation and pulmonary intersitital emphysema. *Pediatrics* 60:273, 1977.
7. Deneke SM, Fanburg BL: Normobaric oxygen toxicity of the lung. *N Engl J Med* 303:76, 1980.
8. Boat TF, Kleinerman JI, Fanaroff AA, et al: Toxic effects of oxygen on cultured human neonatal respiratory epithelium. *Pediatr Res* 7:607, 1973.
9. Fox RB, Halidal JR, Brown DM, et al: Hyperoxia causes a preterminal influx of polymorphonuclear leukocytes (PMN) into the lungs and is associated with increased lung lavage chemotoxin for PMN and death of alveolar macrophages. *Am Rev Respir Dis* 121:340, 1980.
10. Janoff A, Carp H, Lee DK, et al: Cigarette smoke inhalation decreases alpha$_1$-antitrypsin activity in rat lung. *Science* 206:1313, 1979.
11. Bruce M, Boat T, Martin R, et al: Proteinase inhibitors and inhibitor inactivation in neonatal airways secretions. *Chest* 81(Suppl.):44S, 1982.
12. Fox WW, Morray JP, Martin RJ: Chronic pulmonary diseases of the neonate, in Fanaroff AA, Martin RJ (eds): *Behrman's Neonatal-Perinatal Medicine*, ed 3. The CV Mosby Co, 1983, p. 469.
13. Edwards DK: Radiographic aspects of bronchopulmonary dysplasia. *Pediatrics* 95:823, 1979.
14. Halliday HL, Dumpit FM, Brady JP: Effects of inspired oxygen on echocardiographic assessment

of pulmonary vascular resistance and myocardial contractility in bronchopulmonary dysplasia. *Pediatrics* 65:536, 1980.

15. Ehrenkrantz RA, Bonta BW, Ablow RC, et al: Amelioration of bronchopulmonary dysplasia after vitamin E administration. *N Engl J Med* 299:564, 1978.

16. Markestad T, Fitzhardings PM: Growth and development in children recovering from bronchopulmonary dysplasia. *J Pediatr* 98:597, 1981.

17. Smyth JA, Tabachnik E, Duncan WJ, et al: Pulmonary function and bronchial hyperreactivity in long-term survivors of bronchopulmonary dysplasia. *Pediatrics* 68:336, 1981.

18. Owens WC, Owens EV: RLF in premature infants. *Am J of Ophthalmology* 32:1631–37, 1949.

10

Cystic Fibrosis and Its Therapy

Christopher G. Green
Carl F. Doershuk

Cystic Fibrosis involves the mucus-secreting organs and has been recognized as a distinct disorder since 1938. It is a complex, multisystem, ultimately fatal disorder of infants and children; however, increasing numbers are surviving into productive adult life. Cystic fibrosis is the most common, life-threatening genetic trait in whites. It is characterized by an elevated sweat electrolyte content, chronic obstructive pulmonary disease, and exocrine pancreatic insufficiency and is the underlying cause for most chronic lung disease of children. It can occur in a great variety of ways at any age from the neonatal period to adulthood. Lung disease causes most of the serious complications and usually is the ultimate cause of death. Awareness of cystic fibrosis and early diagnosis before serious or irreversible pulmonary damage has occurred are important to improving long-term survival in the great majority of patients. Approximately 18 percent of all known patients with cystic fibrosis are 18 years of age or older. National longevity statistics of all those with cystic fibrosis indicate a median survival expectancy of greater than 19 years.

Cystic fibrosis involves almost all organ systems. Physicians caring for such patients need to be aware of all aspects of the disorder and deal with them effectively. The Cystic Fibrosis Foundation supports more than 125 centers throughout the country to provide expertise in diagnosis and long-term care.

This study was supported in part by grants AM08305, AM27651, and HL07415 from the National Institutes of Health, Cystic Fibrosis Foundation, and United Way Services of Cleveland.

DIAGNOSIS

Cystic fibrosis is a clinical syndrome characterized by elevated sweat electrolyte content, chronic obstructive lung disease, and exocrine pancreatic insufficiency. Virtually all patients have an elevated sweat electrolyte content, although infrequent patients may have intermediate values (between 40 and 60 mEq/L of chloride), and rarely a patient has been reported with classic symptoms and findings but a negative sweat test. The diagnosis of cystic fibrosis is established by a positive sweat test plus at least one of the other diagnostic criteria, such as obstructive lung disease, exocrine pancreatic insufficiency, or a verified family history of cystic fibrosis. Azoospermia is increasingly recognized as an additional positive factor in the diagnosis, since greater than 97 percent of the men are so affected.

GENETICS

The evidence strongly suggests that cystic fibrosis is inherited as an autosomal recessive trait, but no single biochemical defect has been found to provide a unifying hypothesis. The chromosomal location of the affected gene(s) is unknown. There appears to be no correlation with major HLA loci. The combination of cystic fibrosis with other genetic disorders seems to occur by chance. The heterozygote frequency in the white population is estimated to be 5 percent. Estimates of the frequency of cystic fibrosis vary from 1/1000 to 1/4000 live births, with approximately 15,000 to 20,000 persons living in the

United States at present. Some white populations have an incidence as high as 1/620. The incidence in nonwhite populations is much lower; estimates are 1/17,000 in black populations and much less in Oriental populations.

Parents of a cystic fibrosis child are obligate heterozygotes. They have no clinical findings or symptoms of cystic fibrosis. At present no test reliably identifies heterozygotes for genetic counseling.

PATHOPHYSIOLOGIC MECHANISMS

Numerous defects have been postulated, but as yet none clearly explains all aspects of the syndrome. Since Farber's[1] report of widespread mucous obstruction of various organs in cystic fibrosis, mucous glycoproteins have been studied, but there is little evidence that uninfected cystic fibrosis mucus has abnormal chemical properties. The regulation of secretion may be disturbed. Various studies suggest that the mucous secretions, including sputum, meconium, and cervical mucus, are relatively dehydrated. A low water content may explain the excessively tenacious mucus and plugging of gland ducts and acini.

Water secretion is linked secondarily to electrolyte movement across epithelia. Altered electrolyte transport in exocrine systems therefore may also be contributory. High levels of sodium and chloride in cystic fibrosis sweat and, to a lesser extent in salivary secretions, appear to result from inhibition of sodium reabsorption by duct cells as the primary secretory fluid passes from acinar regions to the skin surface. The properties of this inhibitor have eluded definition, although it has been postulated that the inhibitor interacts specifically with the amiloride-sensitive sodium transport system at the luminal membrane of duct epithelium. Although calcium has received considerable attention as a pathophysiologic factor, levels of this divalent cation are, for the most part, appropriate for the protein or glycoprotein content of secretions in cystic fibrosis. There does not seem to be a generalized disturbance of membrane function.

Fatty acid deficiency as the cause of cystic fibrosis does not account for those who retain exocrine pancreatic function (and thus normal fatty acids) but develop other aspects of the syndrome. A number of "cystic fibrosis factors"

have been described, but none have been isolated or completely described, and the assay systems do not yield consistent results from one laboratory to another. Absence of protease (arginine esterase) activity in cystic fibrosis serum and secretions has been reported; however, quantitation has not been uniformly reliable. Cultured fibroblasts have been used in the study of cystic fibrosis, but the results have been either inconsistent or challenged by others. There is no true animal model of cystic fibrosis. One group has used a reserpinized rat model for study, whereas others are employing various animal models to study aspects or the chronic Pseudomonas infection.

Obstruction of exocrine gland ducts or the passageways into which the exocrine secretions are discharged occurs in all, or nearly all, patients with cystic fibrosis. Sites of obstruction include the lung airways, paranasal sinuses, mucus-secreting salivary glands, small intestine, pancreas, biliary system, uterine cervix, and possibly the male genital tract. Inspissation of secretions has been blamed for the obstructive events. Lack of water, alterations of electrolyte concentration, and abnormal organic constituents, especially mucous glycoproteins, have all been implicated in the pathogenesis of inspissated secretions. In addition, it has been suggested that autonomic control of the secretory process is disturbed in patients with cystic fibrosis. Although the eccrine sweat glands and parotid salivary glands, including ducts, are not involved histologically, despite abnormalities in the electrolyte content of their secretory product, striking changes are characteristically observed in the organs affected by abnormal mucous secretions.

The lung usually has a normal macroscopic and microscopic appearance at birth. With development of symptoms and infection, goblet cell hyperplasia and mucous gland hypertrophy occur with subsequent accumulation of mucus in the bronchial airways. Other early lesions are acute and chronic peribronchiolar inflammatory cell infiltrates (bronchiolitis), followed by plugging of small airways with inspissated secretions. Bronchiolar stenosis is a frequent consequence. Infection is the chief cause of progression of the lung involvement and leads to destruction of the airway walls, resulting in bronchiolectasis and bronchiectasis. Bronchiectatic cysts and abscesses become prominent. Squamous metaplasis of ciliated epithelium may occur. As airway involvement advances, bronchiolitis becomes more extensive and areas of fibrosis develop. Bronchitis and bronchiolitis are potentially reversible with therapy, but the fibrosis is essentially irreversible.

Distension of air spaces in an early finding, but little alveolar wall destruction (emphysema) is observed. Areas of segmental or even lobar pneumonitis may follow acute exacerbations of pulmonary disease. Subpleural blebs often develop, and their rupture is responsible for most episodes of pneumothorax. Bronchiectasis results in the development of a rich vascular network in peribronchial granulation tissue. This network shunts blood from bronchial to pulmonary arteries, compounding the problem of uneven ventilation-perfusion distribution.

Endobronchial infection, especially with *Staphylococcus aureus* and *Pseudomonas aeruginosa,* plays a major role in the pathogenesis of chronic lung disease in cystic fibrosis. It is intriguing that this damaging infection is confined to the lung. Furthermore, dissemination, even into the pleural space, is rare. The determinants of lung infection in cystic fibrosis seem to be expressed selectively at the airway surface. Humoral and cellular immunity, as well as complement activity, are generally intact, although functional deficits may occur in cellular immunity and in the alternate pathway of complement as lung infection progresses to an advanced stage. Pulmonary alveolar macrophages display normal phagocytic properties unless exposed to cystic fibrosis serum.

The pancreas is usually small, occasionally cystic, and often difficult to find at postmortem examination. The extent of involvement is variable at birth. Microscopically in infants, the acini and ducts often are distended and filled with eosinophilic material. The acinar epithelium is attenuated. In 85–90 percent of patients the leision progresses to complete or nearly complete disruption of acini and replacement of the pancreas with fibrous tissue and fat. The islets of Langerhans contain normal numbers of β-cells, although they many begin to show some evidence of architectural disruption by fibrous tissue during the second decade of life.

The intestinal tract shows only minimal changes. Esophageal and duodenal glands are often distended with mucous secretions. Goblet cells may be hyperplastic in surface epithelium, especially in the colon and appendix. Concretions may form in the appendiceal lumen or cecum. Rectal biopsy shows dilated crypt lumina and in some cases, increased numbers of goblet cells.

Focal biliary cirrhosis secondary to blockage of intrahepatic bile ducts is uncommon in early life, although it is responsible for occasional cases of prolonged neonatal jaundice. This lesion becomes more prevalent and extensive with age and is found at postmortem examination in 25 percent or more of patients. Infrequently this process proceeds to symptomatic multilobular biliary cirrhosis, with a distinctive pattern of large irregular nodules and contracted bands of fibrous tissue. At autopsy, hepatic congestion secondary to cor pulmonale frequently is observed. The gallbladder may be hypoplastic, filled with mucoid material, and often contains stones. The epithelial lining may display extensive mucous metaplasia.

Mucus-secreting salivary glands are usually enlarged and display focal eosinophilic plugging and ductal dilation. The glands of the uterine cervix are distended with mucus, and copious amounts of mucus collect in the cervical canal. In men the body and tail of the epididymis, vas deferens, and seminal vesicles are completely obliterated or atretic.

DIFFERENTIAL DIAGNOSIS

Because of the frequency and severity of cystic fibrosis, awareness of the many possible manifestations is important to early diagnosis, before irreversible pulmonary disease has occurred. A high degree of suspicion of the symptoms of cystic fibrosis is important. Since it is almost always diagnostic, a sweat test by an experienced laboratory should be performed early in all suggestive cases (Table 10-1).

Incorrect diagnoses such as bronchial asthma, asthmatic bronchitis, chronic bronchitis, whooping cough, tuberculosis, immune deficiency, celiac disease, newborn intestinal obstruction, and failure to thrive have preceded the diagnosis of cystic fibrosis in many cases.

A few other conditions, mostly rare, are associated with elevated sweat electrolytes. These include untreated adrenal insufficiency, ectodermal dysplasia, hereditary nephrogenic diabetes insipidus, glucose 6–phosphatase deficiency, hypothyroidism, mucopolysaccharidoses,

Table 10-1 *Presenting Symptoms of Cystic Fibrosis and Indications for Sweat Testing**

Pulmonary	*Gastrointestinal*	*General*
Chronic or productive coughing	Meconium ileus	Family history of cystic fibrosis
Recurrent bronchitis	Steatorrhea, malabsorption	Failure to thrive
Recurrent or chronic pneumonia or infiltrates	Rectal prolapse	Salty taste when kissed
Recurrent bronchiolitis	Childhood cirrhosis	Heat prostration with unexplained hypochloremic alkalosis
Infection with *Pseudomonas* (mucoid) organisms	Portal hypertension	Nasal polyps
Hemoptysis	Bleeding esophageal varices	Pansinusitis
Staphylococcal pneumonia	Hypoprothrombinemia beyond newborn period	Azoospermia in mature individuals

*Individuals with cystic fibrosis may initially present with any of these signs or symptoms.

fucosidosis, and malnutrition. Most of these conditions can be distinguished from cystic fibrosis by clinical criteria.

KEY DIAGNOSTIC TESTS

The Sweat Test

The sweat test* has remained the single best diagnostic test since first reported in 1957 by Gibson and Cooke[2] (Fig. 10-1). Pilocarpine iontophoresis is used to stimulate the sweat, and subsequent chemical analysis of the chloride content is required for accuracy and reproducibility. It is essential that the amount of sweat collected is measured, preferably 100 mg or more, and reported. Modifications of the test, using variations of the Wheatstone bridge to determine conductivity or an ion-specific electrode to measure chloride concentrations have resulted in errors, both false positive and false negative. These qualitative tests should not be relied on for accurate diagnosis. The approved method (pilocarpine iontophoresis with quantitative chloride analysis) requires care and accuracy. A 3 mA electric current is used to carry pilocarpine into the skin of the forearm and stimulate the sweat glands. In infants it may be necessary to use the upper back to obtain more sweat. After washing the arm with distilled water, pre-weighed filter paper is placed on the stimulated skin, and covered to prevent evaporation. After 30–60 minutes the filter paper is removed and reweighed. The sweat is then eluted from the filter paper and analyzed for chloride. A chloridometer is recommended for the chloride analysis. Cystic fibrosis centers nationwide usually have a laboratory with such equipment and the experience required to obtain reliable results. Positive tests should be confirmed, and negative tests should be repeated if the diagnosis remains questionable. For reliable results, at least 50 and preferably 100 mg of sweat must be collected.

Up to the age of approximately 20 years, more than 60 mEq/L of chloride in sweat is diagnostic of cystic fibrosis when one or more other criteria are present. Values between 40 and 60 mEq/L suggest cystic fibrosis and have been reported in cases with typical involvement. In normal adults sweat chloride values gradually increase, so that a level of 80 mEq/L may be normal. Chloride

*Details are available from the authors.

concentrations in sweat are somewhat lower in individuals with cystic fibrosis who retain exocrine pancreatic function. Their values typically remain within the diagnostic range. Reliable sweat testing may be difficult in the first week or two of life because of difficulty in obtaining adequate amounts of sweat. Placement of electrodes over the back may provide more sweat than forearm skin in newborns.

Pancreatic Function Tests

Pancreatic function tests are useful to document the pancreatic insufficiency present in 80–90 percent of patients. Qualitative stool fat examination may be suggestive but a 3-day collection with controlled fat intake is required for quantitation of steatorrhea. Duodenal intubation is technically difficult, subject to error, and uncomfortable for the patient. With the addition of pancreozymin-secretion stimulation, however, this procedure may help in the diagnosis of borderline cases. Documentation of the trypsin and chymotrypsin in a fresh stool sample has proved an easy and fairly reliable test to screen for pancreatic insufficiency[3]. Serum pancreatic isoamylase is either absent or greatly diminished in patients with documented pancreatic insufficiency. Meconium albumin tests for screening of newborns have not been approved, and those with normal pancreatic function will be overlooked. Stool enzyme analyses and analyses for pancreatic isoamylase in serum are the most widely accepted today, based on patient comfort and reliability of results.

Roentgenographic Examination

Roentgenographic examination may suggest the diagnosis of cystic fibrosis. Generalized hyperinflation alone by chest roentgenography may occur early and may be overlooked in the absence of infiltrates or streaky markings. Bronchial thickening, especially in the apices, and irregular hyperinflation are frequently encountered as symptoms develop. Diffuse patchy areas of atelectasis and infiltration, hilar adenopathy, and more hyperinflation with depression of the diaphragms, anterior bowing of the sternum, and increased anteroposterior diameter of the chest are common with moderate to advanced disease. Often improvement can be noted after intensive treatment. Segmental or

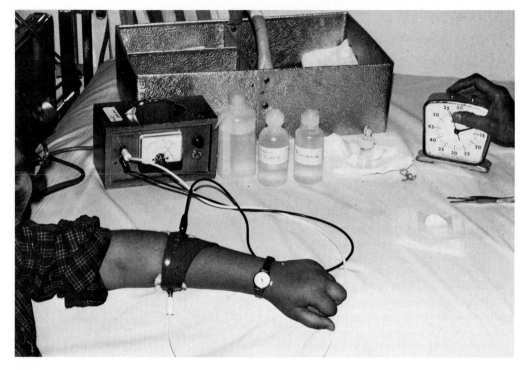

Figure 10-1   Pilocarpine iontophoresis which is part of the sweat test for cystic fibrosis.

lobar atelectasis, cyst formation, extensive bron-chiectasis and infiltrates, pneumothorax, or car-diac enlargement all indicate more irreversible and late involvement. Bronchoscopy and bron-chography are not required for diagnostic evalua-tion.

In older children with cystic fibrosis, roent-genograms of the paranasal sinuses reveal pan-sinusitis and failure of frontal sinus development in almost all cases. These findings are consistent with the diagnosis.

Pulmonary Function Studies

Routine pulmonary function studies cannot be obtained until children are 4–6 years of age. By then most undiagnosed patients will have the typical pattern of obstructive pulmonary involve-ment with decreased vital capacity and flow rates, overinflation (increased residual volume), and a normal or increased total lung capacity. The earliest involvement is believed to occur in the peripheral airways, affecting the distribution of ventilation, and increasing the alveolar-arte-rial oxygen difference. Documentation of ob-structive airway disease in the absence of a response to a bronchodilator is consistent with the diagnosis of cystic fibrosis. Subsequent test-ing once or twice yearly, or more often if needed, can be used to evaluate the effect of therapy and the course of the pulmonary involvement.

CLINICAL MANIFESTATIONS

Expression of the cystic fibrosis defect is highly variable. Manifestations reflect a wide range of pathologic involvement of the lung and pancreas, and a high degree of suspicion is required to make the diagnosis.

Lung Disease

Lung disease accounts for most of the morbid-ity and mortality of cystic fibrosis. Coughing is the most constant symptom of pulmonary in-volvement. It may be dry and hacking, but eventually it becomes loose and then productive. Characteristically in older patients, the cough is most prominent on arising in the morning or after activity. Expectorated mucus is usually purulent. Some patients remain asymptomatic for long periods of time or seem to have slowly clearing acute respiratory tract infections. Others develop a chronic cough or within the first months of life repeatedly develop pneumonia. Extensive bronchiolitis is accompanied by wheezing and frequently occurs during the first years of life. As lung disease progresses to an irreversible degree, exercise intolerance, shortness of breath, and failure to gain weight or grow are noted. Exacerbations of lung symptoms eventually require hospitalization for effective treatment. Finally, repiratory failure, cor pulmonale, and death supervene.

Physical findings include an increased anteroposterior diameter of the chest, generalized hyperresonance, scattered or localized rales, and digital clubbing. Coughing that produces purulent secretions is common in older children. High-pitched expiratory rhonchi may also be heard, especially in young children. Cyanosis is a late sign. Pulmonary complications include atelectasis, hemoptysis, pneumothorax, and cor pulmonale.

Intestinal Tract

Intestinal tract involvement may be apparent even at birth. The ileum is completely obstructed by meconium (meconium ileus) in over 10 percent of newborns with cystic fibrosis. Evidence for obstruction, including abdominal distension, emesis, and failure to pass meconium, appears within the first 24–48 hours of life. Abdominal roentgenograms show dilated loops of bowel with gas-fluid levels and frequently a collection of granular, "ground-glass" material in the lower central abdomen. Meconium plug syndrome may occur more commonly in infants with cystic fibrosis than in other infants. Ileal obstruction with fecal material (meconium ileus equivalent) occasionally occurs in older patients, causing cramping abdominal pain and abdominal distension.

More than 85 percent of children with cystic fibrosis have evidence of maldigestion because of exocrine pancreatic insufficiency. Symptoms include frequent, bulky, greasy stools and failure to gain weight even when the food intake appears to be large. Characteristically, stools will contain readily visible droplets of fat. A protuberant abdomen, decreased muscle mass, poor growth, and delayed maturation are typical physical signs. Excessive flatus may be a problem.

Less common gastrointestinal tract manifestations include intussusception, fecal impaction of the cecum or appendix with an asymptomatic right lower quadrant mass, or epigastric pain due to duodenal inflammation. Cystic fibrosis appears to be the major cause of rectal prolapse in children in temperate zones. Hypoproteinemia with anasarca in infants may result from the use of soy-base formula. Deficiency of fat-soluble vitamins is occasionally symptomatic. For example, hypoprothrombinemia due to vitamin K deficiency may result in a bleeding diathesis.

Other Manifestations

Biliary cirrhosis rarely becomes symptomatic. Manifestations may incude icterus, ascites, hematemesis from esophageal varices, or evidence of hypersplenism. Biliary colic secondary to cholelithiasis may occur in the second decade of life.

Hyperglycemia, glucosuria, polyuria, and weight loss may appear, usually after 10 years of age. In most cases ketoacidosis does not occur, and the other complications of diabetes mellitus are infrequently observed.

Recurrent *acute pancreatitis* occasionally occurs in those adolescents and young adults who have residual exocrine pancreatic function and may be exacerbated by diet or tetracycline.

Sexual development is often delayed by an average of 2–3 years. More than 97 percent of males with cystic fibrosis are azoospermic because of failure of development of wolffian duct structures, but sexual function is generally unimpaired. Adolescent females may experience secondary amenorrhea, especially with exacerbations of pulmonary disease. Cervicitis and accumulation of tenacious mucus in the cervical canal have been noted. The female fertility rate is unknown, but is probably lower than normal. Pregnancy is generally tolerated well by women with good pulmonary function, but may cause progression of pulmonary disease and even death in those with moderate or advanced lung problems.

The *sweat glands* do not show pathologic changes. Parents may note salt "frosting" of the skin or that the child tastes salty when kissed. Excessive loss of salt in the sweat predisposes young children to salt depletion episodes, especially with gastroenteritis, vomiting, or diarrhea. These children present with hypochloremic alkalosis. This complication appears to be more common in warm-weather zones. The decreasing salt content of prepared formulas may result in an increasing incidence of this problem.

THERAPY

Therapy must be comprehensive as well as individualized. At the time of diagnosis most patients have some pulmonary involvement. Because of the serious prognosis, we almost always use a period of hospitalization for accurate diagnosis, overall baseline assessment, initiation of treatment, optimal clearing of the pulmonary involvement, and education of the parents and patient. The patient is hospitalized for as long as is necessary to control the pulmonary involvement and achieve steady weight gain.

General Approach

The general approach to care includes follow-up outpatient visits scheduled every 4–8 weeks, regardless of the patient's status, because many aspects of the condition require careful monitoring. Significant pulmonary progression can occur without acute symptoms. The interval history and physical examination are conducted by an experienced physician. A sputum sample is obtained for culture and antibiotic sensitivities. In patients who cannot expectorate sputum, a deep throat culture is taken during or after a forced cough. Even apparently asymptomatic patients may produce sputum after forced exhalations or stimulation with a pharyngeal swab. Progressive and irreversible loss of function from the low-grade pulmonary infection can occur gradually; therefore emphasis is placed on the pulmonary history, including any change in the cough. Exacerbation of pulmonary infection is indicated by a change in cough frequency or productivity, the appearance of a nocturnal cough, or onset of paroxysmal coughing with or without vomiting or hemoptysis. The appearance of new rales, irritability, decreased activity, decreased appetite, or failure to gain weight also may reflect increased pulmonary infection and suggest the need for increased or altered antibiotic and physical therapy.

Adequate time should be reserved at each visit for experienced physician contact that may change in emphasis from visit to visit and include other caretakers as required. The goal of therapy is to maintain a stable condition for long periods of time. This can be accomplished for the majority of patients with interval evaluation and adjustments to the home treatment program. Some patients, however, never reach a stable condition or have episodic acute or low-grade chronic lung infections (usually with *P. aeruginosa*) that steadily progress. For these patients, rehospitalization for 2 or more weeks of intensive inhalation and physical therapy and intravenous antibiotics is indicated. Such admissions may be required infrequently or as frequently as every 2–3 months. Significant improvement in pulmonary function and patient well-being are usually achieved until late in the course.

The *basic daily care program* varies somewhat, depending on the age of the patient, degree of pulmonary involvement, other system involvement, and time available for therapy. The major components of this care program include digestive therapy and pulmonary therapy. Immunizations for rubeola, pertussis, and influenza are also important.

Pulmonary Therapy

Measures to control or combat the pulmonary obstruction and infection play a major role and are the most time consuming and expensive. These include aerosol therapy, segmental postural drainage, and antibiotic therapy. Although infants usually receive intermittent aerosol therapy two to four times daily for 5–10 minutes followed by 20–30 minutes of postural drainage, by school age the available time often limits therapy to two sessions daily. Maintaining a balance requires a great deal of understanding, education, and encouragement by those providing care.

Pulmonary therapy is empiric and symptomatic. Its objective is to clear airway secretions and control infection. Although there may be a divergence of opinion about various aspects of therapy, the effectiveness of the overall approach to therapy (including close supervision, continuity of care, aggressive interaction, and an optimistic outlook) is more important than variations in the use of individual measures. Furthermore, each available measure may not be effective for every patient. Iatrogenic complications are always possible and must always be considered.

Intermittent medication aerosol therapy is used to deliver decongestant, bronchodilator, mucolytic, antibiotic, or anti-inflammatory agents to the lower respiratory tract. The basic aerosol solution consists of 2 ml of 0.125 percent phenylephrine, in 10 percent propylene glycol, or 0.45 percent saline and is administered two to four times daily, usually before chest physiotherapy. In patients with hyperreactive airways, isoetharine or isoproterenol can be added.

When secretions are very thick and difficult to clear, a mucolytic agent such as N-acetylcysteine may be useful. A dose of 2 ml of 20 percent acetylcysteine in 2 ml of basic aerosol solution can be used before postural drainage. Because of the potential for irritation of respiratory epithelium, usage of mucolytic agents should be limited.

When bacteria resistant to oral antibiotics are present or when the infection is difficult to control at home, aerosolized antibiotics may reduce symptoms of tracheitis or bronchitis. It is probably most effective to administer antibiotics by aerosol after postural drainage has been given. Colistimethate, gentamicin, or tobramycin, 20–40 mg in 2 ml of saline, have been used two to four times daily in home therapy and also in the hospital in conjunction with intravenous therapy. Some have used carbenicillin, 1 g, or ticarcillin, 0.5 g, in the aerosol. There is concern that more frequent sensitization or resistance to these agents might occur as a result of this usage.

For intermittent aerosol therapy, a nebulizer is driven by a small compressor. Aerosol equipment should be cleaned, rinsed, and air dried daily. As soon as the patient can reliably breathe through the mouth and not through the nose, mouth breathing of aerosols should be encouraged, with occasional breath-holding after inspiration, in an effort to increase deposition. The patient's position should not restrict diaphragm movement during aerosol therapy. Nebulization therapy of any sort can provoke irritation or intolerance. If either is suspected, the therapy should be discontinued.

Direct inhalation therapy, is used when thick or copious secretions are difficult to mobilize. Direct inhalation from an ultrasonic nebulizer with .22 percent saline for 10–20 minutes can be used before postural drainage.

Mist tent therapy has been used overnight in an effort to enhance humidification and deposit water droplets in the lower respiratory tract. It may be beneficial for selected patients. Either a pneumatic-type nebulizer or an ultrasonic nebulizer can be used to generate mist. Ultrasonic units are quiet and have a large water output but are more difficult to maintain and are more easily contaminated. The choice of unit is best determined by availability of service. A small tent should be used to achieve a relatively dense mist. For ultrasonic units, the solutions most commonly nebulized are 5 percent propylene glycol by volume in distilled water, a dilute (.22 percent) saline solution, or distilled water. In pneumatic units, 10 percent propylene glycol by volume in distilled water is used. The solution should be sterile and free from organic matter to minimize bacterial growth. Nebulizers should be washed at least every other day with a disinfectant detergent A-33 (Airwick Industries Inc., Seacaucus, NJ 07094) or 2 percent acetic acid solution, followed by rinsing and thorough drying. Gas sterilization is preferable in the hospital.

Antibiotic therapy is central to the pulmonary therapy of cystic fibrosis. Infection and resulting tissue injury play a major role in the progression of the pulmonary lesion. The goal of antibiotic therapy is to reduce the intensity of infection and to minimize or delay the inflammatory reaction and progressive lung damage. Although some organisms such as *S. aureus* can be eradicated temporarily from sputum, others such as *P. aeruginosa* rarely are eliminated, even for short periods. Patients vary considerably in their past history, the type and quantity of organisms present in their respiratory tract secretions, and the amount of damage already incurred. The usual guidelines for acute infections such as fever, tachypnea, or chest pain are usually absent. Consequently, all aspects of the patient's history and examination are used to guide the frequency and duration of antibiotic therapy. Antibiotic treatment varies from intermittent short courses of one antibiotic, for example, a semisynthetic penicillin for a 2-week period, to continuous treatment with one or more antibiotics for weeks at a time. Dosages are often two or three times the amount recommended for minor infections, because patients with cystic fibrosis have proportionately more lean body mass and higher clearance rates for many antibiotics than do other individuals. In addition, it is difficult to achieve effective drug levels of many antimicrobials in respiratory tract secretions.

Outpatient antibiotic therapy is used for at least 2 weeks for many patients during each 6–8 week interval. The most common cystic fibrosis–related organisms recovered are *S. aureus* and *P. aeruginosa,* but *Pneumococcus* organisms and

Haemophilus influenzae a may be found also. When acute symptoms develop, the initial antibiotic selection should include appropriate therapy for these organisms. For patients with acute symptoms, treatment should be continued for a number of days after the symptoms are under control, usually for 2 or more weeks. If improvement is not observed in 5–7 days, the antibiotic therapy should be adjusted. If symptoms reappear after successful therapy, the course of antibiotic therapy should be repeated. Some recommend continuous semisynthetic penicillin therapy in full dosage from the time of diagnosis in an effort to prevent or minimize staphylococcal infection. Low-dosage, continuous antibiotic therapy is not recommended because achievement of adequate airway levels is difficult and because of the tendency for *Pseudomonas* and other organisms to develop resistance. Patients in good condition may culture only *S. aureus, H. influenzae,* or even normal flora. Sputum of those with more advanced involvement usually contains *P. aeruginosa,* including the mucoid form. More recently a number of other species of *Pseudomonas,* notably *maltophilia* and *cepacia,* have been encountered. These organisms, along with *P. aeruginosa,* may develop resistance to most or all available antibiotics. Whenever possible, choice of antimicrobials should be guided by in vitro sensitivity testing. Sulfisoxazole or trimethoprim are the only oral agents that appear effective in vitro, and they may be effective clinically. Chloramphenicol sodium succinate can be extremely valuable when symptoms are uncontrolled by other agents. These antimicrobials may be effective, even when the in vitro sensitivities appear negative. Tetracyclines should be avoided, if possible, in children under 9 years of age, but may be useful thereafter. Young children may be colonized with *Pseudomonas* organisms relatively early. If they seem to be doing well clinically, antibiotic therapy is concentrated on other organisms present. If symptoms develop and are not controlled, however, every effort is made to treat the *Pseudomonas* infection as well.

Inpatient antibiotic therapy is required for the patient who has progressive or unrelenting symptoms or signs despite the most intensive measures at home. Then hospitalization for intensive intravenous antibiotic and physical therapy is recommended. Although many patients improve measurably within 7 days, we usually extend the hospital treatment period to 14 days or longer if there is continued improvement. Some patients have a return of symptoms after discharge and require further intensive hospital therapy. The development of the "heparin lock" has permitted frequent daily infusions with minimal discomfort to the patient and freedom for activities between infusions. A 23-gauge scalp vein needle with a resealing cap or an indwelling intravenous cannula can be used. The scalp vein needle can be maintained for periods up to 10–14 days with rare evidence of local phlebitis or infection. The heparin lock system is flushed and filled between infusions with a solution containing 10 units of heparin for each milliliter of normal saline. In some cases requiring chronic home antibiotic therapy, a Broviac catheter has been surgically placed and used for periods up to 2 years without complications.

The antibiotics selected for intravenous use are determined from the sputum culture and susceptibility studies. Two agents are frequently used against *Pseudomonas* organisms. A frequent combination is ticarcillin, 200–400 mg/kg/24 hours, or carbenicillin, 300–500 mg/kg/24 hours administered every 4 hours, and tobramycin or gentamicin. The aminoglycosides have a relatively short half-life in many patients with cystic fibrosis. The initial dosage is 8 mg/kg/24 hours, given every 8 hours. Toxicity can be minimized if blood levels are monitored. Trough levels should be kept below 1.5–2 mg/L.

In some cases an antistaphylococcal antibiotic is added even if the organism is not recovered on a recent culture, especially in those with hemoptysis or those not responding as anticipated. Changes in therapy should be guided by culture results. In patients who do not improve, other factors should be considered, such as infection with *Aspergillus fumigatus* or mycobacteria, heart failure, or hyperreactive airways.

Chest physical therapy consists of segmental posture drainage in each of 12 positions with associated clapping for at least 1-minute periods followed by chest vibration for five exhalations in each position. This form of therapy is most effective when used in conjunction with inhalation and antibiotic therapy. Each family and older patient is instructed in the use of all 12 positions at the time of diagnosis. Postural drainage therapy can be initiated even in the young infant. When old enough to cooperate, children are encouraged to extend exhalations using pursed-lip breathing to prevent airway collapse and permit better emptying of the lungs. Because localized mucous plugging has been described even in patients with little or no clinical evidence of active pulmonary infection, a minimum of one aerosol followed by 20–30 minutes of postural drainage is recommended daily for every patient. Young infants with pulmonary symptoms receive this therapy three or four times a day. Flare-ups of the pulmonary infection or periods of acute respiratory illness require additional treatment periods to bring the exacerbation under control. Although infants and children can be treated effectively on the lap, the use of a tilt board or folding therapy table* facilitates this treatment for older individuals. Effective coughing should be encouraged after each segment is clapped. The clapping and vibrating should be repeated in positions that are productive. Older individuals are encouraged to do their own therapy. This can be facilitated by the use of mechanical percussors or vibrators. On occasion chest physical therapy may contribute to hemoptysis and may need to be discontinued or modified temporarily. Physical activity and forced deep breathing frequently result in significant expectoration of mucus and should be encouraged. A regular program of exercise appears to maintain a feeling of general well-being.

Bronchodilator therapy is effective in some patients. Reversible airway obstruction has been documented in up to one third of patients with cystic fibrosis. Some of these cases occur in conjunction with allergic bronchopulmonary aspergillosis. The reversible obstruction is suggested by improvement of 15 percent or more in pulmonary function, especially the flow rates, after inhalation of a bronchodilator aerosol. Treatment should include regular use of a bronchodilator aerosol and sustained-release oral theophylline, with the dosage adjusted after blood levels are obtained. In some cases aerosol or a systemic steroid is required, at least briefly.

Endoscopy and lavage are sometimes used in the treatment of obstructive airway disease, especially if atelectasis or mucoid impaction is present. The flexible fiberoptic bronchoscope has simplified endoscopy but it decreases ventilating space and thus has limitations in smaller patients. Evidence for sustained benefit from lavage procedures in cystic fibrosis is lacking.

*Available from the Cystic Fibrosis Foundation, 3091 Mayfield Road, Cleveland, Ohio 44118.

Expectorants, such as iodides and glyceryl guaiacolate, in recommended doses do not increase water secretion into the respiratory tract, change the rheologic properties of the secretions, or provide clinical improvement. Goiter formation with prolonged use of iodides has been documented.

Treatment of Pulmonary Complications

Hemoptysis is more frequent with increasing numbers of older patients. When small amounts (less than 20 ml) of blood are lost, postural drainage should be continued and the antibiotic regimen reviewed to be certain that coverage is adequate. Some patients who do not have *S. aureus* on sputum culture still may improve with the addition of antistaphylococcal therapy. With more persistent or increased hemoptysis, hospital admission is advised for intravenous antibiotic therapy. Massive hemoptysis (total blood loss of 250–500 ml or more in a 24-hour period) requires close monitoring. The sputum should be cultured and blood obtained and cross-matched for later use. Chest physical therapy is often discontinued until 12–24 hours after the last bleeding episode and then is gradually reinstituted. Vitamin K, 5 mg daily, may be helpful. Hemoptysis in cystic fibrosis invariably stops, but a great deal of reassurance may be needed. Hemoptysis is aggravated when the person is lying flat and may be relieved by use of the semierect position. Bronchoscopy usually fails to reveal the exact bleeding site. Ticarcillin and perhaps other drugs may interfere with platelet function and aggravate diffuse pulmonary bleeding. In most cases, a lobectomy should be avoided if at all possible. Bronchial artery embolization has been used successfully to control significant hemoptysis but carries the risk of emboli to the vessels supplying the spinal cord.

Pneumothoraces are increasingly encountered in the second and third decades. The onset may be relatively mild but some chest pain or shortness of breath are usually present. Whenever symptoms suggest a pneumothorax, chest roentgenography is advised. The small, less than 5–10 percent, pneumothorax may resolve under hospital observation. A larger pneumothorax or one under tension requires at least a tube thoracostomy immediately. We usually elect open thoracotomy via a small incision with plication of blebs, apical pleural stripping, and basal pleural abrasion to prevent delayed closure of the air leak and to avoid the otherwise high rate of recurrence. This procedure has been well tolerated, and recurrence has been extremely rare. Intravenous antibiotics and aerosols are begun on admission and postural drainage resumed as soon as possible. Others use only tube thoracostomy, despite the greater recurrence rate, or add a sclerosing agent such as tetracycline.

Allergic aspergillosis may present with wheezing, increased coughing or shortness of breath or with notable hyperinflation on pulmonary function testing. In some there are localized infiltrates on the chest roentgenogram. Recovery of *Aspergillus* organisms from the sputum, the presence of brown sputum, several serum precipitin bands to *Aspergillus fumigatus* extract, or the presence of eosinophils in fresh sputum samples support the diagnosis. The IgE level may be within the normal limits or elevated. Bronchodilators are used to control the bronchospasm and systemic and possibly aerosol corticosteroids also may be needed. This is usually a limited complication, which will subside with several weeks of therapy. Remissions should be similarly treated. In some cases, aerosolized amphotericin B or systemic flucytosine may be considered.

Lobar atelectasis occurs relatively infrequently. It may be asymptomatic and noted only at the time of routine chest roentgenography. Aggressive therapy is warranted with intravenous antibiotics and increased chest physical therapy for the affected lobe. If there is no improvement in 7–10 days, bronchoscopy may result in the removal of a mucous plug, but this does not necessarily enhance resolution. If the atelectasis does not resolve, the patient should be discharged with continued intensive home therapy to the involved lobe. There should be no early decision for a lobectomy, since the atelectasis may still resolve over a period of weeks or months. Even if the lobe does not expand, it may not be a source of symptomatic infection. If the patient has progressive difficulty from fever, anorexia, unrelenting coughing, or sputum production, a lobectomy should be considered. Such a procedure should be performed only after a period of intensive hospitalization to improve the status of all remaining portions of the lung.

Hypertrophic pulmonary osteoarthropathy results in elevation of the periosteum of the distal portions of the long bones on the roentgenogram and may cause bone pain, edema, and joint effusions. The use of acetaminophen, ibuprofen, or zomepirac sodium may provide relief. Control of lung infection may be most helpful.

Acute respiratory failure is rarely encountered and is usually the result of a severe viral illness such as influenza. All available and necessary intensive therapy measures are given in anticipation of recovery to previous status. Oxygen therapy usually is required to maintain the PaO_2 above 50 mm Hg. A rising $PaCO_2$ may required a period of ventilator assistance. Endotracheal or bronchoscopic suction may be necessary and repeated daily. Right ventricular failure requires diuretics and a reduced salt intake. Recovery does not begin until after the acute illness has subsided. Intensive intravenous antibiotic therapy and postural drainage should be continued for several weeks after the patient has regained baseline status.

Chronic respiratory failure develops either as a result of incomplete recovery from an acute episode or from prolonged slow deterioration. Although this can occur at any age, it is more frequently seen in adolescent and adult patients. Because a long-standing PaO_2 of less than 45–50 mm Hg increases the development of right ventricular failure, these patients usually benefit from low-flow oxygen therapy. Increasing hypercapnia may prevent the use of optimal FiO_2. These patients do not benefit from ventilator assistance or a tracheostomy. Most patients will improve somewhat with intensive antibiotic and pulmonary therapy and can be discharged again after gradual weaning from the supplemental oxygen. In some cases it will be necessary to provide low-flow oxygen therapy at home. These patients nearly always have cor pulmonale and should maintain a reduced salt intake.

Right ventricular failure may develop in individuals with long-standing advanced pulmonary disease, especially those with severe hypoxemia (PaO_2 less than 50 mm Hg). Some may develop acute right ventricular failure as a result of complications such as acute viral infection or a pneumothorax. Some combination of cyanosis, increased shortness of breath, gallop rhythm, increased liver size with a tender margin, ankle edema, jugular venous distension, increased heart size on a chest roentgenogram, or an unusual increase in weight help to confirm the diagnosis. Furosemide is the diuretic of choice in most instances of acute, severe cor pulmonale. For chronic therapy spironolactone is preferable because of its potassium-sparing effects. Electrolytes should be monitored after changes in diuretic dosages. Potassium deficiency may occur, and magnesium depletion may accompany concomitant aminoglycoside therapy. The effectiveness of digitalis has not been documented in cases of pure right ventricular failure. When there is associated left-ventricular failure, however, digitalis may be useful. As with chronic respiratory failure, supplemental oxygen therapy is also important but may be limited by increasing hypercapnia. Sodium intake should be decreased and fluid overload avoided. Intensive pulmonary therapy as described previously is most important. Antibiotics should be monitored for sodium content. Pulmonary vasodilator therapy does not seem to provide long-term benefit. In the past, cardiac failure usually meant death within several months. More recently, a number of older patients have survived for 3 years or more after an initial episode.

Gastrointestinal Therapy

Consideration of diet, vitamin supplements, and pancreatic enzyme replacement are important for the 85–90 percent of patients who have inadequate pancreatic function. Despite vigorous supervision, many will evidence inadequate weight gain even when lung infection is minimal.

Pancreatic enzyme replacement through use of the recently developed pH-sensitive, enteric-coated enzyme microspheres has improved efficacy so that most patients now tolerate an average fat intake with infrequent oily stools or abdominal cramps. Stool fat and nitrogen losses are not fully corrected, however. The enzyme product and dosage must be individualized for each patient. One to three capsules of pancrelipase (Cotazym-S, Pancrease) during each meal are sufficient for most patients. Infants may need only one third to one half a capsule with each meal or may do better with pancreatin powder (Cotazym). Preparations containing bile salts may be helpful for some. Some older patients have noted a decrease in enzyme requirement. Rarely, family members may experience allergic rhinitis, watery eyes, or bronchospasm when exposed to pancreatin powders.

Vitamin and other supplements have been recommended. Vitamins A, D, E, and K are fat soluble, and extra amounts are usually provided. A and D are replaced in the usual multivitamin preparations. A water soluble preparation of vitamin E is given in 50 IU daily dosages in infants and young children and 100 IU or more after that. Vitamin K, 5 mg orally, may be used in the newborn period and during episodes of hemoptysis, intense antimicrobial therapy, or surgery. Some patients with cheilosis benefit from riboflavin or local steroid-antifungal therapy.

It is difficult to force the young child to consume more food. Some older children and adolescents fail to eat properly, and an increase in caloric intake will result in weight gain. Medium-chain triglycerides (MCT) are more readily absorbed without digestion and have been useful with infants. Many older patients find MCT and artificial diets unpalatable and usually give them up after a short time. There is no direct evidence to support selenium supplementation. Selenium toxicity is enhanced in the presence of vitamin E deficiency in animals.

When *meconium ileus* is suspected, a nasogastric tube is placed for suctioning to prevent vomiting and aspiration, and the infant is hydrated with intravenous fluids. An enema of diatrizide meglumine and diatrizoate sodium solution (Gastrografin) with a reflux of contrast material into the ileum has resulted in passage of a meconium plug and clearing of the obstruction in a number of cases. Use of the hypertonic solution requires careful replacement of water losses into the bowel. An atretic segment of the ileum requires surgery with resection and anastomosis. Survivors generally have a prognosis similar to that of other patients. Infants with a suspected meconium ileus should be treated as having cystic fibrosis until adequate sweat testing can be carried out, usually after 1–2 weeks of life.

Meconium ileus equivalent and intussusception may occur. In some patients an accumulation of fecal material in the terminal portion of the ileum and cecum results in intermittent or complete obstruction (meconium ileus equivalent). For intermittent obstruction, pancreatic replacement should be continued or even increased, and a laxative or stool softeners (milk of magnesia, dioctyl sodium sulfosuccinate, or mineral oil) should be given along with increased fluid intake. For complete obstruction, Gastrografin enema, accompanied by large amounts of intravenous fluids, can be therapeutic. Hypertonic Gastrografin can draw water into the ileum and loosen the inspissated fecal material. Intussusception and volvulus also must be considered in the differential diagnosis. Intussusception, usually ileocolic, can occur at any age in these patients and often follows a 1- or 2-day history of "constipation." If present, it can be both diagnosed and reduced by a Gastrografin enema. If a nonreduceable intussusception or volvulus is present, laparotomy is required. Repeated episodes may be an indication for cecectomy. Once or twice daily dosages of mineral oil (1 tablespoon) may prevent repeated episodes of meconium ileus equivalent.

Chronic appendicitis with or without periappendiceal abscess occurs occasionally in patients receiving long-term antibiotic therapy and may present with recurrent or persistent abdominal pain. Lack of acid buffering in the duodenum appears to promote duodenitis and ulcer formation in some.

Rectal prolapse occurs frequently before diagnosis and is usually related to steatorrhea, malnutrition, and a repetitive cough. It usually can be replaced manually by continuous gentle pressure with the patient in the knee-chest position. Sedation may be needed. To prevent an immediate recurrence, the buttocks can be taped closed. Adequate pancreatin replacement, decreased fat and roughage in the diet, and control of pulmonary infection result in improvement. Infrequently a patient may continue to have rectal prolapse and require surgery (a subcutaneous sling of silicone rubber [Silastic] placed around the rectum).

Biliary cirrhosis infrequently results in portal hypertension with esophageal varices, hypersplenism, or ascites. The acute management of bleeding esophageal varices includes nasogastric suction and cold saline lavage. Intravenous or celiac artery infusion of vasopressin (Pitressin) has been tried. An episode of significant bleeding is an indication for portal systemic shunting. A splenectomy and splenorenal anastomosis decrease portal pressures and also effectively treat hypersplenism when present, but adequate pressure and vessel size are necessary for a successful shunt. Portacaval anastomosis may be used. Ascites is best managed conservatively, with a low-sodium diet and diuretics as necessary. These patients may require a shunt for long-term management. Rarely, biliary cirrhosis progresses to hepatocellular failure, which should be treated as in other patients with hepatic failure. A cholecystectomy is frequently necessary for relief of symptoms when gallstones are found.

Pancreatitis may be precipitated by fatty meals, alcohol ingestion, or tetracycline therapy. Serum amylase and lipase levels may remain elevated for some time. Treatment is symptomatic and includes analgesia, intravenous fluids, and nasogastric suctioning. An occasional patient may have mild symptoms and improve with several days of clear liquids. Once the pain and amylase level decrease, the patient can resume oral intake, but animal fat may need to be avoided for some time.

Hyperglycemia can develop at any age, and the occurrence is not related to the severity of the disease. Ketoacidosis is rarely encountered. If blood glucose levels are only moderately elevated and there is no glucose in the urine, no treatment is necessary. A greater elevation of blood glucose level results in calorie and water losses into the urine, and insulin treatment should be instituted. Oral antidiabetic agents are usually not effective in these patients. Exocrine pancreatic insufficiency and malabsorption make strict dietary control of hyperglycemia more difficult. The development of hyperglycemia does not appear to change the prognosis significantly; however, it is at least a nuisance and may precipitate psychologic problems.

Other Therapy

Nasal polyps occur in 15—20 percent of patients with cystic fibrosis and may be a recurrent problem. Corticosteroid and decongestant nasal sprays occasionally provide relief. Allergy skin testing and possible hyposensitization may be helpful in a few with allergic symptoms. With complete obstruction or constant rhinorrhea, surgical removal is indicated. Polyps may recur promptly but frequently do not grow to the point of obstruction for long periods.

Salt depletion and hypochloremic alkalosis can occur from sweat salt losses, especially on hot days. Infants, and less frequently, older patients may present with hyponatremic hypochloremic dehydration requiring 10—15 ml/kg of normal saline to reestablish an adequate circulating volume. Prevention is the best approach. Children should have free access to salt. Infants may need salt supplementation. Precautions against overdressing infants in hot weather should be observed.

Delayed sexual maturation occurs fairly frequently in cystic fibrosis and may be associated with short stature. Although many have severe pulmonary infection or poor nutrition, delayed puberty also occurs in patients with otherwise mild disease and is not well explained. Individuals with cystic fibrosis have the same adolescent and development concerns as others. Each should receive specific counseling concerning sexual development and potential reproductive problems through the developing years.

Men are almost always azoospermic but have normal sexual function. Explanation and later support are important. Women occasionally have problems with cervical polyps. Pregnancy often results in premature delivery and progression of the pulmonary disease. Patients with mild pulmonary disease often tolerate pregnancy successfully. Antibiotic therapy presents risks to the fetus (e.g., tetracycline, chloramphenicol, and aminoglycosides).

Surgical procedures of a minor nature, including dental work, should be performed under local anesthesia if possible. Those with good or excellent pulmonary status can tolerate general anesthesia without intensive pulmonary measures before the surgery. Patients with moderate or severe pulmonary infection, are better off with a 1- to 2-week course of intensive antibiotic treatment before surgery. If this is not possible, initiation of intravenous antibiotic therapy is useful as soon as it is recognized that major surgery will be required. Aerosol and postural drainage treatments immediately before anesthesia are advisable. The anesthesia time should be kept to a minimum. Tracheal suctioning is useful and should be repeated at the end of the operation. When necessary, even patients in respiratory failure or right ventricular failure can undergo anesthesia and major surgery without intraoperative or postoperative mortality. Such patients require frequent monitoring of their blood gases and may require ventilatory assistance in the immediate postoperative period. A tracheostomy does not appear necessary.

After major surgery, coughing should be encouraged as a routine. Postural drainage treatments should be reinstituted as soon as possible, usually within 24 hours, and gradually intensified until full treatments are completed. For those with significant pulmonary involvement, intravenous antibiotics are continued for at least 2 weeks postoperatively. Early ambulation and intermittent deep breathing are important and an incentive spirometer can be helpful.

After an open thoracotomy for treatment of a pneumothorax or lobectomy, the chest tube quickly becomes the greatest single obstacle to effective pulmonary therapy and should be removed as soon as possibile so that full postural drainage therapy can resume.

PERSPECTIVE ON NEW AND FUTURE DEVELOPMENTS

Currently, there are no generally accepted tests for cystic fibrosis heterozygosity, prenatal detection, or newborn screening. Also, the basic pathophysiologic defect in cystic fibrosis is unknown. This section will briefly review some of the promising lines of investigation aimed at developing such tests and increasing our knowledge of cystic fibrosis.

Since some 5 percent of American whites are estimated to be carriers of the cystic fibrosis gene, a test to detect heterozygotes would have widespread applicability. In the late 1960s, a serum fraction from heterozygotes was found to cause abnormalities in the ciliary motion of rabbit tracheal explants and oyster gills. Subsequent investigators have met with mixed success in attempts to duplicate this work. Researchers continue efforts to isolate and characterize a "cystic fibrosis protein" that causes ciliary dyskinesia using isoelectric focusing and counterimmunoelectrophoresis.

In 1981 evidence for a difference between normal and cystic fibrosis heterozygotes and homozygotes was published. The difference was in sodium transport in cultured fibroblasts. Later the same investigators were unable to reproduce their results in a blinded study but are continuing this work.

Nadler and Walsh have found deficiences of serine protease activity in midtrimester amniotic fluid from women carrying infants later diagnosed as having cystic fibrosis. Further studies of amniotic fluid may yield a reliable method for prenatal detection of cystic fibrosis.

The sweat test may be inaccurate in the first few weeks of life. Some believe that the study of meconium albumin or a blood test for trypsin will be effective as a newborn screening test. The latter test is under study.

The basic gene defect in cystic fibrosis remains unknown. Recently, Knowles et al. found that the bioelectric potential difference across respira-

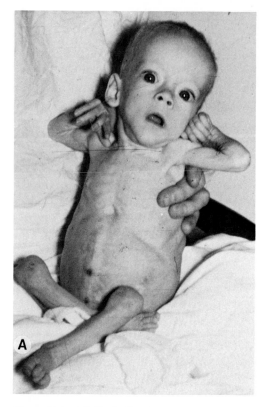 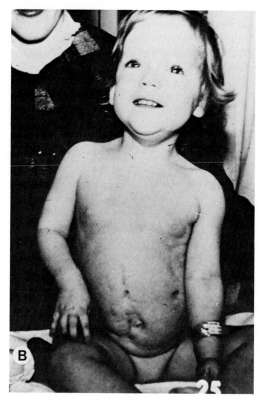

Figure 10-2 (A) Cystic fibrosis patient at diagnosis. (B) Same patient at 19 months of age.

tory epithelium is significantly greater in persons with cystic fibrosis than in normal persons. They presented evidence that this is secondary to increased sodium transport away from the airway secretions. This may lead to increased loss of water from the lumen, resulting in more viscous mucous secretions and perhaps decreased mucous clearance and obstructive lung disease. Further studies are needed in all of these areas to finally provide definite answers.

CASE REPORTS

The following two cases are meant to illustrate the presentation, diagnosis, therapy and course of infants with cystic fibrosis. There are many other clinical presentations of infants with cystic fibrosis. Also cystic fibrosis is sometimes diagnosed in later childhood and occasionally diagnosed in adults.

A 16-month-old white male was referred for evaluation of chronic colds, coughing, and rhinorrhea beginning at a few weeks of age. He was treated with cough medicines, decongestants, and courses of oral antibiotics, but the cough persisted.

He had frequent, oily, bulky, foul-smelling stools. He was thin, despite a good appetite and several diet changes, chronically pale, and increasingly listless.

Physical examination showed a thin, blond toddler with raspy breathing and a protuberant abdomen. He was afebrile and had mild tachypnea. His length and weight were below the third percentile, whereas the head circumference was greater than the fiftieth percentile. Clear rhinorrhea was present. The anteroposterior diameter of the chest was increased, and moderate retractions were noted. Diffuse rhonchi were present. Mild clubbing was present. The skin was pale but without cyanosis.

At 16 months of age a sweat test was performed and found to be positive at 104 mEq/L of chloride. The stool trypsin level was 56 μg/g, and chymotrypsin was 58 μg/g the (normal level is 80 μg/g for both). A chest roentgenogram showed minimal peribronchial thickening. A deep throat culture grew normal flora and *Haemophilus* species. The hemoglobin level was 11.6 g/dL, and the white blood cell count was 4600/mm³ with 33 neutrophils, 3 bands, 60 lymphocytes, and 4 monocytes. The serum sodium level was 135 mEq/L; potassium, 4.9 mEq/L; chloride, 106 mEq/L; and bicarbonate, 18 mm/L.

The patient was hospitalized and given a regular diet, pancreatic enzyme replacement therapy, oral vitamins, chest physical therapy, aerosol therapy, and intravenous tobramycin and ticarcillin. After the throat culture results were available, he was changed to oral trimethoprim and sulfamethoxazole. A month later he had gained 800 g (the fifth percentile), his chest was clear to auscultation, coughing was minimal, and he was having one or two formed stools a day.

During the hospital period, his parents were taught about cystic fibrosis and its treatment. By the day of discharge they were able to do the aerosol and chest physical therapy and give the oral medications. Participants in the educational process included physical therapists, a social worker, a dietician, ward nurses, a pulmonary nurse specialist and pulmonary physicians.

Routine outpatient follow-up was scheduled every 6 weeks. At these visits the interval history focuses on respiratory and gastrointestinal tract symptoms and general activity. Physical examination includes careful measurement of growth parameters. Other evaluation includes a sputum or deep throat culture at every visit, chest roentgenogaphy every 6–12 months, and pulmo-nary function testing twice a year over age 5 years. Therapy is modified appropriately afer each visit.

An 11-month-old girl was diagnosed at birth as having a meconium ileus and meconium peritonitis. Her birth weight was 2.6 (kg 5 pounds, 12 ounces). Despite surgical recovery, she had progressive coughing and wheezing, but the diagnosis of cystic fibrosis was not made until she was 3 months old. Her symptoms could not be controlled, and at 11 months she weighed only 3 kg ($6\frac{1}{2}$ pounds) (Fig. 10-2, A). She was afebrile, had an increased anteroposterior chest diameter, a productive-sounding cough, and a suggestion of clubbing. Rales and mild wheezing were present on auscultation.

She was hospitalized for 2 months for evaluation and control of her many problems. Discharge therapy included pancreatin replacement, vitamins, a high-caloric diet, aerosols, postural drainage, and oral antibiotics as indicated by the culture results. Follow-up was at 4- to 6-week intervals. By 19 months of age (10-2,B) she weighed 7.5 kg (17 pounds), her cough was minimal, and the chest was clear to auscultation.

REFERENCES

1. Farber S: Experimental production of achylia pancreatica. *Amer J Dis Child* 64: 953–954. 1942.
2. Gibson LE and Cook RE: A test for concentration of electrolytes in sweat in cystic fibrosis of the pancreas utilizing pilocarpine by iontophoresis. *Pediatrics* 23: 545–549 1959.
3. Barbero GJ, Sibinga MS, Marino JM et al: Stool trypsin and chymotrypsin. *Amer J Dis Child* 112: 536, 1966.

SUGGESTED READINGS

Chase HP, Long MA, Lavin MH: Cystic fibrosis and malnutrition. *J Pediatr* 95:337, 1979.

Denning CR, Huang NN, Cuasay LR, et al: Cooperative study comparing three methods of performing sweat tests to diagnose cystic fibrosis. *Pediatrics* 66:752, 1980.

di Sant'Agnese PA, Davis PB: Research in cystic fibrosis. *N Eng J Med* 295:481–485, 534–541, 597–602, 1976.

Doershuk CF, Reyes AL, Regan A, et al: Anesthesia for cystic fibrosis patients. *Anesth Analg, 51:413, 1972.*

Handwerger S, Roth J, Gorden P, et al: Glucose intolerance in cystic fibrosis. *N Eng J Med* 281:451, 1969.

Oppenheimer EH, Esterly JR: Pathology of cystic fibrosis: review of the literature and comparison with 146 autopsied cases. *Perspect Pediatr Pathol* 2:241, 1975.

Orenstein DM, Boat TF, Stern RC, et al: The effect of early diagnosis and treatment in cystic fibrosis: a seven-year study of 16 sibling pairs. *Am J Dis Child 131:973, 1977.*

Stern RC, Boat TF, Doershuk CF, et al: Course of ninety-five patients with cystic fibrosis. *J Pediatr* 1976; 89:406.

Stern RC, Stevens DP, Boat TF, et al: Symptomatic hepatic disease in cystic fibrosis: incidence course and outcome of portal systemic shunting. *Gastroenterology* 70:645, 1976.

Stern RC, Boat TF, Abramowsky CF, et al: Intermediate range sweat chloride concentration and *pseudomonas* bronchitis: a cystic fibrosis variant with preservation of exocrine pancreatic funtion. *JAMA* 239:2676, 1978.

Stern RC, Boat TF, Matthews LW, et al: Treatment and prognosis of massive hemoptysis in cystic fibrosis. *Am Rev Respir Dis.* 117:825, 1978.

Stern RC, Borkat G, Hirschfeld SS, et al: Heart failure in cystic fibrosis: treatment and prognosis of cor pulmonale with failure of the right side of the heart. *Am J Dis Child* 134:267, 1980.

Stowe SM, Boat TF, Mendelsohn H, et al: Open thoracotomy for pneumothorax in cystic fibrosis. *Am Rev Respir Dis.* 111:611, 1975.

Taussig L: *Cystic Fibrosis.* New York, Thieme-Stratton, Inc., 1982.

Wood RE, Boat TF, Doershuk CF: State of the art: cystic fibrosis. *Am Rev Respir Dis* 113:833, 1976.

11

Croup and Epiglottitis

James W. Bass
Paul F. Wehrle

Croup is a disease that results from acute obstruction of the larynx. It is caused by allergy, foreign body, infection, or new growth and occurs predominately in infants and children. The characteristic symptoms are a resonant barking cough, hoarseness, and persistent stridor. This discussion will be limited to those causes of acute upper airway obstruction associated with croup shown in Table 11-1. Few conditions are as frightening for the patient or have such a dramatic response to appropriate therapy as those associated with croup.

MORBIDITY AND MORTALITY

Table 11-2 lists the deaths attributed to acute upper respiratory tract infection in the United States for the period of 1970–1978. These deaths were presumably due to acute infections producing obstruction of the upper airway, primarily viral laryngotracheobronchitis (a common disease with low mortality) and acute epiglottitis (an uncommon disease with high mortality). A clear reduction in deaths from acute upper respiratory tract infection has been seen since 1973. Before 1973 more than 500 deaths were reported annually; since 1973 fewer than 400 have been reported annually, and the downward trend continues. This trend probably reflects the evolution of improved diagnosis and treatment of these disorders. Changes include lateral neck roentgenography as a diagnostic aid, "prophylac-

The opinions or assertions contained herein are the private views of the authors and are not to be construed as official or as reflecting the views of the Department of the Army or the Department of the Defense.

tic" nasotracheal intubation for acute epiglottitis, racemic epinephrine and corticosteroids for the treatment of subglottic virus croup, refinements in clinical and blood gas monitoring, and nasotracheal intubation with assisted ventilation for respiratory failure complicating subglottic virus croup. With the exception of laryngeal diphtheria, reporting of the diseases listed in Table 11-2 is not required in the United States; thus it is not possible to document the morbidity attributed to them. Croup is clearly a problem often seen in pediatric practice, particularly in the winter months when these infections are most prevalent.

ACUTE LARYNGOTRACHEOBRONCHITIS (LTB)

Etiology and Epidemiology

Acute laryngotracheobronchitis (LTB) is a term used almost interchangeably with acute laryngotracheitis, depending on clinical evidence of bronchial involvement. It is almost always viral in etiology. LTB is seen year-round, but it is highly seasonal in incidence, occurring mostly in the colder winter months. Although croup is associated with many respiratory viral pathogens, it is caused primarily by parainfluenza viruses 1 and 3, influenza viruses A and B, less frequently by respiratory syncytial viruses, and possibly by rhinoviruses. Adenoviruses, coxsackieviruses A and B, and echoviruses are infrequent causes of croup. There may be much variation in the severity of illness, depending upon the etiology. Croup associated with epidemic influenza A virus

Table 11-1   *Classification of Croup Syndromes*

- Acute laryngotracheitis or laryngotracheobronchitis

    Subglottic laryngitis
    Nondiphtheritic croup
    Virus croup

- Spasmodic croup

    False croup
    Spasmodic laryngitis

- Acute epiglottitis

    Supraglottitis

- Supraglottic and laryngeal angioedema

    Allergic and hereditary angioedema

- Laryngeal diphtheria

- Membranous laryngotracheobronchitis

    Bacterial tracheitis
    Membranous croup

- Retropharyngeal abscess

- Hypopharyngeal or laryngeal foreign body

infection may be more severe than with other viral pathogens. The greatest incidence is at ages 1 or 2 years, but it may be seen in infants as young as 1–2 months of age or in children several years of age. It is more frequent and severe in boys than in girls.

Clinical Manifestations and Diagnosis

Virus croup usually develops after 2 or 3 days of prodrome involving nasal congestion, mucinous rhinorrhea, fever, and coughing. Fever may be absent or greater than 40° C, but usually ranges from 39–40° C. The cough becomes more severe and develops a coarse rasping or barking quality. The voice is often hoarse and as inflammatory edema of the larynx and vocal cords progresses, the airway is obstructed. A musical, inspiratory stridor, first heard during and immediately after cough paroxysms, may become persistent and continuous. When stridor is continuous the airway may be reduced to only 1–2 mm in the larynx, and hypoxia soon develops. Tachypnea and depression of the soft tissues in the substernal, suprasternal, supraclavicular, and intercostal areas become evident with each inspiratory effort. Pallor and sweating appear. In severe cases, the child looks frightened and rolls about searching for a position that may relieve the obstruction; however, most children with virus croup do not progress to this degree of severity. More typically the barking cough persists for 1 or more days and resolves slowly without the development of stridor. In contrast to acute epiglottitis, virus croup evolves slowly and seldom, if ever, is there abrupt obstruction of the airway. Other contrasting features between subglottic virus croup and acute epiglottitis are listed in Table 11-3.

On examination, the child with virus croup usually is moderately febrile. Nasal congestion, a clear mucinous nasal discharge, and a barking cough are present. There may be hoarseness, and, in severe cases, a musical, inspiratory stridor with labored inspirations and soft tissue retractions is present. The pharynx is often diffusely injected and patchy tonsillar exudates are sometimes seen. There may be mild edema of the tonsillopharyngeal tissues but, aside from injection, the epiglottis and aryepiglottic folds are normal. Obstruction is due to edema of the larynx. This can best be determined by auscultation over the larynx and detailed examination of the posteroanterior and lateral neck roentgeno-

Table 11-2   *Acute Upper Respiratory Tract Infection Mortality in United States (1970–1978)*

Year	Deaths
1970	574
1971	522
1972	504
1973	453
1974	377
1975	342
1976	384
1977	368
1978	321

Data from Center for Disease Control: Annual summary 1979: reported morbidity and mortality in the United States, 28(54):101, 1980.

Table 11-3   *Clinical Differentiation Between Subglottic Virus Croup and Epiglottitis*

Clinical Feature	Subglottic Virus Croup	Epiglottitis (Supraglottitis)
Onset	Insidious	Abrupt
Progression	Slow	Rapid
Fever	Moderate	High
Toxicity	Rare	Common
Anxiety	Not characteristic	Often great
Prostration	Rare	Common
Pallor	Not characteristic	Common
Position	Any—young infants prefer knee-chest position	Erect, on side, or prone
		Chin forward, neck extended, tongue protruded on inspiration (late)
Shaking chills	Absent	Frequent
Voice	Often hoarse	Clear but muffled
Cough	Frequent, barking	Only with choking or gasping episodes
Stridor	Smooth, musical, not positional	Coarse, raspy, fluttering, worse supine
Throat	Nontender	May be tender
Neck	Usually supple	May resist flexion and rotation
Respiratory obstruction	Gradual	Often abrupt
Respiratory failure	Rare	Frequent
Dysphagia	Absent	Frequent
Drooling	Absent	Frequent (late)

grams (Fig 11-1). The latter is helpful in the diagnosis and localization of upper airway obstructing lesions, including epiglottitis, retropharyngeal abscess, and other causes.

Therapy

Cool mist and cough suppressants are most helpful in an outpatient setting. Children who have intermittent or continuous stridor, tachypnea, and labored respiration with soft tissue retractions should be hospitalized. They should be given oxygen in a mist tent, or by nasal prongs or a face mask. Intravenous fluids should be administered to maintain good hydration. Although it is widely accepted that this type of croup is due to virus infection, secondary bacterial infections may rarely occur.

Consequently, children who are toxic and have a high fever are often treated with antibiotics, usually ampicillin. In children with virus croup severe enough to warrant hospitalization who do not respond to these measures, treatment with racemic epinephrine and corticosteroids should be considered.

Treatment of virus croup with these two modes of therapy is controversial. A review of the studies evaluating their effectiveness has recently been reported in Bass, 1981[1]. Although the literature addressing these issues is vast, most of the studies were not properly controlled. Experimental design features permitting evaluation include the following:

- Prospective study design
- Well-defined criteria for subject inclusion

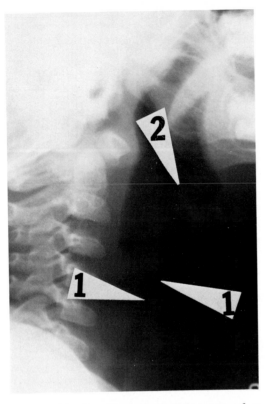

Figure 11-1. Lateral neck roentgenogram of a 2-year-old boy with subglottic virus croup. The hypopharynx is overdistended with air with each inspiratory effort against the narrowed laryngeal air passage. The tracheal air column becomes narrowed and less lucent (*1*) as it is observed in the larynx where it should be wider and more lucent. The epiglottic (*2*) and arytenoid folds are normal in size and configuration.

- Well-defined criteria for monitoring data and measuring response to treatment
- Random assignment of patients to treatment and control groups
- Appropriate controls, comparable to study patients, except for specific treatment
- Blind assessment of response
- Appropriate statistical methodology used in data analysis

When analysis of treatment with racemic epinephrine or corticosteroids is limited to those which fulfill these criteria, the number of studies meriting review is sharply reduced.

Although treatment of croup with racemic epinephrine has been advocated since the early 1960s, most reports have been anecdotal. Only

the three listed in Table 11-4 approach the design requirements specified.

The first study by Gardner and associates[2] compared the response of 10 children treated for 15 minutes with nebulized saline through a face mask with the response of a comparable group of 10 children who received the same treatment but with the addition of 0.5 ml of racemic epinephrine. The course of the disease was not altered in duration or severity by treatment with racemic epinephrine. Half of both the treated and placebo groups showed improvement within 20 minutes after treatment. The conclusion supported by this study is that saline mist through a face mask brings transient improvement for about half of the patients, and the addition of epinephrine neither increases the number responding nor enhances the benefit.

Taussig and his coworkers[3] evaluated six children treated in a tent with saline mist given in a moderately elevated oxygen atmosphere and compared them with seven similarly treated children who had, in addition, an intermittent positive pressure breathing (IPPB) treatment in which racemic epinephrine in nebulized saline was given. The dose of epinephrine was based upon each patient's weight. The response in each group was assessed by defined objective signs that were compiled into a croup score; however, the scorer knew whether or not the IPPB epinephrine treatments had been used, so this study cannot be considered adequately controlled or blind in assessment of outcome. Again, the overall course was not changed by the treatment. The IPPB and epinephrine group did show significant improvement at 20 minutes to 2 hours after IPPB administration, which suggests that IPPB with racemic epinephrine results in transient improvement when compared with saline mist alone. It was not clear whether IPPB, the epinephrine, or both were responsible for improvement.

This question was answered by Westley and associates in 1978.[4] Ten patients were placed in high humidity and given normal saline by oxygen propelled (40 percent) IPPB treatment without epinephrine. Ten other patients had the same treatment, but racemic epinephrine was added. As in the studies previously cited, the overall course of the disease was not found to be different in the two groups. At 10–30 minutes, however, the epinephrine-treated group showed significant improvement over the group that received IPPB without epinephrine.

Table 11-4 *Three Controlled Studies Evaluating Racemic Epinephrine in the Treatment of Croup*

Study	Placebo/Treatment	Placebo	Racemic Epinephrine	Results
Gardner (1973)[2]	10/10	Face mask, 15 min, Saline, 4 ml	Face mask, 15 min, Epinephrine, 0.5 ml, saline to = 4 ml	Overall course unchanged, 5/10 in both improved at 20 min to 4 hr
Taussig (1975)[3]	6/7	Mist tent, 30–40% O_2	Mist tent, 30–40% O_2 IPPB, 8–12 min, with epinephrine, 0.25–1.5 ml,[†] saline to = 3 ml	Overall Course unchanged, epinephrine group had greater improvement ($P = 0.011$) at 20 min to 2 hr
Westley (1978)[4]	10/10	Cool mist, 15–30 min, IPPB,* 10–15 min, With half normal saline, 4 ml, 40% O_2	Cool mist, 15–30 min, IPPB, 10–15 min, with 0.5 ml epinephrine, saline to = 4 ml, 40% O_2	Overall course unchanged, epinephrine group had greater improvement ($P < 0.01$) at 10–30 min

*IPPB was by face mask at 10–15 cm H_2O in all studies.
†Dosage adjusted by child's weight.

Although these studies were well designed and carefully, conducted, they involved small numbers of patients. Despite these reservations, however, critical analysis of these three studies does suggest the following conclusions:

- There appears to be a transient benefit lasting from 10 minutes to 2 hours when epinephrine is administered in aerosol by face mask *with* IPPB. This benefit is greater than that seen with IPPB alone.
- The effective dosage of 2.25 percent racemic epinephrine solution is 0.5 ml in 3–4 ml of water or saline, administered by IPPB with 10–20 cm of water pressure, for a 10 to 15-minute period.
- Repeat therapy is often necessary within 1–2 hours, with decreasing effectiveness of subsequent treatments noted in some patients.
- Because of tachyphylaxis, epinephrine treatment is not recommended for mild croup or as an outpatient procedure in patients with more severe croup in an effort to avoid hospitalization.
- Epinephrine IPPB therapy does not change the overall course of the illness.
- Epinephrine IPPB treatment given once or repeated in severely ill hospitalized patients with impending respiratory failure may "buy time" and avoid the need for endotracheal intubation or a tracheostomy to secure an airway.

Over the past 30 years there have been more than 30 published reports regarding corticosteroids in the treatment of patients with croup. Of these, only seven conform to the criteria listed for optimal experimental design.[5–11] These seven studies are listed in Table 11-5. An exception is apparent in the study by Martensson, since patients were assigned to the treatment or placebo groups alternately rather than randomly.

Of the seven studies listed, only Eden and his associates concluded that no benefit occurred with conticosteroid therapy. The dose of corticosteroids used in Eden's studies was significantly less than that in the others, except for that of Martensson, who in 1960 used prednisolone at a dose of 2–5 mg according to weight. The other investigators, including Skowron, James, Massicotte, and Leipzig, who used significantly higher doses of methylprednisolone or dexamethasone, and Martensson, concluded that patients treated

with corticosteroids benefited significantly when compared with patients treated with placebos. They observed a reduction in retractions, stridor, cyanosis, dyspnea, respiratory rate, heart rate, and sometimes fever. The larger corticosteroid doses used in these studies ranged from 0.3 to 0.5 mg/kg of dexamethasone or its equivalent of methylprednisolone. Based upon the observations of these investigators, the following points may be concluded:

- Corticosteroid treatment of patients with croup appears to be effective in reducing the severity and possibly the duration of illness.
- The effective dose appears to be 0.3–0.5 mg/kg of dexamethasone or the equivalent dose of prednisolone or methylprednisolone.
- Although a single dose is effective, it probably should be repeated at 6-hour intervals for four doses.
- Corticosteroid treatment of croup patients may decrease the need for endotracheal intubation or a tracheostomy to secure an airway.

It is unusual for a child with virus croup to be unresponsive to these treatment measures and progress to respiratory failure. Close clinical observation is necessary to differentiate the child who appears to be improving as evidenced by a decrease in respiratory effort, good color, and clear mental status from the child whose respiratory effort is decreased from exhaustion and impending respiratory failure. The latter children are pale, sometimes cyanotic, and often obtunded, and upon close examination there is little air exchange. Arterial blood gas determination in these patients confirms impending respiratory failure with severe hypoxemia, carbon dioxide retention, and mixed respiratory and metabolic acidosis. Subsequent management of the rare virus croup patient whose disease does progress to this point should be a team effort involving the primary care physician, otolaryngologist, and anesthesiologist. Nasotracheal intubation should be performed; if unsuccessful, a tracheotomy is required to relieve obstruction. For this reason intubation should be performed in the operating room or in an intensive care setting using anesthesia. After intubation the child should be sedated, and assisted respiratory ventilation should be available if needed. Corticosteroid therapy, if not already instituted for treatment of the croup, should be considered to minimize the

Table 11-5 *Seven Controlled Studies Evaluating Corticosteroids in Treatment of Croup*

Study	Placebo/Treated	Treatment	Benefit ($P < 0.05$)	Signs Evaluated
Eden (1964)[5]	14/16	Methylprednisolone, 1 mg/kg, Q6H × 4	No	Cyanosis, Dyspnea, Stridor Retractions
Eden (1967)[6]	25/25	Dexamethasone, 0.1 mg/kg, Q6H × 8	No	Cyanosis, Dyspnea, Stridor Retractions
Martensson (1960)[7]	139/149	Prednisolone, 2–5mg, Q6H until well	Yes	Cyanosis, Dyspnea, Stridor Retractions
Skowron (1966)[8]	97/97	Dexamethosone, 0.5 mg/kg, Q6H × 4	Yes	Respiratory rate, Stridor Fever
James (1969)[9]	43/45	Dexamethasone, 0.5–1 mg/kg, single dose	Yes	Cyanosis, Dysponea, Stridor Retractions
Massicotte (1973)[10]	17/25	Methylprednisolone, 4 mg/kg, Q6H × 2	Yes	Respiratory rate, Retractions, heart rate, Stridor Coughing*
Leipzig (1979)[11]	14/16	Dexamethasone 0.3 mg/kg, Q2H × 2	Yes	Respiratory rate, Stridor heart rate, cyanosis, retractions

*Respiratory rate, heart rate, and other factors combined into a scoring system.

inflammatory reaction to intubation and decrease the complication of postintubation tracheal stenosis. After intubation, respiratory distress is relieved immediately, and the child appears to rest comfortably. Extubation may be achieved after 3 to 5 days, and the patient can be discharged 1–2 days later.

Prognosis

At most, about 1 of 20 children with virus croup are sick enough to require hospitalization, and few hospitalized patients require intubation for respiratory failure. Even in the latter patients the process is relatively slow and insidious so that the intubation is successful. Some children tend to have repeated episodes of croup with subsequent viral infections of the respiratory tract; these become less severe and less frequent as the child grows older.

ACUTE SPASMODIC CROUP

Etiology and Epidemiology

The cause of acute spasmodic croup is unknown, and the pathophysiologic mechanism is not well understood. Viruses, allergy, psychologic factors, and familial predisposition have all been implicated. The peak age incidence is 1–3 years, but it may be seen throughout the preschool-age years. Acute spasmodic croup is known to occur in families and is often recurrent. It is seen more frequently in boys, and, although it occurs at any season, it is seen most often in winter.

Clinical Manifestations and Diagnosis

Acute spasmodic croup usually occurs in the night. The child typically will appear perfectly normal or have a mild cold. One to two hours after going to sleep, or in the middle of the night, the coughing begins. It persists and within a matter of minutes becomes severe. The child is awakened, frightened and anxious, as are the parents, at the rapid progression of the disease. The cough quickly becomes barking and hoarse. Intermittent or continuous inspiratory stridor soon develops, with accompanying labored respirations and soft tissue retractions. Gagging, retching, and vomiting then occur as the other symptoms grow more severe. After vomiting, or sometimes with gagging and retching alone, there may be dramatic relief of what appears to have been laryngospasm; inflammatory reactions are not likely to subside so quickly. The child remains afebrile throughout, and, aside from the croupy cough and respiratory distress, the physical examination is completely normal. The whole incident may last only minutes to, at most, a few hours, after which the child relaxes and soon goes back to sleep. The next day the child appears completely normal but may have a similar episode again during the next two or three nights.

Therapy

The course of acute spasmodic croup is so rapid and changes in severity occur so quickly that it is difficult to properly assess what modes of treatment are effective. Warm or cool mist as may be generated by the bathroom shower has been associated with dramatic relief in many instances. Notable improvement often occurs in the cool night air when the child is taken for medical help. The observation that spontaneous retching and vomiting is almost always immediatley followed by significant improvement has led some clinicians to treat patients with spasmodic croup with syrup of ipecac. A preparation containing 0.5 ml of syrup of ipecac to 4.5 ml of glyceryl guaiacolate in subemetic doses appears to be effective.

Prognosis

The outcome of spasmodic croup is usually uneventful. Although the disease is frightening in both the apparent severity and particularly the rapidity of its progress, nearly all episodes resolve spontaneously. Nasotracheal intubation or a tracheostomy for respiratory failure are seldom, if ever, necessary with this variety of the croup syndromes. Because acute spasmodic croup comes on abruptly in otherwise asymptomatic children, special attention should be given to rule out a pharyngeal or laryngeal foreign body as the cause of obstructive symptoms.

ACUTE EPIGLOTTITIS

Etiology and Epidemiology

Acute epiglottitis, or supraglottitis, is a life-threatening and often fulminating disease of the supraglottic tissues, including the epiglottis, aryepiglottic folds, arytenoid cartilages, and ventricular bands. It is caused almost exclusively by *Haemophilus influenzae* organisms; rarely group A β-hemolytic streptococci and *Staphylococcus*

aureus have been implicated. It occurs primarily in older infants and preschool-age children, but it has been reported in infants as young as 5 months, as well as school-age children and occasionally adults. It occurs in all seasons, with a slight increase in incidence in the winter and spring months. In temperate climates the incidence approximates 0.9 cases/1000 pediatric hospital admissions.

Clinical Manifestations and Diagnosis

Children with acute epiglottitis appear much sicker than those with virus croup, and the disease is much more rapid in progression. Epiglottitis patients often have been sick only 1 or 2 days, frequently less than several hours before the child's condition prompts the parents to seek medical help.

Fever is commonly present and is usually high, ranging up to 40–41°C. The examination may be normal early in the course of the disease. As the illness progresses, prostration, pallor, and shaking chills may appear, reflecting the customary coexisting *H. influenzae* bacteremia. Unlike virus croup in which coryza and a cough are usually present, fewer than 50 percent of patients with epiglottitis have a cold or rhinitis, and less than one third have a cough. Even in this group the cough is more of a reaction to choking and gagging on pharyngeal secretions. The resonant, barking cough so characteristic of virus croup is not present in epiglottitis. Older children may complain of a sore throat with pain and difficulty on swallowing. This may result in drooling of excessive saliva accumulations from the corners of the mouth. Stridor varies in severity with time and position. The child with epiglottitis prefers to sit erect on the mother's lap or lie on the side face down. If the tongue is depressed to visualize the epiglottitis while the child is supine, sudden abrupt complete obstruction of the airway may occur. This examination should never be attempted if epiglottitis is suspected until provisions have been made for immediate nasotracheal intubation or a tracheostomy if intubation is unsuccessful.

The child who develops acute onset of high fever, toxicity, pallor, cyanosis, labored respirations with significant soft tissue retractions on inspiration, coarse fluttering inspiratory stridor, protrusion of the tongue with each inspiratory effort, and accumulation of pharyngeal secretions with drooling almost certainly has acute epiglottitis. This classic picture of the disease occurs late, and death may be imminent unless immediate treatment is instituted. Since successful outcome depends upon early diagnosis and treatment, the presence of any of these findings should alert the physician to acute epiglottitis. If the diagnosis is in doubt and the child's condition permits, the lateral neck roentgenogram is often helpful to confirm or rule out this diagnosis (Fig. 11-2).

Therapy

Approximately one half of all patients with epiglottitis will require an artificial airway for survival; in half of these the obstruction will be abrupt. For these reasons patients with suspected epiglottitis should be regarded as medical emergencies with a potential for death if an artificial airway is not provided promptly, as soon as the diagnosis is made. If the diagnosis is certain and the condition is stable enough, the child should be taken to the operating room immediately. The attending physician should stay with the child at all times, and an endotracheal tube, laryngoscope, and emergency tracheotomy set should be at hand. An otolaryngologist and anesthesiologist should be alerted to receive the child in the operating room. Using general anesthesia, the hypopharynx and larynx can be examined under direct visualization with a laryngoscope (Fig. 11-3) and a nasotracheal tube can be positioned to secure the airway. After the airway is assured, cultures of the epiglottitis and blood should be obtained, and intravenous antibiotic therapy should be started. Ampicillin (200 mg/kg/day) and chloramphenicol (75 mg/kg/day) in divided doses at 4- to 6-hour intervals are recommended until culture and antimicrobial sensitivity results are known. At this time chloramphenicol can be discontinued if the strain of *H. influenzae* recovered is ampicillin sensitive. Some *H. influenzae* organisms may be β-lactamase negative but ampicillin resistant. Ampicillin can be discontinued if it is resistant. An acceptable alternative would be intravenous cefamandole (100 mg/kg/day) in divided doses at 4- to 6-hour intervals. Corticosteroids and racemic epinephrine have no place in the treatment of epiglottitis; however, corticosteroids may be used in the intubated patient for the same reasons as in the rare patient intubated for virus croup.

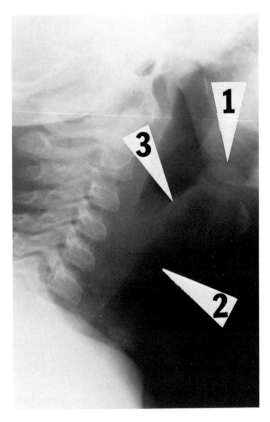

Figure 11-2. Lateral neck roentgenogram of a 3-year-old girl with acute epiglottitis. The hypopharynx is overdistended with air with each inspiratory effort against the edematous obstructing epiglottis and arytenoid folds. The swollen epiglottis (*1*) exhibits a rounded, thumblike configuration (normal configuration resembles the end of the little finger on the lateral projection). The tracheal air column becomes wider and more lucent as it is observed in the larynx (*2*), indicating a normal laryngeal air passage up to the swollen and thickened arytenoid folds (*3*) and epiglottis.

Once the airway is secured, antibiotic therapy initiated, and intensive care monitoring provided, the outlook for epiglottitis patients is good. Sedation may be required and adequate restraints used to ensure against accidental extubation. Septic shock may still ensue, and evaluation is required to detect early signs of this complication. If respiratory obstruction is severe and prolonged, some patients may still develop pulmonary edema even after the obstruction is relieved. This complication has been seen most often with epiglottitis, but it has also occurred with severe subglottic virus croup. It is believed

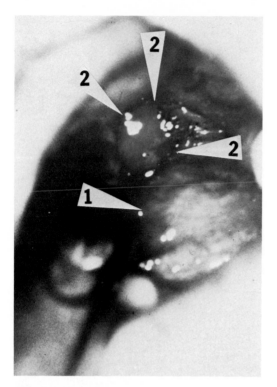

Figure 11-3. Direct laryngoscopic view of the hypo-pharynx of a 3-year-old boy with acute epiglottitis. The laryngoscope displaces the tongue downward (*1*), and the greatly edematous, rounded epiglottis is seen filling the entire hypopharyngeal space (*2*). This photograph was taken in the operating room just before nasotracheal intubation.

to be mediated by alveolar hypoxia, increased alveolar-capillary transmural pressure gradient, and a catechol-mediated shift of blood volume from the systemic to the pulmonary circulation. Successful management of this complication includes mechanical ventilation with high oxygen concentrations and positive end expiratory pressure, diuretics (preferably furosemide), and support of the intravascular volume with colloid infusions. If septic shock or pulmonary edema are to occur, they usually develop within the first 24 hours after hospitalization. Edema of the supraglottic structures subsides after 2 or 3 days and the patient can be extubated. Again this is best accomplished by the intubating team in the operating room using anesthesia. Under direct visualization edema of the supraglottic structures can be confirmed to have subsided, and the child

can be safely extubated. The child may then be discharged after an additional 1- or 2-day period of observation with a total hospitalization course of only 5–7 days.

Prognosis

Epiglottitis patients treated as outlined have an excellent prognosis. With "prophylactic" intubation as soon as the diagnosis is made, the morbidity and mortality from this disease have drastically declined. Only in those patients in whom the diagnosis was not considered or prolonged medical management and observation was attempted do disastrous results still occur (Fig. 11-4). Abrupt obstruction under compromising circumstances so that intubation or a tracheostomy cannot be achieved before death or hypoxic brain injury results is still encountered in these patients.

SUPRAGLOTTIC AND LARYNGEAL ANGIOEDEMA

Etiology and Epidemiology

Angioedema is a painless swelling of the subcutaneous tissues in a localized area that may occur anywhere in the body. The edema is not pitting, erythematous, or tender. It may develop within a few minutes or over 1 or 2 days and measure up to several centimeters in diameter. The dorsum of the hands and feet or the genitalia are sometimes involved, but angioedema most often occurs on the face and may be isolated to the eyelids, cheek, nose, ears, lip, or tongue. It is most serious when it involves the base of the tongue, supraglottic structures, or larynx, producing acute life-threatening airway obstruction. Two types of this reaction are recognized: sporadic or allergic angioedema, which is caused by hypersensitivity to specific "allergens," and hereditary angioedema, which is transmitted as an autosomal dominant trait and is associated with a decrease in the serum of inhibitor to the activated first component of complement, C1 esterase. Neither type is associated with fever or other signs of infection.

Clinical Manifestations and Diagnosis

The allergic type of angioedema usually is associated with hypersensitivity to certain foods, such as shellfish, strawberries, or nuts, or it may

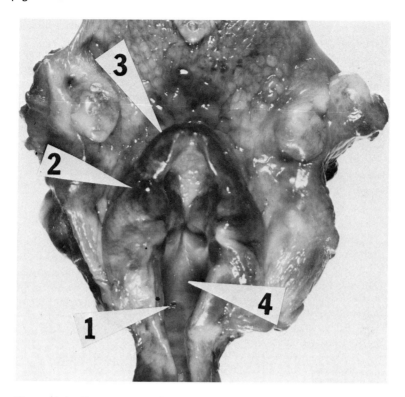

Figure 11-4. Postmortem specimen of the larynx and supraglottic structures of a 2-year-old boy who died of acute epiglottitis. The death occurred before 1973 and before "prophylactic" nasotracheal intubation became accepted as the management for this disease. The correct diagnosis had been made, and the child was hospitalized. He received intravenous ampicillin and was observed in a mist tent with oxygen. An endotracheal tube, laryngoscope, and tracheostomy set were at the bedside. Two pediatricians were immediately available, and an otolaryngologist had been alerted. Two hours after admission the child was believed to be doing well, when he developed sudden, abrupt, and complete airway obstruction. All attempts at endotracheal intubation were unsuccessful. A large-bore needle was passed through the cricothyroid-trachea interspace (*1*), but adequate ventilation could not be achieved. An emergency tracheostomy was attempted but the child died before an airway could be established. Significant edema of the arytenoid folds (*2*) and epiglottis (*3*) with little or no involvement of the larynx (*4*) is shown in this specimen.

be precipitated by specific inhalants or contactants. Drugs (particularly aspirin or penicillin), contrast media containing iodides, and insect stings have been implicated. Sometimes the patient may experience several episodes and never become aware of what is causing them, although frequently the offending allergen is known and avoided. Allergic angioedema may occur with no other sign of allergy or hypersensitivity, or its appearance may coincide with generalized urticaria. When it develops within

minutes after exposure and the angioedema involves the supraglottic structures and larynx, frequently there is an associated generalized urticaria, acute bronchospasm, and rarely anaphylaxis with cardiovascular collapse and death unless treatment is initiated promptly.

Hereditary angioedema associated with C1 esterase deficiency leads to formation of vasoactive mediators from the complement sequence that cause leakage of fluid and colloid into the tissues. This type of angioedema frequently is associated with gastrointestinal symptoms, including vomiting and severe abdominal pain due to involvement of the abdominal viscera. Supraglottic and laryngeal involvement is more common with hereditary angioedema than with the allergic type, and it is usually more severe. Acute airway obstruction is responsible for death in nearly one third of patients with this disorder. The diagnosis is established by clinical history and demonstration of low levels of the fourth component of complement (C4) and low C1 esterase inhibitor activity in the patient's serum.

Therapy

Patients with rapidly developing airway obstruction from supraglottic and laryngeal allergic angioedema often respond dramatically to treatment with epinephrine, antihistamines, and corticosteroids, particularly if there is an associated urticaria, bronchospasm, or cardiovascular collapse. Allergic angioedema that has evolved more slowly and is not associated with other symptoms is less responsive to these modes of therapy. Intramuscular epinephrine is recommended, 0.01 ml/kg administered as a 1:1000 aqueous solution. This may be repeated in 15 minutes, or if the initial dose appears effective, a longer acting preparation containing aqueous crystalline epinephrine 1:200 (Sus-Phrine) may be given along with diphenhydramine hydrochloride (Benadryl), 1 mg/kg every 4 hours. In severe cases prednisolone, 2 mg/kg/day, may be added for 3–4 days.

Hereditary angioedema is not an allergic or hypersensitivity response, and epinephrine, antihistamines or corticosteroid therapy will not be beneficial. No form of treatment has been found to be effective for acute episodes causing airway obstruction. Endotracheal intubation or tracheostomy is lifesaving in these patients. In controlled clinical trials in adults, prophylactic treatment with methyltestosterone or more recently danazol, a less virulizing new synthetic androgen, or aminocaproic acid may reduce the incidence of these acute life-threatening episodes in patients with hereditary angioedema. Experience with these modes of treatment in children has been limited.

Prognosis

The outlook for patients with allergic angioedema is good. It is rare in young children, and in older individuals the offending allergen can usually be identified and avoided. Patients who have had attacks of allergic angioedema causing airway obstruction should carry an emergency kit containing an epinephrine injection for self-administration and an antihistamine. These are lifesaving should an episode occur when no immediate medical help is available.

The outlook is less favorable for patients with hereditary angioedema. First attacks usually occur in early childhood, nearly half before a child is 6 years old, when the airway is relatively small. Fatal attacks from acute airway obstruction have resulted in association with minor trauma such as dental extraction, so that contact sports and other activities that may cause injury to the head and neck should be avoided. Prophylactic treatment with one of the newer synthetic androgens or treatment with aminocaproic acid may be considered in patients with severe life-threatening hereditary angioedema.

LARYNGEAL DIPHTHERIA

Etiology and Epidemiology

Diphtheria is an acute infection caused by *Corynebacterium diphtheriae* that is usually localized to the tonsils, pharynx, larynx, nares, and occasionally skin. Infection of the mucous membranes is associated with membrane formation with notable erythema and edema of the adjacent tissues due to the production of a potent soluble exotoxin by the organism. Airway obstruction caused by swelling of the supraglottic tissues or larynx due to localized infection and inflammation in these areas may be life threatening. Also, the absorption of toxin, with its direct effect on major organ systems, particularly the heart, nervous system, and kidney, represents the other major hazard from this disease process. Diphtheria is worldwide but its incidence has significantly declined in highly industrialized and developed countries where immunization with diphtheria toxoid has been widely achieved. It occurs more frequently in developing countries with poor socioeconomic conditions, crowding, and inadequate immunization practices. It also frequently is recognized in temperate climates, where it may be seen year-round, although the prevalence is greater in the fall and winter months.

Clinical Manifestations and Diagnosis

Clinical findings vary greatly with the location and severity of infection. Isolated nasal or skin infection may be protracted with few other symptoms. Tonsillar diphtheria, the most frequent form, may remain localized to the surface of the tonsils and have a benign course with proper treatment. This type of diphtheria is often without membrane formation, or the membrane may be mistaken for tonsillar exudate, and the diagnosis of diphtheria may not be considered unless other circumstances are suggestive and a culture is obtained. Membrane formation may progress to involve the soft palate, uvula, pharyngeal walls, and larynx, with notable enlargement of the cervical lymph nodes and confluent cellulitis of the surrounding soft tissues of the neck (bullneck or malignant diphtheria). Such membrane extension may cause airway obstruction and is associated with massive toxin absorption. The diagnosis in these patients is obvious, but even with immediate appropriate therapy many of these patients die.

Since diphtheria may occur in any of several forms, diagnosis early enough for therapy to be effective depends upon recognition by the treating clinician that *diphtheria should always be considered in any patient with membranous pharyngitis in which the membrane extends off of the tonsils onto the surrounding tissues.*

Patients with diphtheria may have isolated involvement of the larynx or laryngotracheal area without involvement of the supraglottic tissues or pharynx. The illness in these individuals is usually indistinguishable from other croup syndromes with fever, hoarseness, a barking cough, and stridor as the only clinical manifestations. If the history reveals no past immunization against diphtheria or travel to any area where the disease remains prevalent, this diagnosis should be more strongly considered. Direct larynogoscopy and bronchoscopy may be indicated to substantiate the diagnosis in these patients. Isolated laryngeal or laryngotracheal involvement usually is associated with relatively low levels of toxin absorption; airway obstruction with these types of diphtheria is the main threat to life.

Therapy

Appropriate treatment of diphtheria requires both neutralization of circulating unbound toxin with antitoxin and eradication of *C. diphtheriae* organisms with an appropriate antibiotic. In addition, with bullneck tonsillopharyngeal and laryngeal diphtheria, an airway may be required if airway obstruction is severe.

Antitoxin should be given as soon as the clinical diagnosis is established. Delay until culture studies are reported is associated with an increase in both morbidity and mortality. The recommended dose varies with the location and extent of infection. Mild skin and nasal diphtheria may be treated effectively with 40,000 units, moderately severe tonsillopharyngeal infections with 80,000 units, and bullneck or malignant diphtheria with extensive involvement of the pharynx and larynx should be treated with 120,000 units after skin testing to rule out sensitivity to horse serum. This should be administered as a single intravenous dosage of equine antitoxin in a 1:20 dilution in isotonic saline over a 20-minute period.

Penicillin and erythromycin have been shown to be effective in the eradication of *C. diphtheriae* from patients infected with this organism. Procaine penicillin, 600,000 units daily, or oral erythromycin, 50 mg/kg/day in divided doses at 6-hour intervals for 10 days, is recommended.

Prognosis

The widespread use of diphtheria toxoid vaccine that has been achieved in the United States over the past three decades has been associated with a hundredfold drop in reported cases from 5796 in 1950 to 3 in 1980. During most of this period the case fatality ratio remained unchanged at approximately 10 percent. The major progress in this disease has been in its prevention. With prompt diagnosis and treatment, patients with skin or nasal diphtheria have an excellent outcome. Tonsillar diphtheria without involvement of the adjacent pharyngeal mucosa, significant enlargement of the cervical lymph nodes, and cellulitis of the subcutaneous and deep tissues of the neck is also responsive to therapy. Early diagnosis and treatment of patients with this type of involvement are associated with a mortality of less than 2 percent. Patients with extensive membranes over the tonsils, soft palate, lateral or posterior pharyngeal wall, and larynx who have bullneck cellulitis involving the cervical lymph nodes and neck tissues still have a grave prognosis, even with intensive therapy. Mortality in these patients remains around 30–40 percent.

Death is less often due to airway obstruction, since this is now more effectively managed than in the past, than to systemic and major organ toxicity. Myocarditis is currently the major cause of death in these patients.

MEMBRANOUS LARYNGOTRACHEOBRONCHITIS

Etiology and Epidemiology

Membranous LTB (membranous croup, bacterial tracheitis) was more common in the preantibiotic era than in recent years. Two current reports suggest, however, that it is still being seen in some areas. In one report[12] eight patients with bacterial tacheitis were observed over a 14-month period. In this report bacterial tracheitis was said to be seven times less frequent as a cause of croup syndrome prompting hospitalization than virus croup but one and a half times more frequent than epiglottitis. In the second report[13] 28 patients with membranous LTB were seen and treated from 1973 to 1977. In both reports the patients had signs and symptoms of virus croup but were more sick, toxic, and unresponsive to racemic epinephrine and other usual modes of therapy for virus croup. Purulent secretions obtained from tracheal aspiration revealed pus and bacteria.

Membranous LTB is characterized by a diffuse inflammation and edema of the larynx extending into the trachea and bronchi, with accumulation of copious mucopurulent secretions. Frequently scattered patchy purulent membranes or crust may be loosely adhered to the mucosa. The infection is most often due to *S. aureus* but group A streptococci, pneumococci, and *H. influenzae* also have been implicated. Most patients with this type of croup are under 2 years old, but sporadic cases have been reported in children as old as 15 years. The disease occurs primarily in the winter. Viral respiratory pathogens, including types A and B influenza, parainfluenza and enteroviruses have been recovered together with bacterial pathogens in up to half of patients where virus studies were performed. The association of virus croup symptoms and the high frequency of isolation of viral respiratory pathogens from patients with membranous LTB have led the authors in both reports to speculate that the disease may be due to secondary bacterial infections in patients with virus croup.

Clinical Manifestations and Diagnosis

Patients with membranous LTB have many features in common with patients with virus croup, acute epiglottitis, and laryngeal diphtheria. As in virus croup, children with membranous LTB have signs of a respiratory tract infection with rhinorrhea, hoarseness, and a cough that soon becomes brassy, and inspiratory stridor may develop. Unlike virus croup and more like epiglottitis, the disease moves on rapidly with high fever, toxicity, leukocytosis with an elevated band count, and severe life-threatening airway obstruction. The mean duration of illness before hospitalization has varied from 12 to 72 hours, although in some patients it has been less. Severe stridor with notable inspiratory soft tissue depression is progressive and unrelenting. Auscultation of the chest frequently reveals numerous loose rattling rhonchi and coarse wet rales. The lateral neck roentgenogram shows narrowing and decreased lucency of the tracheal air column as it is observed up into the larynx and is indistinguishable from the findings of subglottic virus croup. Opacities caused by patches of exudate or membrane may sometimes be seen on the inner wall of the trachea. When due to exudate rather than membranes, they may change in location because of coughing or a change in position. The lateral neck roentgenogram is most helpful in differentiating membranous LTB, which involves the subglottic area, from epiglottitis, which usually involves only the supraglottic structures. It cannot differentiate patients with membranous LTB from those with severe subglottic virus croup or isolated laryngeal diphtheria. In patients with membranous LTB progressive airway obstruction usually mandates that an artificial airway be secured for survival. Notable relief of airway obstruction occurs as the endotracheal tube or bronchoscope is passed through the edematous larynx. With subglottic virus croup the obstruction is caused by nonsuppurative erythematous edema of the larynx. In patients with membranous LTB there are copious purulent secretions below the larynx that must be frequently removed in order to maintain an open airway. Patients with membranous LTB must be differentiated from those with isolated laryngeal diphtheria. In diphtheria the membrane is firm and adheres tightly to the mucosa; it bleeds profusely upon attempted removal. The membrane or exudate in membranous LTB is more often soft and buttery. It is loosely attached and easy to remove without bleeding and usually with only suctioning.

Therapy

As with epiglottitis, patients with membranous LTB should be managed in an intensive care setting by a team that includes the primary care physician, an otolaryngologist, and a pulmonologist. An intensivist or anesthesiologist also would be helpful. A secure airway is essential for effective treatment. In most patients this can be achieved by endotracheal intubation, although a tracheostomy may be required. Repeated suctioning of the rapidly reaccumulating purulent secretions is essential. Immediate examination of the gram-stained secretions may guide proper antibiotic therapy. If gram-positive cocci are seen, an intravenous penicillinase-resistant penicillin in a daily dosage of 150 mg/kg given in divided doses at 4- to 6-hour intervals is recommended. If gram-negative rods are seen, antimicrobial therapy directed against *H. ifluenzae* as outlined for epiglottitis should be initiated.

Prognosis

The outlook for patients with membranous LTB was poor in the preantibiotic era. Currently, it is good if it is recognized early and treated with appropriate antibiotics, a secure airway, and effective suctioning. The diagnosis should always be considered in patients presumed to have virus croup who do not respond to traditional treatment, have a high fever, and are toxic.

RETROPHARYNGEAL ABSCESS

Etiology and Epidemiology

In early chidhood there is a potential space between the prevertebral fascia and the posterior pharyngeal wall that contains lymphatics and several lymph nodes which drain the nasopharyngeal and tonsillopharyngeal tissues. Suppurative infection in these areas may spread to involve this space and lead to cellulitis or abscess formation. These infections are almost always caused by group A β-hemolytic streptococci or *S. aureus*. They are encountered most often in the winter and spring months in association with upper respiratory tract infection. Retropharyngeal abscess is seen most frequently in young children. Children younger than 6 years make up 96 percent of the cases, and 50 percent of all cases are seen in infants 6–12 months of age[14]. Less commonly, retropharyngeal abscess may occur as a complication of a penetrating injury of the posterior pharyngeal wall such as may occur when a child falls or is hit while there is something in the mouth, frequently a sucker stick, pencil, or toy. Rarely, retropharyngeal abscess can occur from anterior extension of vertebral osteomyelitis.

Clinical Manifestations and Diagnosis

In older children and adults retropharyngeal abscess usually is associated with a number of specific signs calling attention to the pharynx. In infants and young children the diagnosis is often difficult. In these children the infection usually complicates an apparent viral respiratory tract infection with the gradual or rapid onset of high fever, toxicity, and difficulty in feeding. Difficulty in swallowing and noisy, gurgling, labored respirations develop along with drooling. The patient prefers to keep the head hyperextended, which makes the symptoms seem less severe. Examination of the posterior pharynx may show bulging, but this is difficult to observe in small infants by direct visualization. Also, the abscess may be below the area that can be visualized directly. Palpation of the posterior pharynx is difficult and dangerous. Care must be taken not to cause rupture and permit aspiration of purulent material into the lungs. If manual examination is attempted, it should be done under general anesthesia in Trendelenburg's position with adequate suction at hand, and the airway should be secured by endotracheal intubation with a cuffed tube to prevent aspiration.

The lateral neck roentgenogram has proven invaluable in the diagnosis of patients suspected of having retropharyngeal abscess (Fig. 11-5). The film should be taken during inspiration with the head hyperextended. The normal prevertebral space under these conditions should not be wider than the contiguous vertebral bodies. The lateral neck roentgenogram may, in addition to substantiating the clinical diagnosis of oral retropharyngeal abscess, show an abscess that is too low to be seen by direct examination of the

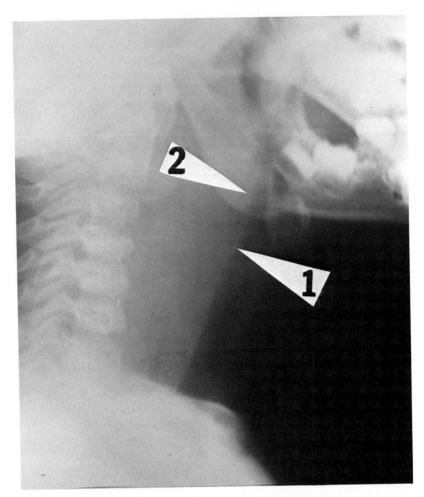

Figure 11-5. Lateral neck roentgenogram of a 5-year-old boy with a retropharyngeal abscess. The prevertebral space is greatly widened as it is observed up the neck to the pharynx. (*1*). The abscess displaces the pharyngeal air space and impinges on the airway at the level of the larynx and supraglottic structures (*2*), which are displaced forward.

oropharynx. Although it is invaluable in detection of retropharynheal space disease, it cannot differentiate between cellulitis and abscess formation.

Therapy

Patients with obvious retropharyngeal abscess who have fluctuance and "pointing" of the abscess should have surgical drainage under the conditions described for diagnosis using anesthesia. Often there is no evidence of fluctuance or pointing, and the cause of retropharyngeal fullness or distension cannot be differentiated between cellulitis and abscess. In these patients treatment with an intravenous penicillinase-resistant penicillin as recommended for membranous LTB should be initiated. Favorable response to this treatment is usually evident within 24–48 hours, and in individuals who do not show clinical improvement during this period abscess formation and the need for surgical drainage become apparent.

Prognosis

As with the other causes of airway obstruction caused by infectious processes of the upper respiratory passages, the outlook of patients with retropharyngeal abscess is determined by early diagnosis and initiation of appropriate therapy. This diagnosis should always be considered in any illness in early childhood involving difficulty with respiration and swallowing.

HYPOPHARYNGEAL OR LARYNGEAL FOREIGN BODY

Etiology and Epidemiology

A foreign body in the hypopharynx or larynx should always be considered in any child with croup, particularly those whose symptoms grow progressively worse and are unresponsive to therapy. The peak age incidence is 1–2 years as with most of the other croup syndromes. If the foreign body is undiagnosed for a significant period, a secondary infection with fever may develop. This may be misleading, since the diagnosis of infectious croup is then more readily accepted and the possibility of a foreign body is less likely to be considered.

The most common objects involved in older children and adults are food particles, particularly peanuts or pieces of meat. In infants and young children food particles may also be involved, but more commonly they are small metal (radiopaque) or plastic (frequently nonradiopaque) objects such as coins, safety pins, nails, screws, rocks, or pieces of toys that the toddler is prone to mouth if they are within reach.

Clinical Manifestations and Diagnosis

The clinical manifestations vary widely and reflect the size, shape, and consistency of the object and where it is lodged. There may be complete abrupt obstruction of the airway, causing death within minutes, unless the object is dislodged, removed, or an emergency tracheostomy performed. Often the child was known to be playing with the object and may have been seen putting it into the mouth when signs of airway or esophageal obstruction developed. If the object lodges posteriorly in the hypopharynx or upper cervical esophagus, there may be little or no airway obstruction but only apparent

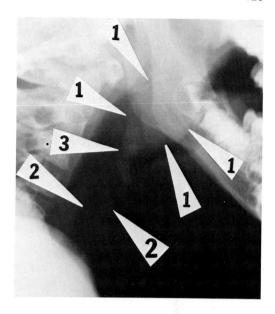

Figure 11-6. Lateral neck roentgenogram of a 4-year-old girl with notable tonsillar hypertrophy due to infectious mononucleosis. There is mild airway obstruction produced by the hypertrophy of the palatine tonsils (1). The tracheal and laryngeal air column (2) and supraglottic structures (3) are normal.

difficulty in swallowing with pooling of pharyngeal secretions and drooling. This may cause gurgling or rattling noisy respirations but little or no other signs of airway involvement. This type of foreign body is usually soon spontaneously expelled or swallowed.

The most dangerous foreign body is one that lodges over or in the larynx, particularly if it has sharp penetrating projections that allow it to be fixed to adjacent structures. This type of foreign body may produce fulminant disease with rapid secondary infection, local cellulitis, edema, and airway obstruction, prompting the need for a secure airway. Sometimes no history is obtained, suggesting the possibility of a foreign body, and it comes as a surprise to the endoscopist who may be attempting to place a nasotracheal tube for what had been presumed to be severe virus croup. If the foreign body is lodged in the larynx and is small enough to permit good air passage around it initially, the subsequent course may be almost identical to severe virus croup with fever due to secondary infection, with symptoms such as increasing obstruction, hoarseness, and stridor, all of which are unresponsive to therapy. This type of course may evolve quickly in just several hours, or it may proceed more slowly over several days. The development of hemoptysis or infection with gram-negative enteric organisms in any patient with croup should always suggest a foreign body.

The lateral neck roentgenogram is most helpful in the diagnosis of airway and esophageal obstruction due to a foreign body. The exact type and location of the object can be readily shown if it is radiopaque. If it is not, the diagnosis may still be made or suspected by the character and pattern of displacement of the soft tissues adjacent to it.

Therapy

Obviously, foreign bodies in the esophagus or upper air passages should be removed as soon as possible by an experienced and skilled endoscopist. With abrupt life-threatening obstruction attempts to manually dislodge the object with the finger may force it into a more obstructing position. Direct examination with a laryngoscope or bronchoscope is preferred. If the patient's condition is rapidly deteriorating and there is no skilled help at hand, an attempt at the Heinlich maneuver may be undertaken to dislodge the object and open the airway. If the object has been in place for a significant time, and particularly if there is evidence of local or systemic

infection with fever, antiobiotic therapy should be initiated to cover those organisms which usually cause infection secondary to a retained foreign body in respiratory passages (such as *S. aureus* and a wide range of gram-negative enteric rods). Intravenous penicillinase-resistant penicillin as previously described for staphylococcal infections and intramuscular gentamicin, 5 mg/kg/day in three divided doses at 8-hour intervals, is also recommended.

Prognosis

If the foreign body is located in the posterior hypopharynx or in the upper cervical esophagus, there is little threat to life unless it is dislodged forward into the larynx. It is usually thrown up or swallowed without causing airway obstruction. When it causes persistent symptoms of esophageal obstruction, the diagnosis is usually suspected and the foreign body is removed by an endoscopist. When the object causes abrupt complete obstruction of the airway, death often occurs before medical help can be reached. The outlook for patients who have a foreign body with croup symptoms consistent with the diagnosis of the other more common croup syndromes depends upon the constant concern and vigilance of the treating clinician to consider this diagnosis in all patients who have croup.

REFERENCES

1. Bass JW: Racemic epinephrine and corticosteroids for croup. *J Respir Dis* 2:57, 1981.
2. Gardner HG, Powell KR, Roden VJ, Cherry VD: The evaluation of racemic epinephrine in the treatment of infectious croup. *Pediatrics* 52:52, 1973.
3. Taussig LM, Castro O, Beaudry PH, et al: Treatment of laryngotracheobronchitis (croup): Use of intermittent positive pressure breathing and racemic epinephrine. *Am J Dis Child* 129:790, 1975.
4. Westley CR, Cotton EK, Brooks JG: Nebulized racemic epinephrine by IPPB for treatment of croup. *Am J Dis Child* 132:484, 1978.
5. Eden AN, Larkin VD: Corticosteroids in croup. *Pediatrics* 33:768, 1964.
6. Eden AN, Kaufman A, Yu R: Corticosteroids in croup. *JAMA* 200:403, 1967.
7. Martensson B, Nilsson G, Torbjar JE: The effect of corticosteroids in the treatment of psuedocroup. *Acta Otolaryngol* 158(suppl):62, 1960.
8. Skowron RN, Turner JA, McNaughton GA: The

use of corticosteroids in the treatment of acute laryngotracheitis. *Can Med Assoc J* 94:528, 1966.
9. James JA: Dexamethasone in croup. *Am J Dis Child* 117:511, 1969.
10. Massicotte P, Tetreault L: Evaluation de la methylprednisolone dans le traitement des laryngites aidqües de l'enfant. *Union Med Can* 102:2064, 1973.
11. Leipzig B, Oski FA, Cummings CW, et al: A prospective randomized study to determine the efficacy of steroids in treatment of croup. *J Pediatr* 94:194, 1979.
12. Jones R, Santos JI, Overall JC: Bacterial tracheitis. *JAMA* 242:721, 1979.
13. Han BK, Dunbar JS, Striker TW: Membranous laryngotracheobronchitis (membranous croup) *AJR* 133:53, 1979.
14. Seid AB, Dunbar JS, Cotton RI: Retropharyngeal abscesses in children revisited. *Laryngoscope* 89:1717, 1979.

SUGGESTED READINGS

Bass JW, Steel RW, Wiebe RA: Acute epiglottitis: A surgical emergency. *JAMA* 229: 671, 1974.

Bates JR: Epiglottitis: Diagnosis and treatment. *Ped Rev* 1:173, 1979.

Battaglia JD, Lockhart CH: Management of acute epiglottitis by nasotracheal intubation. *Am J Dis Child* 129:133, 1975.

Fried MF: Controversies in the management of supraglottitis and croup. *Pediatr Clin North Am* 26:931, 1979.

Milko DA, Marsak G, Striker TW: Nasotracheal intubation in treatment of acute epiglottitis. *Pediatrics* 53:674, 1974.

Rapkin RH: Tracheostomy in epiglottitis. *Pediatrics* 52:426, 1973.

Rowe LD: Advances and controversies in the management of supraglottitis and laryngotracheobronchitis. *Am J Otolaryng* 1:235, 1980.

Travis KW, Todres ID, Shannon DC: Pulmonary edema associated with croup and epiglottitis. *Pediatrics* 59:695, 1977.

12

Chronic Cough in Children

Hyman Chai

Coughing is caused through a series of mechanisms, commencing from the smallest of airways and eventually involving the entire respiratory tract. This chapter will attempt to outline the pathophysiologic mechanism of coughing.

MECHANISMS

The production of a cough is a normal physiologic response whereby the body attempts to defend itself from injury. The initiating factor can vary from an inhaled foreign body to the "nervous" cough that is unassociated with organic disease.

ANATOMIC ASPECTS

Coughing involves (1) mechanisms that will assist in moving air, foreign bodies, mucus, or bacteria toward the mouth; (2) the anatomic structure working in unison to allow "pressure buildup," which can be released as an "explosive" force; and (3) providing "safeguard" mechanisms whereby this explosive force can be used voluntarily or involuntarily.

Closure of the vocal cords allows air pressure distal to the cords to build up. They are ideally suited to very rapid opening and therefore ensure rapid expulsion of air, foreign body, or physiologic substance (e.g., mucus) from the lung and trachea.

Below the larynx and vocal cords, the trachea and bronchial tree down to the twelfth generation, is supported by cartilage thus allowing rapid transfer of air. The production of a cough depends much more on these structures than on the bronchi and alveoli below the twelfth to thirteenth generation. There is evidence to support the view that the bronchial ducts and alveoli do play a role, albeit a passive one.

Nerve Supply

The need for "sudden" coughing requires stimulation of various structures. It is highly unlikely that any chemical mediators could achieve this objective with the rapidity necessary for effective coughing. The parasympathetic (vagal) system, glossopharyngeal nerves, and nerve supply to the diaphragm are also critical. The abdominal muscles are involved in forcing the diaphragm upward into the chest and are part of this process. Finally, the cough center in the medulla, which controls involuntary and voluntary coughing, is an integral part of the cough mechanism.

Bronchi and Bronchioles

The epithelium of these structures is important. Mucus rests on a watery layer of fluid over the surface of the bronchial and bronchiole epithelium. The cilia, with their inherent ability to "beat as one" in a rhythmic fashion, will move any foreign body, bacteria, or other substance up toward the mouth, where it is either swallowed or expectorated. Mucus is derived from epithelial cells and muscous glands situated below the epithelial basement membrane.

Mucus

The viscosity of mucus is very important. This aspect of the physical properties of mucus is called *rheogenicity*. The glycoproteins and lipids

129

contained in the mucus have notable effects on its physical properties. The more viscous the mucus is, the more difficult it will be for the cilia to escalate the mucus toward the mouth. Mucus is produced by the Clara cells, as well as the epithelial cells. Production also occurs in the submucosal cells and by the submucous glands. These submucous glands are controlled by the parasympathetic and sympathetic nervous systems; the former reduces mucus production, the latter stimulates it.

A variety of irritants may cause a rapid increase in mucus production, either via tracheal and bronchial receptors or direct action on the mucus-producing cells.

Cilia

The magnitude of the ciliary output (the strength and rapidity of their movement) depends on their length, density at any one site, and frequency and cohesion of the beat. The efficiency of this "escalator" thus will depend on all these factors, as well as the amount of mucus that is required to be moved at any one time. The cilia are susceptible to some infections (e.g., influenza A). These infections tend to destroy the cilia, and it may take a month or more for such cilia to regenerate.

PATHOPHYSIOLOGIC MECHANISM OF COUGHING

A cough is produced by a sequence of events: (1) an initial rapid deep inspiration; (2) a forced expiration against a closed glottis, hence no exhalation of inspired air during that time; (3) the sudden opening of the closed glottis; and (4) an almost simultaneous respiratory effort (voluntarily or involuntarily) that involves contracture of the diaphragm, the muscles of the abdominal wall, and to some degree the muscles of the thoracic cage (the intercostal muscles). A "blast" of rapidly moving air is created that expels relatively large quantities of air, and any "movable" substance will accompany it.

A number of receptors throughout the lung respond to multiple and variable stimuli. Evidence for these are based on animal experiments and therefore may not necessarily be applicable to the human lung in all respects. Some receptors respond to mechanical stimulation, and others respond to a variety of chemicals (e.g., citric acid and sulfur dioxide). There are probably other more complex mechanisms such as immune complexes and an increasingly large number of mediators (histamine, prostaglandins, and leukotrienes).

Data available at present suggest that these receptors have a limited distribution. They appear to be confined to the area of the larynx and down to the large bronchi. The anatomic distribution and makeup of these fibers vary. Some are myelinated, some are not, some are near the epithelial surface, some are deep. Some of the anatomic structures, especially the most sensitive areas, have a nerve supply that is extremely sensitive and near the surface, whereas others are much less sensitive and have a much deeper nerve supply. In regard to the various stimulants that may affect these receptors and associated nerves, it appears that the major factor is stretching the deflation of the lung itself.

It is interesting that the larynx does not appear to be an essential anatomic structure contributing to an effective cough. Patients with tracheostomies are able to cough, although it may be less effective. Although cough "receptors" have been discussed as anatomic entities, there is no evidence to substantiate their existence as receptors in the anatomic or molecular sense. Their presence is suggested by responses elicited at these sites by mechanical, chemical, irritative, and other mediators.

DISEASES ASSOCIATED WITH COUGHING

It is not the intent of this chapter to discuss every disease involved with the production of a cough. Other chapters in this book will have covered the major elements involved in the diseases of which coughing is only a symptom. Asthma, cystic fibrosis, and a variety of chronic lung diseases have been discussed earlier. Furthermore, it is not the intention of the author to discuss the therapy of a cough, since it is essentially a symptom associated with a vast array of diseases and psychologic problems. Intermittent or continuous coughing is part of the pathologic process, and therefore its treatment should be focused on the underlying disease.

ANATOMIC ABNORMALITIES AND COUGHING

Congenital Laryngeal Stridor

The defect associated with congenital laryngeal stridor is usually an excessively long epiglottis, the coughing being the result of local stimulation of the peripheral nerves in the upper airway system. The epiglottis has an "omega-like" shape. It is also associated with abnormal aryepi-glottic folds or very mobile aryentoid cartilages. Stridor is the prominent symptom, but this is often accompanied by a chronic cough. No therapy is usually necessary, since the cough is a secondary problem. Fortunately, in general, the problem is self-limiting and disappears over time.

Laryngeal Web

This defect is a web of tissue in the larynx that attaches to the vocal cords. Again, stridor is the major event; chronic coughing is a secondary feature of no major importance compared with the stridor. Dilation of the larynx, using appropriate dilators, is the therapy required. This may alleviate the cough.

Cysts and Laryngoceles

Cysts are filled with fluid, whereas laryngoceles are not. Both may require surgical removal if airway obstruction is significant.

Enlarged Tonsils and Adenoids

A chronic cough can be associated with enlarged tonsils and adenoids, although the serious problem is not the cough. The abnormal sleep patterns and abnormal ventilation associated with upper airway obstruction require attention. Children may develop a cough when lying supine and infrequently develop pulmonary hypertension due to alveolar hypoventilation and hypoxia. A tonsillectomy and adenoidectomy relieve upper airway obstruction with subsequent improvement in alveolar oxygenation and resolution of cor pulmonale.

Tumors

The tumors involved will be glottic or subglottic in nature. They are commonly angiomas or papillomas, and stridor and coughing are the major symptoms. Surgical removal is the therapy of choice.

Foreign Bodies

Foreign bodies are common causes of a chronic cough. It should always be a first consideration when there is either a sudden onset of unexplained coughing or wheezing, which then settles into a chronic cough without any obvious clinical disease or symptoms. Secondary infection is not uncommon and may be complicated by a localized abscess. There appears to be little interference with respiration or physical capabilities, unless the foreign body lies in the trachea or large airway.

Clinical Course

The acute phase of initial inspiration of the foreign body will depend on where the foreign body lodges. A foreign body in the trachea constitutes an acute emergency; if it is pulled into the large bronchi, then excessive coughing, wheezing, and atelectasis may follow. If a foreign body is lodged in the smaller subdivisions of the bronchi, a chronic cough will dominate the picture. A prolonged recovery period and "repeated" infections in the same lung area must alert the pediatrician to a potential foreign body. For suspected foreign body aspiration, bronchoscopy is mandatory.

Roentgenographic Techniques

If the foreign body is radioopaque, an ordinary roentgenogram of the chest will make the diagnosis. If the lesion is not radioopaque, a special roentgenographic procedure may identify the foreign body. For older children, a forced inspiratory and expiratory film will delineate the obstruction, even though the actual foreign body is not seen. The same is achieved with young children by taking a film during a normal inspiration and thereafter compressing the abdomen manually to provide an adequate deep expiration. A shift in the mediastinum is diagnostic. Therapy is removal of the foreign body, achieved through bronchoscopy.

Chronic Sinusitis

Chronic sinusitis is common in children. The problem may well be infection by a variety of organisms but also may reflect an "allergic" origin involving the nose and often associated with serous otitis media. The cough has always been assumed to be due to the postnasal mucous drip (and reasonably so, since much of the coughing takes place in a recumbent position and especially during sleep). It may also be related to the irritation of the vagal nerve supply along its fibers in the sinuses and then through the vidian nerve, ending finally in collateral involvement with the parasympathetic and glossopharyngeal nervous systems.

The use of vasoconstrictors, either oral or directly into the nasal mucosa as drops or a spray, together with an oral antihistamine (for allergic causes) may work well enough. Some severe cases may need a gamut of therapy, however. This would include a vasoconstrictor and an inhaled (nasal) steroid such as beclomethasone or Nasolide (Funisolide). If this is considered to be purely infection, then appropriate therapy would be amoxicillin or cefaclor (Ceclor) for a period of 10–14 days, together with the local or oral vasoconstrictors. Antihistamines may be useful if a true allergic (IgE antibody) cause exists.

Whooping Cough

Whooping cough is dominated by the classic paroxysmal cough and the associated inspiratory "whoop." Vomiting after the paroxysm supports the diagnosis.

Asthma

Asthma has been dealt with in more detail elsewhere in this book. A condition often called "hidden asthma" exists much more frequently than one thinks, however. The common form consists of a repeated cough, often in an allergic person and therefore often seasonal, but can also occur in perennial nonallergic asthmatic patients even though this is less common. It may only become evident after exercise-induced broncho-spasm in some cases. Diagnosis of this cough as being an asthmatic variant is usually relatively simple. The cough will respond dramatically to inhaled bronchodilators of the β_2-sympatho-mimetic format (metaproterenol, albuterol, or isoetharine). Pulmonary function tests per-formed during the coughing period will demon-strate reduction in large airway function, such as the forced expiratory volume in 1 second (FEV_1) or the peak expiratory flow rate (PEFR). Cough-ing is much less prominent in regard to small airways, demonstrated by abnormal forced expi-ratory flow (FEF_{25-75*}). Therapy will be directed to proper investigation of the asthmatic patient and the entire gamut of therapeutic modalities varying from environmental control to bron-chodilators such as cromolyn.

Cystic Fibrosis

The subject of cystic fibrosis has been dealt with elsewhere. The cough is fairly characteristic. It is usually productive and may be associated with a wheeze.

Chronic Rhinitis

The cough associated with chronic rhinitis falls into the same category as that previously dis-cussed for chronic sinusitis. It may be "mechani-cally induced" by postnasal mucous drip or stimulation of the parasympathetic fibers or both. The rhinitis can be of two major types: a true allergy and so-called vasomotor rhinitis. In a true allergy, such as found in hay fever, there is a definitive allergen with a specific antibody (most often IgE but occasionally IgG_1 or IfG_4) and a seasonal history. Diagnosis is more difficult if the history is perennial with no seasonal exacerba-tions. Vasomotor rhinitis is a term that merely indicates our inability to find a cause that would be acceptable. Therapy for allergic rhinitis consists of either medication or immunotherapy or both. There is increasing acceptable evidence that immunotherapy (hyposensitization or desensit-ization or even "shots") is an effective treatment for many allergic individuals. The demonstration of blocking IgG, an increase in T-suppressor cells with a reduction in T-helper cells after immuno-therapy, is a possible mechanism of immunother-apy. Difficulties arise when selecting the correct allergens, the quality of the injectable material, the presence or absence of overriding nonallergic factors, and the fact that T-helper and T-suppres-sor cells have not as yet been shown to be related to a specific antigen. In regard to medication, antihistamines are useful for the allergic child with rhinitis but unnecessary and unhelpful for the child who has rhinorrhea not of allergic origin. For both allergic and nonallergic forms, however, oral or nasal vasoconstrictors such as pseudoephedrine work very well. It is unusual to require inhaled vasoconstrictors with or without inhaled nasal steroids, but severe cases may well need such therapy.

α-1-Antitrypsin Deficiency

α-1-Antitrypsin deficiency is not a very com-mon illness but there is increasing evidence that it may well start in childhood, even though clinical symptoms may be delayed to the later years. The author has seen three children ages 14, 11, and 7, who have had all of the physiologic and pulmon-ary function evidence of "emphysema," which is characteristic of α-1-antitrypsin deficiency. In-vestigation will include proteinase inhibitor typ-ing to demonstrate the heterozygous state (MZ or SZ usually) for those who are not usually symptomatic (this is not a total certainty; some of them may be symptomatic but this is unusual) and have α-1-antitrypsin protein levels of 100 and higher. The homozygotes are always symptomatic (ZZ type) if the protein level is low (50 or less).

Coughing is a prominent symptom, and, in the inability to find an acceptable cause, α-1-antitrypsin should always be evaluated. This applies to any child with a cough and bilateral basal emphysema.

OTHER COUGH-RELATED ILLNESSES

Tuberculosis

Tuberculosis will be dealt with elsewhere in this book, but coughing can be a prominent symptom of the disease. The presence of blood in the sputum should arouse suspicion.

Kartagener's Syndrome

Kartagener's syndrome is associated with abnormalities of the cilia. (See immotile cilia syndrome.)

Pulmonary Edema

Pulmonary edema can arise from a variety of pulmonary diseases if the pathophysiologic mechanism results in an increase in vascular or osmotic pressure, which causes fluid effusion from the vessels. Coughing can be one of the symptoms, but dyspnea is by far the most prominent symptom and sign. Therapy will depend on the cause of the pulmonary edema and hence may cover cardiovascular, as well as pulmonary, pathologic conditions.

IMMOTILE CILIA SYNDROME

The ciliary apparatus is a tubular arrangement of nine outer "doublet" microtubles and two central tubules that have dyenein arms and radial "spoke" linkages. It is essential that cilia "beat" in unison and therefore use mucus as part of the escalator system to remove bacteria and foreign bodies. Cilia appear to be the same from the nasal mucosa down to the bronchi.

Immotile cilia syndrome (which includes Kartagener's syndrome) is relatively new, having been discovered or at least described in 1975. Since that time, periodic case reports appear in the journals. The initial description concerned immotile spermatozoa and demonstrated that the abnormality resided in the axoneme, which is the name given to the central core, whether it be the spermatozoal tail or cilia found in the respiratory system. After this report, additional cases have been published with different variants of abnormal cilia. These relatively isolated reports testify that not many suffer from this apparently genetic abnormality; however, it is a cause of chronic coughing and may occur at any age. Abnormal cilia are often associated with other abnormalities such as Kartagener's syndrome (dextrocardia, IgA deficiency, male sterility, and corneal malformations). Some cases have had variants with this combination but not the dextrocardia associated with Kartagener's syndrome, which only occurs in about half the patients (who may have other characteristic cilia malformations).

The term immotile cilia syndrome has been questioned because some of the cilia may not be totally immotile but only very sluggish. For all practical purposes, both are physiologically ineffective and might just as well be considered as a single entity.

Anatomy

Ciliated epithelia is found in the nasal cavity, paranasal sinuses, middle ear, respiratory tract, epididymis, and oviducts. The role of the cilia in the respiratory system is to promote movement of the mucus "blanket" resting on the fluid moiety in the respiratory tract. It therefore follows that if such movement is to be effective, it needs to beat in unison and with the desired strength to move whatever has to be moved toward the mouth. Any abnormality in the cilia, either no movement or erratic movement, will result in obstructive problems in the lungs. In microscopic examination of a cross section the cilia appear as a wheel, with spokes and a central axel. Around the circular outer edge are fibrous sheets. Below this area and in a concentric circle are nine arms, numbered clockwise from one to nine, the ninth arm being followed by the first arm. There is an inner and an outer arm and nine spokes (one each from the arms) that end in a central axon which consists of two tubelike substances closely attached to each other. Ab-

Table 12-1 *Diseases Associated with Chronic Cough in Children*

Larynx and Pharynx

Chronic laryngitis
Chronic pharyngitis
Parasitic infections (*Ascaris* sp., hookworm)
Anatomic adnormalities
Various tumors

Trachea and Bronchi (essentialy large and medium bronchi)

Chronic tracheitis
Chronic bronchitis
Foreign bodies (undetected, radiotranslucent)
Bronchiectasis
Cystic fibrosis
Tumors, malignancies
Chronic exposure to irritants

Lungs

Chronic asthma
Tuberculosis (not common as cough in children)
Edema from a variety of causes
Alveolitis
Emphysema
Effusion into pleura

Mediastinum

Transposition of vessels
Masses of various origin

General

Irritation of external auditory meatus
Subdiaphragmatic lesions, especially Gastroesophageal reflux
Psychosocial factors
Nervousness
Immotile ciliary syndrome
Kartagener's syndrome
Chronic sinusitis
Chronic allergic rhinorrhea
Chronic vasomotor rhinitis
Whooping cough
α1-Antitrypsin deficiency
Pulmonary edema
Chronic lung abscess
Emotional factors
Habit
Gastroesophageal reflux

normalities of any of these structures result in abnormal cilia function (as it does with sperm tails), which may be immotile, sluggish, or display totally incoherent movment.

Diseases Associated with Abnormal Cilia

Rhinitis, chronic sinusitus, asthma, recurring bronchitis, and infections may adversely affect the cilia even though they are normal. Examples are rhinovirus and myxovirus infections. Other mechanisms may result in the same outcome, such as cilia destruction by inhalation of destruction or corrosive gases. Actual destruction of the cilia (and hence the syndrome) also has been demonstrated in *Mycoplasma* infections in which the replacement membrane on healing is not ciliated, but stratified. It also has been described with pollinosis, but the evidence is questionable because the abnormaility may have existed before exposure.

A chronic cough will result from any abnormalities or destruction of the ciliated epithelium in the respiratory system. Although coughing is a prominent symptom, the presence of an effective cough may be advantageous because it is probably the only effective manner of removing mucus from the lung. In practice, the cough may not be sufficient, and postural drainage treatment will be indicated.

EMOTIONAL OR NERVOUS COUGH

Some children develop an unproductive cough that is often repeated and short lived; it occurs in stress situations. Problems arise from family and friends who notice this repetitious cough and are worried about its medical implications. The cough continues without the usual "stress" associated with pathologic coughs, relates to no evidence of upper or lower respiratory tract disease, is essentially ineffectual, and appears to continue without effort or tiredness. It is usually absent at night. The treatment for this cough obviously relates to psychosocial stresses, either continuous or intermittent (such as being asked to read a report at school) and may require psychologic assistance, not so much for the cough, but for the underlying problems.

Table 12-2   *Cough Suppressants* *

Medication: Codeine
Site of Action: Central nervous system
Comments: Effective but addicting

Elixer: usually with 85 mg/5 ml of terpin hydrate 10 mg/5 ml of codeine

Tablets: 15, 30, and 60 mg

Antitussive dosage: 1–1.5 mg/kg/24 hours qid (maximum in 24 hours, 30 mg)

Side effect: central nervous system depression, constipation, respiratory depression, and sometimes intestinal cramps

Medication: Dextromethorphan
Site of Action: Same as codeine
Comments: Same as codeine

Available as syrups in varying doses from 2.5 mg/5 ml to 15 mg/5 ml

Also may be combined with glyceryl guiaicolate, 100 mg/5 ml

Dosage: Children, 1 ml/kg/24 hours tid or qid

Other Cough Mixtures and General Comments

Other cough mixtures consist of liquids or tablets, mostly in combination formats of an antihistamine and a vasoconstrictor if a "postnasal drip" is considered the basic cause of the cough. Acetylcysteine has been advocated as a mucolytic. In my opinion it is very irritating to mucous membranes and may even necessitate administrtion of a bronchodilator.

*In my view, treatment of a cough is treatment of the abnormality producing the cough. The following limited medications have been used as cough suppressants, however.

INVESTIGATION OF THE CHRONIC COUGH

Investigation of the chronic cough is obviously the investigation of diseases that could be associated with the history and physical findings. Some final points could apply to the chronic cough, which, despite routine investigations, still appears to elude a definable cause. Two special investigations in particular are involved. The simpler of these is the flow-volume loop taken in expiration and inspiration. The former is performed as a maximal effort from residual volume (the amount of air left in the lung after a maximal complete expiration) and the latter from maximal inspiration. Changes in the shape of the curve will delineate the presence of an extrabronchial or tracheal obstruction or an intrabronchial obstruction, depending on an alternation in the shape of the curve developed by the XY plotter attached to the flow-volume instrumentation. It follows that any such abnormality will require bronchoscopy; most pediatric pulmonologists and otolaryngologists believe that bronchoscopy is indicated in every case of chronic cough where a clear-cut diagnosis cannot be made.

There are many causes of a cough associated with the lung and tracheobronchial system. In general, few medications effectively control a cough. Codeine is the only drug this author has found helpful in suppressing significant coughing. Most cough mixtures are palliative at best, and the essential therapy must be of the underlying disease.

Pulmonary alveolar proteinosis, idiopathic pulmonary hemosiderosis, Wegener's granulomatosis, Goodpasture's syndrome (type II immunologic disease affecting the basement membranes of the alveoli), cardiovascular problems such as mitral stenosis and congestive cardiac failure, fungal infections (histoplasmosis, *Monilia,* and coccidiooidomycosis) may also produce coughing because of the inflammatory reaction in the airways, especially the larger airways. A lung abscess will produce coughing regardless of the organism involved. *Aspergillus* is one of the fungi that might be involved, especially where exposure is high. Finally, a variety of parasites such as *Ascaris* and *Stronglyoides* organisms, hookworms, and visceral larva migrans, pass through the lung as part of their life cycle.

REFERENCES

Afzelius BA: A human syndrome caused by immotile cilia. *Science* 198:317–319, 1976.

Eliasson R, et al: The immotile ciliary syndrome: a congenital ciliary abnormality as an etiologic factor in chronic airway obstruction and male senility. *N Engl J Med* 297:1–6, 1977.

Exertional dyspnea and cough as preludes to acute attack of bronchial asthma. *N Engl J Med* 292:555–8, 1975.

Godfrey RC: Diseases causing cough. *Eur J Respir Dis* 110(suppl 61):57, 1980.

Immotile ciliary syndrome and ciliary abnormalities induced by injury and infection. *Am Rev Respir Dis* 124:107–9, 1981.

Karlin JM: The use of antihistamines in allergic disease. *Pediatr Clin North Am* 22:157-62, 1975.

King M: Rheological requirements for optimal clearance of secretions: ciliary transport vs. cough. *Eur J Respir Dis* 110(suppl 61):39, 1980k.

Lopez-Vidriero MT, Reid L: Respiratory tract fluid—chemical and physical properties of airway mucus. *Eur J Respir Dis* 110(suppl 61):25, 1980.

Mossberg: Muco-ciliary clearance by cough: *Eur J Respir Dis* 110(suppl 61):245, 1980.

Mossberg B, Camner P: Mucociliary transport and cough as tracheo-bronchial clearance mechanisms in pathological conditions. *Eur J Respir Dis* 110(suppl 61):47, 1980.

Newhouse M, et al: Lung defense mechanisms. *N Engl J Med* 295:990–8, 1976.

Phipps RJ: Physiological control of airway mucus secretion. *Eur J Respir Dis* 110(suppl 61):33, 1980.

Proctor—, et al: Receptors in the trachea bronchi in the cat. *J Physiol* 123:71–104, 1954.

Sturgess J, et al: Transportation of ciliary microtubules. *N Engl J Med* 303:318, 1900.

Widdicombe JG: Reflex control of breathing, in Widdicombe JG (ed): *International Review of Science,* London, Butterworth & Co, 1900, series 1, vol 2: *Respiratory Physiology.*

Widdicombe JG: Mechanism of cough and its regulation. *Eur J Respir Dis* 110(suppl 61):11, 1980

13

Lower Respiratory Tract Infections

Terrence L. Stull
Paul M. Mendelman
Christopher B. Wilson
Arnold L. Smith

Children have approximately six to eight respiratory illnesses a year. These illnesses constitute one of the most common problems in general pediatrics, accounting for more than half of the pediatric office visits.[1] The incidence of lower respiratory tract illnesses, including croup, bronchiolitis, and pneumonia, is approximately 50 illnesses /1000 individuals each year for children less than 6 years of age. Most of these episodes are pneumonia. Table 13-1 shows the age-related and seasonal epidemiology of the most common causes of nonbacterial pneumonia. The incidence of pneumonia is greatest in the first year of life with a gradual decline in incidence after this initial peak. Boys are affected approximately 25 percent more frequently than girls. In addition to the morbidity of the acute illness, it has been suggested that lower respiratory tract infections, especially with influenza virus, may be a risk factor for the development of obstructive airway disease in adulthood.[2]

VIRAL PNEUMONIA

The most common cause of lower respiratory tract infection in children is a viral agent. Pneumonia is more common in children under 4 years old, but even in this age group viruses are the most frequent etiologic agents.

Clinical Manifestations and Epidemiology

The clinical manifestations of viral pneumonia depend on the host's age and immune status and the etiologic agent. Respiratory Syncytial Virus (RSV) is the most important cause of pneumonia in infants.[1] Three fourths of the isolates are from infants less than 3 years of age. Fever and coughing are almost constant features; otitis media, pharyngitis, conjunctivitis, and rhinitis are frequently present. Pneumonia may be present with or without bronchiolitis.[3] RSV infections occur in yearly epidemics in midwinter to early spring. Older siblings with mild illness are usually the index case in families; infants less than 1 year of age have the highest secondary attack rate. The risk of acquisition of RSV and its severity is related to family size. Hospitalization is more common in patients from low-income and rural homes. In hospitalized infants, the severity of illness correlates with the duration and titer of viral shedding. These infants are therefore an important source of nosocomial infections.

Parainfluenza virus types 1, 2, and 3 are most commonly associated with upper respiratory tract infections, but the second most common clinical manifestation is pneumonia.[1] Of parainfluenza virus types 1 and 3, 85 percent of the infections occur in children less than 7 years of age,[2] and the age distribution for parainfluenza type 3 infections is similar to RSV. Parainfluenza virus type 1 rarely infects children less than 6 months of age. Parainfluenza infections occur endemically from fall to spring.[4] Fever, coughing, pharyngeal erythema, and rhinorrhea are common clinical findings.

Influenza type A viral infections occur in epidemics every 2–4 years, usually in winter. Sequential epidemics occur when antigenic variants emerge. Although sore throat and systemic

Table 13-1 *Epidemiology of Nonbacterial Pneumonia*

Agent	Season	Age (years) of Incidence*		
		< 1	1–5	> 6
RSV	Winter to early spring	+ + + +	+	−
Parainfluenza virus type 3	Fall to spring	+	+ + +	+ +
Parainfluenza virus type 1	Fall to srping	+	+ +	+ + +
M. pneumoniae	Year-round	−	+ +	+ + + +

*− indicates lowest incidence; + to + + + + indicate increasing incidence.

symptoms are most common in adults and older children, young children frequently present with fever (91 percent), vomiting or diarrhea (49 percent), severe croup (13 percent), bronchiolitis (6 percent), or pneumonitis (29 percent). Influenza type A infection occurs most commonly in children less than 2 years of age.[5] Although influenza type B is not considered a common respiratory pathogen,[1] the incidence of influenza type B pneumonia may be similar to the incidence of influenza type A pneumonia.[2]

Adenoviruses can be isolated from the upper respiratory tract of well children; thus isolation of such an agent from the nasopharynx of an ill child does not establish its causative role in pneumonia. Using antibody response as evidence of infection, however, Foy et al .[4] showed a peak incidence at 1 year of age; the overall incidence was 3 cases/1000 children each year. This rate declines to approximately 0.4 cases/1000 when the children reach 7 years of age.[4] Adenovirus infections occur throughout the year without a seasonal trend.[4] Types 1, 2, 3, and 5 account for approximately 80 percent of the isolates from children with respiratory tract diseases. Although type 7 is much less frequently isolated, it can cause more severe illness than the other types. In addition to the symptoms associated with pneumonia, adenovirus infections may have more diverse manifestations, including myocarditis and meningoencephalitis.

Rhinoviruses and reoviruses are most frequently associated with upper respiratory tract infections, but they occasionally cause pneumonia. Enteroviruses can also cause lower respiratory tract disease; pneumonitis with pleuritis has been reported to be associated with coxsackie A

and B viruses and ECHOvirus.[1] Cytomegalovirus may cause pneumonia in very young infants.

Pathophysiologic Mechanism

Initiation of infection is enhanced by overcrowded living conditions that presumably lead to a higher inoculum of virus.[3] Infection with viruses that commonly infect the upper respiratory tract mucosa can also cause pneumonia, which may occur despite previous host experience with the virus. The symptoms, however, are usually milder and of shorter duration.

The effects of viral infection on other respiratory tract flora are poorly understood. Viruses may potentiate bacterial infections by providing growth nutrients from cellular damage and by damaging ciliated epithelial cells that constitute a barrier to penetration of the lower respiratory tract. In uncomplicated infections, destruction of the ciliated cells, goblet cells, and bronchial mucous glands leads to sloughing of the epithelium at the basement membrane throughout the respiratory tract. Bronchial walls become edematous and infiltrated with mononuclear cells. More severe infections progress to localized or generalized hemorrhagic pulmonary edema.[6]

Differential Diagnosis

Acute viral pneumonia is difficult to distinguish from early bacterial pneumonia. Although epidemiologic, clinical, and laboratory features are helpful, the distinction still may not be clear. Other etiologies that may mimic viral pneumonia are aspiration of stomach contents or a foreign body, fungi, mycobacteria, parasites, mycoplasma, and neoplasms.

Key Diagnostic Tests

Leukocytosis with a preponderance of immature granulocytes is commonly seen in viral pneumonia, although notable leukocytosis is more frequently associated with bacterial illnesses. The elevation of serum levels of C-reactive protein is as sensitive or more sensitive than leukocytosis, an elevated erythrocyte sedimentation rate, or a fever greater than 40°C in detecting bacterial pneumonia.

The most common pattern seen on chest roentgenograms of children with viral pneumonia is a peribronchial infiltrate radiating from the right hilum. Localized and general hemorrhagic pulmonary edema and mixed parenchymal-pleural reactions have been described.

Although isolates from tracheal aspirates, lung aspirates, or pleural fluid provide the most definitive diagnosis, viral isolates from the nasopharynx generlly correlate with the etiologic agent of the pneumonia. Exceptions are the adenoviruses and herpes simplex virus.[1] Approximately 25–30 percent of children with pneumonia have nasopharyngeal cultures that grow one of the viruses commonly associated with pneumonia. Serologic diagnosis is possible by demonstrating a specific rise in antibody level in convalescent sera (by comparing it to the acute specimen). Cultures and serologic diagnosis are not helpful in uncomplicated cases of viral pneumonia, but are important for epidemiologic purposes and selected cases.

Therapy

Although antibiotic therapy has not been studied in all viral pneumonias, it does not prevent bacterial superinfection in Influenza A pneumonia. The dilemma of whether to initiate antibiotic therapy because of the difficulty in distinguishing viral from bacterial pneumonia must be resolved by clinical judgement after careful evaluation of the epidemiologic features, physical examination, and results of the laboratory tests.

Mist tent therapy adds little to the treatment of viral pneumonia. Very little of the moisture reaches the lower airway, which normally receives humidity from the upper airway. The most important therapy of viral pneumonia is the administration of oxygen and ventilatory assistance in severe cases based on the physical examination and arterial blood gas pressures.

New and Future Developments

The most important clinically related advance in viral infections has occurred in the field of rapid diagnosis. The presence of viruses in nasopharyngeal secretions can be ascertained within hours by the fluorescent antibody test. The direct fluorescent antibody test uses fluorescein-conjugated antiviral antibodies (e.g., anti-RSV) to attach to the epithelial cells obtained from the patient. The presence of the antibodies can be detected by fluorescence microscopy.

In the indirect fluorescent antibody test, antiviral antibodies bind to the epithelial cells; these antibodies are detected by a second fluorescein-labeled antibody directed against the first antibodies. The sensitivity and specificity of the fluorescent antibody test may be improved in the future with the use of monoclonal antibodies.

Prevention of selected viral infections is being actively investigated. Killed-virus vaccine is partially effective in preventing Influenza type A infections, but repeated doses are necessary, and the long-term effectiveness has not been established. Unfortunately, emergence of new antigenic strains requires periodic changes in vaccine composition. Killed-virus vaccine against RSV has been administered to infants, but more severe disease resulted when natural infection subsequently occurred. A shortcoming of killed-virus vaccines is the lack of mucosal IgA antibody response. Surface immunity may be more important than serum antibody in protection against viral infections.

Enteric capsules containing adenovirus types 3, 4, and 7 produce a subclinical infection of the lower gastrointestinal tract; vaccinated military volunteers have been resistant to subsequent disease. Because of the oncogenic potential of adenoviruses, this approach has not been used to vaccinate children against the adenoviruses that cause childhood pneumonia.

Temperature-sensitive mutants have been investigated as vaccine candidates, but they have, thus far, proven to be genetically unstable. More complex DNA manipulation is being investiated to produce attenuated, genetically stable viruses to use for vaccines. Purified protein antigens developed with recombinant DNA technology also are being investigated.

MYCOPLASMA PNEUMONIAE PNEUMONIA

Mycoplasma are the smallest free-living organisms; they are classified separately from viruses and bacteria. Because they have no cell wall, they are not seen with a gram stain. Correspondingly they are not susceptible to antibiotics that attack the cell wall, such as penicillins and cephalosporins. Infection of volunteers with respiratory secretions occurs after removal of the bacteria by filtration; therefore Mycoplasma infections were initially associated with viral infections.

The epidemiologic pattern of *M. pneumoniae* pneumonia is different from viral pneumonia. Although mild or asymptomatic infections may be common in very young children, the peak incidence of *M. pneumoniae* infection is 5–15 years of age; it accounts for 75 percent of pneumonia in this age group.[2] *M. pneumoniae* pneumonia occurs throughout the year with a broad peak in fall and early winter.[1] Smoldering epidemics that last for months may occur ever 3–5 years. *M. pneumoniae* is spread by droplets, but close contact usually is required. The incubation period is approximately 2–3 weeks, and carriage may continue for up to 5 months. The age and season-related epidemiology of viral and *M. pneumoniae* pneumonia are shown in Table 13-1.

Clinical Manifestations

M. pneumoniae infections characteristically begin insidiously with fever, headache, and anorexia, which is followed by a sore throat and dry cough.[7] Rales and rhonchi are common physical findings. Fever, headache, and malaise usually last 3–10 days, but coughing and rales may continue for months.[7] Coryza, sore throat, and headaches are significantly more common with *M. pneumoniae* infections than with viral infections.

Other organs may be involved in the presence or absence of respiratory symptoms.[7] The rare fatalities are usually due to meningoencephalitis or hemolytic anemia. Carditis occurs in approximately 5 percent of patients hospitalized with *M. pneumoniae* infection, and antibiotics do not seem to alter the duration or sequelae. A wide variety of rashes, including urticarial, maculopapular, bullous, and scarlatiniform rashes, also have been associated with *M. pneumoniae* infections.[7] Myalgias, migratory polyarticular arthralgias, and arthritis may occur in large or medium-size joints 3–8 days after the onset of respiratory symptoms. Articular erosions and synovial hypertrophy occur infrequently.

Autoimmune phenomena are commonly associated with *M. pneumoniae* infections.[8] Cold agglutinins, usually anti-I antibodies of the IgM class, occur less frequently in adults than children.[7] The Coombs' test may be positive, and antibodies to lung, liver, and brain have been detected. [4,6]

There is no pathognomonic chest roentgenographic pattern, but unilateral pneumonitis with subsegmental consolidation 5–9 days after the onset of illness is common, although bilateral involvement also may occur (Fig. 13-1). Pleural effusions may be detected in approximately 20 percent of patients if decubitus chest roentgenograms are taken. The severity of the disease as judged from roentgenograms is often significantly different from the clinical appearance of the patient.

Laboratory investigations during acute infections also are not diagnostic. The white blood cell count is usually normal, but it is elevated in approximately one third of patients.[7] Low titers of cold agglutinins may occur in viral infections, but titers greater that 1:64 indicate a greater probability of *M. pneumoniae* infection.[9] Confirmation of the diagnosis requires a fourfold or greater increase of serum complement-fixing antibodies or isolation of the organism, which usually requires a week or more.

Antibiotic therapy shortens the duration of the cough if initiated within 5 days of onset of the illness. Erythromycin is preferable in children, although tetracycline may be used in adolescents; resistance to erythromycin has been described. Prophylactic administration of antibiotics to contacts does not prevent colonization, but it does prevent disease.[1]

CHLAMYDIA PNEUMONIA

Chlamydia pneumonia was first described by Schachter and Grossman[10] in 1975. Beem and Saxon[11] published the first series of cases with this disease 2 years later. Several groups have subsequently corroborated their observations.[12–14] Although the majority of cases have been diagnosed on the basis of clinical findings and by isolation of the organism from upper respiratory tract secretions or by serologic methods, the most convincing evidence of its etiologic role is provided by isolation of *Chlamydia* organisms as the sole agent from lung biopsies of three cases.[10]

The Organism Pathogenesis and Pathologic Mechanism

Chlamydia trachomatis is an obligate intracellular bacterium with a unique life cycle. The infectious extracellular form of the organism, the elementary body, is ingested by host cells. Within the phagosome of the host cell, the organism transforms into a replicative form, the reticulate body. At the end of an approximately 48-hour replicative cycle, reticulate bodies reorganize into elementary bodies and are released from the cell. Serotypes D through K cause inclusion-body conjunctivitis and pneumonia in infants and urethritis and cervicitis in adults.

Adult infections with *C. trachomatis* are sexually transmitted. Infections occur in approximately two thirds of infants born to mothers with cervical infection. Organisms are inoculated into the eyes or nasopharynx of the infant during parturition or rarely by the ascending route in utero. In approximately 10 percent of infants born to infected mothers, direct spread of organisms from the upper respiratory tract to the lung occurs within 2 weeks to 4 months and results in pneumonia.

Histologically both interstitial and alveolar involvement and necrotizing bronchiolitis have been observed. The inflammatory response is usually a mixture of polymorphonuclear and mononuclear cells; typical intracytoplasmic inclusions are not usually observed in lung tissue.

Concomitant infection with viruses occurs in approximately 40–50 percent of infants; cytomegalovirus followed by RSV infections are most common. Clinical findings in patients with concomitant viral infections are not different from those with *Chlamydia* infection alone.

Incidence and Epidemiology

In prospective studies, 2–18 percent of pregnant women have *Chlamydia* cervical infection at term, and 28–70 percent of their infants become infected; thus *Chlamydia* infection occurs in 14–85/1000 live births. Of such infants 11–20 percent develop pneumonia; approximately half of these

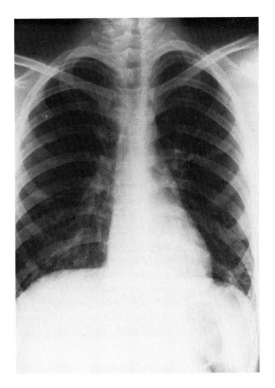

Figure 13-1. *M. pneumoniae* infection in a 13-year-old child. Reticulonodular infiltrates are present in both lower lobes.

infants also have or have had conjunctivitis. Of infants who have pneumonia in the first 6 months of life, 15–50 percent of the cases are associated with *Chlamydia* infection. Mortality is very rare but protracted respiratory distress is common in untreated patients.

Clinical features

Principal clinical features are indicated in Table 13-2. A typical roentgenogram is shown in Figure 13-2. Viral pneumonitis and recurrent aspiration pneumonitis due to gastroesophageal reflux are the chief entities that must be ruled out.

Diagnosis

The diagnosis should be strongly suspected in any child with onset of pneumonia between the age of 2 weeks and 4 months. The absence of fever and the presence of a staccato cough, eosinophilia (greater than or equal to $300/mm^3$),

Table 13-2 *Features of Chlamydia Pneumonia*

• Age of onset	Two weeks to four months
• Physical signs	Afebrile, staccato cough, tachypnea, good aeration, rales; occasionally wheezing and apnea; conjunctivitis in ~50%; occasionally serous otitis media, other signs of upper respiratory tract infection
• Roentgenographic findings	Hyperinflation; bilateral interstitial infiltrates; diffuse patchy atelectasis or infiltrates; lack of lobar consolidation or pleural effusion
• Duration	Two weeks to four months

and elevated total IgG and IgM levels are strongly suggestive of the diagnosis. Definitive diagnosis requires isolation of the organism from respiratory secretions or the presence of IgM anti-*Chlamydia* antibodies in a titer of greater than or equal to 1:64. The organism presently can only be isolated in cell culture, which requires several days and is not widely available.

Treatment

Uncontrolled data suggest that treatment with erythromycin (40 mg/ kg/day) or sulfisoxazole (150 mg/kg/day) for 2 weeks shortens the duration of symptoms and decreases the duration of shedding of the organism. Erythromycin is considered to be the drug of choice. Recently strains with decreased susceptibility to erythromycin have been observed.

COMMON BACTERIAL PNEUMONIAS

Pneumococcal Pneumonia

Streptococcus pneumoniae, first described 100 years ago, remains the most common bacterial pathogen in childhood pneumonia. It is a gram-positive coccus with a minimum of 84 capsular serotypes. The exact incidence of pneumococcal pneumonia in children is unknown, but it represents over one third of the hospital admissions for pneumococcal disease in childhood. The currently estimated rate in the United States for adults and children combined is 68–260 cases/ 100,000 population each year. Other epidemiologic features are shown in Table 13-3.

The morbidity of uncomplicated pneumococcal pneumonia is negligible. Pulmonary compli-

cations, pleural effusion, and empyema, however, are often associated with protracted fever, a prolonged hospital stay, and the need for surgical intervention. The case fatality rate for uncomplicated pneumococcal pneumonia is 5–7 percent in the United States. Associated meningitis has a significantly higher mortality and more severe sequelae, however.

The exact pathophysiologic mechanism is unknown but a viral upper respiratory illness is a common primary event. The organism gains access by aerosolization or aspiration of nasopharyngeal contents into the bronchi with subsequent proliferation in the alveoli. Unlike staphylococcal pneumonia, pneumococcal pneumonia rarely causes tissue necrosis. Progression through the four classic stages of congestion, red and gray hepatization, and resolution rarely occurs today due to the earlier institution of effective antibiotic therapy.

The epidemiologic characteristics are listed in Table 13-3. The peak incidence is early in the second year of life. Pneumococcal pneumonia with sepsis in the newborn has been reported. It is rare in the first 3 months of life, however. Although the racial incidence has not been well studied, black children with sickle cell disease are at increased risk because splenic function deteriorates. The typical patient is the child less than 2 years of age with a viral upper respiratory tract illness for 1 week who has the abrupt onset of high fever, tachypnea, mild to moderate dyspnea, a leukocytosis of greater than 25,000 cells/ mm^3, and a lobar infiltrate on chest roentgenography. A less common presentation is the infant with occult pneumococcal bacteremia who returns with a clinically apparent pneumonia.

The roentgenographic features (Fig. 13-3) are

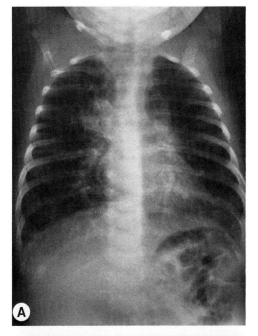

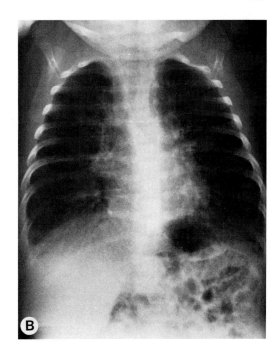

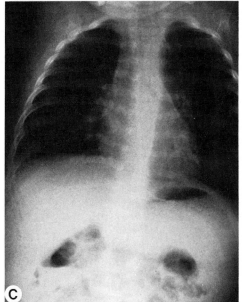

Figure 13-2. *C. trachomatis* pneumonia in a 6-week-old child. (**A**) Diffuse interstitital and patchy alveolar infiltrates are present. The lungs are hyperinflated. (**B**) Two weeks later the infiltrates have cleared substantially but the lungs remain hyperinflated. (**C**) The process has nearly resolved $2\frac{1}{2}$ months later. There is a residual infiltrate in the left upper lobe.

Table 13-3 *Epidemiologic Characteristics of* S.
pneumoniae *Pneumonia*

• Age of onset	First 4 years of life; median age is 14 months
• Sex	Male/female, 2:1
• Season	Winter to spring

listed in Table 13-4. An interstitial pattern has
not been described. The pneumococcus caused
64 percent of the cases of childhood empyema in
the preantibiotic era. In the immediate postan-
tibiotic era (1944), it was responsible for only 17
percent of cases and currently accounts for 10
percent.

The most accurate diagnostic test is the blood
culture. Although one fourth to one third of
adults have associated bacteremia, the data in
children are limited. In those children with
severe illness, the reported bacteremia rate is 15
percent. Upper respiratory tract cultures are
unreliable for diagnosis because one third of
infants and children carry the pneumococcus in
their upper airway. Diagnostic theoracentesis
may be quite helpful. A gram stain and a
precipitin (quellung) reaction of the pleural fluid
are rapid diagnostic tests. Moreover, even
though empyema fluid in the presence of prior
antibiotic therapy may be sterile, antigen detection by counterimmunoelectrophoresis (CIE) is
reliable and sensitive. In addition to pleural fluid,
concentrated urine is an appropriate fluid for
CIE investigation, since it contains capsular
antigen in culture-negative cases.

The therapy of pneumococcal pneumonia is
quite straightforward. Penicillin G is the drug of
choice; the child with severe disease, underlying
illness, or complications requires parenteral therapy. Oral therapy with phenoxymethylpencillin
(penicillin V) may be used for mild to moderate
disease. The number of penicillin-resistant
strains reported in 1978–1980 is less than 2
percent. Surgical drainage of small effusions is
unnecessary, and large effusions should respond
to needle thoracentesis. A persistent fever or
pneumatoceles require patience in the child who
is improving; neither should delay discharge.
Followup studies reveal an excellent prognosis as
measured by roentgenographic resolution and
normalization of pulmonary function tests.

The currently licensed pneumococcal vaccine
contains 14 of the 84 capsular serotypes.[15,16] Since
these are responsible for 80 percent of pneumococcal disease in children, and the vaccine is
approximately 80 percent effective, the vaccine
offers approximately 60 percent protection in the
immunized patient. Antibody levels persist for a
minimum of 3–5 years. This is of particular value
for those populations at increased risk of overwhelming pneumococcal disease. These include
children with sickle cell disease; functional,
congenital, or surgical asplenia; nephrosis; and
immunosuppression. All children over 2 years of
age in these categories should receive the vaccine. Unfortunately, polysaccharides are poor
antigens in children less than 2 years old, and
efficacy rates in this age group are low. Modification of the vaccine is needed to improve its
immunogenicity in this high-risk population.

Haemophilus **pneumonia**

Haemophilus influenzae is a gram-negative
pleomorphic rod. There are six known capsular
serotypes (a through f), as well as nontypable,
unencapsulated strains. Tissue invasive disease,
including pneumonia, is due to the type b
serotype. The true frequency of *H. influenzae*
type b pneumonia is unknown; a reasonable
estimate is that approximately 2 percent of all
pneumonias in children are caused by this pathogen. Of documented cases of patients hospitalized with bacterial pneumonia, however, *H.
influenzae* type b represents over one third of the
cases, and pneumonia is the second most common presentation of systemic *H. influenzae*
disease (second to meningitis).

In the past 5 years 155 cases[17–20] of *H.
influenzae* type b pneumonia have been documented in four retrospective studies. These
reports more than double the number of cases
described in the prior two decades and probably
relect both an increase in incidence and recognition of the disease.

The overall mortality in these series is 5.8
percent, divided equally among patients with
pneumonia alone and those with pneumonia
associated with meningitis. Of these cases 50
percent have additional foci infected with *H.
influenzae* (Table 13-5). The mortality in these
cases reflects the associated disease since the
morbidity of uncomplicated *H. influenzae* type b
pneumonia is negligible.

The pathogenesis of the disease is not clear;
one hypothesis suggests bacterial invasion of the

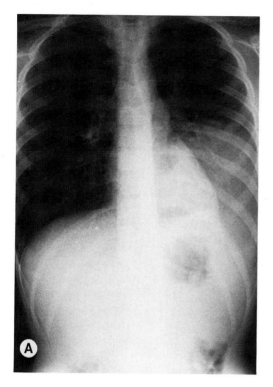
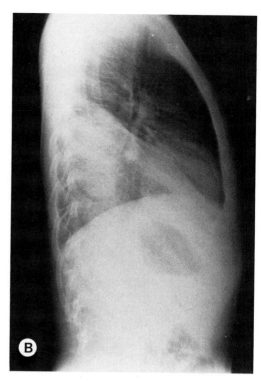

Figure 13-3. Pneumococcal pneumonia in an 8-year-old child. There is consolidation of the lateral and anterior basal segments of the left lower lobe. (**A**) Postero anterior view. (**B**) Lateral view.

nasopharyngeal mucosa with subsequent bacteremic spread to the lungs. The exact mode of entry of the organisms into the vascular compartment is unknown, but it is assumed that phagocytic cells carry organisms via the lymphatics into the bloodstream. Alternatively, the bacteria may spread from the upper airway to the lower respiratory tract.

The clinical characteristics of *H. influenzae* pneumonia are listed in Table 13-5. The age distribution parallels that for *H. influenzae* meningitis. There have been several case reports of *H. influenzae* pneumonia in premature neonates who developed disease on the first day of life with an illness clinically similar to group B streptococcal pneumonia.

The roentgenographic features are listed in Table 13-6. Of these cases 50 percent have evidence of pleural involvement, and 90 percent yield fluid by thoracentesis (Fig. 13-4). Four cases of pneumatoceles have been reported.

The differential diagnosis includes pneumonia due to *S. pneumoniae,* which can be clinically

indistinguishable and staphylococcal pneumonia, which occurs in the younger child (median age of 3 months) and characteristically causes more respiratory distress, tuberculosis, and congenital lobar sequestration.

The single best diagnostic test is the blood culture (Table 13-7). There is a poor correlation between upper airway culture results and lower respiratory tract pathogens. In infants, 70 percent are colonized with *H. influenzae* and 5 percent carry type b organisms. A gram stain of the pleural fluid may be helpful, although it is misinterpreted in 46 percent of the examinations. Detection of the type b capsular polysaccharide in pleural fluid, serum, or urine is a rapid and reliable means of establishing the diagnosis. The enzyme-linked immunosorbent assay is the most sensitive technique, followed by latex agglutination and CIE. Concentrations of capsular polysaccharide of 0.1 ng/ml, 1 ng/ml, and 20 ng/ml are detectable by these methods respectively. The concentration of this antigen at the site of the infectious focus is at least a thousand times

Table 13-4 *Roentgenographic Features of* S. pneumoniae *Pneumonia*

Symptoms	Overall Incidence (%)	Age (years) of Incidence (%)	
		<2	>2
Lobar involvement	72	62	92
Bronchopneumonia	23	38	8
Empyema	10		
Pneumatocele	Rare (7 cases reported)		
Pneumothorax	Very rare (1 anecdotal case)		

greater than that in the serum. A pleural fluid aspiration therefore may be helpful in diagnosis. The fluid ranges from a few drops to 150 ml. Late in the disease, the consistency has been noted to resemble chicken fat and therefore will be difficult to drain. Ultrasound may be helpful when pleural reaction and fluid density cannot be resolved by examination of plain films.

Initial therapy should include both ampicillin and chloramphenicol, since the current inci-dence of ampicillin-resistant strains is 18–30 percent. Once the sensitivity of the organism is known, therapy may be completed with the single most appropriate agent. One fourth of hospitalized cases will show persistent pleural reaction at discharge, and restrictive pulmonary function may be present for 12–18 months; long-term follow-up reveals no residual abnor-malities in lung function or in roentgenographic appearance.

Table 13-5 *Characteristics of* H. influenzae *Type b pneumonia*

Age	75% <2 years of age; 88% <4 years of age; range, 2 weeks to 15 years; median age, 14 months
Sex	Male/female, 2:1
Season	Winter to spring (80%)
Mean number of symptomatic days before hospitalization	<4 days (range 2–21 days)

Preceding symptoms
  URI*   82%
  Fever   98%
  Cough   75%
Abnormal lung examination   73%
  Median white blood cell count   19,500/mm^3
  mean polymorphonuclear cell count   14,200/mm^3

Additional foci of *H. influenzae* infections
  Otitis media   22%
  Meningitis   16%
  Epiglottitis   5.8%
  Pericarditis   2.6%

Mean duration of fever
  Without associated disease   3.2 days
  With associated disease   6 days
Mean hospital stay 12½ days

*Upper respiratory infection

Table 13-6 *Roentgenographic Findings in* H. influenzae *Type b Pneumonia*

Features	Percentage (%)
Segmental and lobar involvement	35
Segmental involvement alone	35
Lobar involvement alone	12.4
Involvement of one lobe	68
Involvement of two lobes	26.4
Involvement of three lobes	5.7
Bronchopneumonia	15
Unilateral	70
Bilateral	30
Interstitial pneumonia	2
Pleural reaction	50
Pleural fluid	89
Pneumatoceles	0.0065
Pleural thickening at discharge	23

Staphylococcal pneumonia

Staphylococcus aureus is the third most common cause of bacterial pneumonia in childhood. An increased incidence occurred in the late 1950s due to the epidemic of the virulent phage type 80/81, but currently *S. aureus* pneumonia occurs infrequently and represents approximately 1 percent of all childhood pneumonia.

The mobidity and mortality of *S. aureus* pneumonia is the highest of all the common bacterial pneumonias. Available data precede the introduction of the penicillinase-resistant β-lactam antibiotics, however, and must be interpreted in this light.[21–22] Data on the outcome with current management techniques are lacking. The seriousness of the disease in young infants is striking; of infected childen who died, 86 percent were less than 12 months of age and 75 percent were less than 4 months of age. Of the hospitalized patients, 35 percent died within hours of admission, and an additional 20 percent died within the first 48 hours. The overall case fatality rate was 15 percent; however, the rate is 18 percent for infants less than 12 months of age and 20 percent for infants less than 6 months of age. The average hospital stay was 28 days, suggesting significant morbidity in survivors.

There are two distinct roentgenographic patterns of *S. aureus* pneumonia that reflect a different route of entry; it may be airborne or hematogenous. The airborne route is primary or associated with an antecedent viral respiratory tract infection. Entry is by aspiration of nasopharyngeal secretions or aerosolization directly into the tracheobronchial tree. Experimental infection requires a high density of organisms. Associated cutaneous infections are present in 15 percent of cases. The hematogenous route is associated with soft tissue infection in over 80 percent of cases, excluding drug addicts, those with vascular prostheses, and hemodialysis patients. The mechanisms by which staphylococci invade tissues are not known. Most pathogenic strains elaborate enzymes and toxins that facilitate tissue invasion by damaging tissues and the host defense. These include an exotoxin (α-toxin), a Δ-toxin, leukocidins, and coagulase. The production of coagulase correlates with virulence. Coagulase is believed to protect the organism from phagocytosis, inhibit bacteriostatic substances in serum, and promote abscess formation. Some pathogenic staphylococci can survive within human leukocytes; this may prevent them from being killed by certain antibiotics. Tissue necrosis is the hallmark of staphylococcal infection. In contrast to the classic roentgenographic pattern of staphylococcal pneumonia (Fig. 13-5), the hematogenous variety characteristically has single or multiple, central or peripheral, small round densities (less than or equal to 3 cm) that may not initially cavitate.

The clinical characteristics of *S. aureus* pneumonia are listed in Table 13-8. There is an apparent association with preceding upper respiratory tract viral illnesses, most strikingly influenza type A and measles. Children with cystic fibrosis have an increased incidence of staphylococcal pneumonia. Twenty-two percent of the cases are nosocomially acquired. Colonization of term and preterm newborns is common (5–10 percent) and places them at an increased risk. The typical patient is a very young infant who develops fever and a cough for 1–3 days. The child then experiences an abrupt increase in toxicity manifested by grunting respirations, subcostal retractions, and cyanosis. An occasional child will have gastrointestinal signs such as emesis, diarrhea, or abdominal distension, suggesting an intra-abdominal illness.

The roentgenographic features of staphylococ-

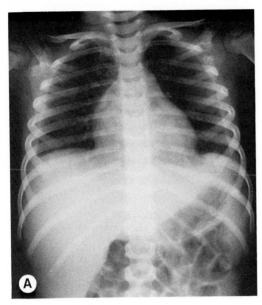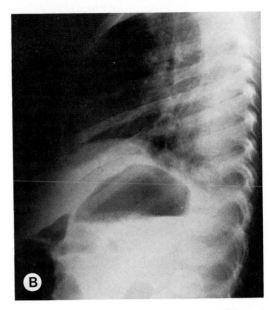

Figure 13-4. *H. influenzae* in a 3-year-old child. There is a left lower lobe retrocardiac infiltrate and bilateral pleural effusions. **A,** Postero anterior view. **B,** Lateral view.

cal pneumonia are listed in Table 13-9. The chest roentgenogram on admission may show a minimal or nonspecific infiltrate with little, if any, pleural reaction. The roentgenographic hallmark is significant change within hours to consolidation of multiple lobes, empyema, and pneumatoceles (Fig. 13-5). Roentgenographic findings may be particularly helpful, since 40 percent of all reported cases were not bacteriologically confirmed, and diagnosis was based on the pathognomonic finding of a pyopneumothorax and a consistent clinical course.

The differential diagnosis includes the necrotizing pneumonias due to gram-negative organisms, specifically *Klebsiella pneumoniae, Escherichia coli,* and *Pseudomonas* organisms. In addition, tuberculosis, hydrocarbon ingestion, measles, and other viral pneumonias may be infrequently associated with pneumatoceles. Often the early phase of the illness will be misdiagnosed as bronchiolitis. The best diagnostic test is pleural fluid culture (Table 13-10). Because of the low incidence of bacteremia, most patients do not have detectable serum antibody to teichoic acid by CIE or passive gel diffusion.

The therapy for *S. aureus* pneumonia includes β-lactam antibiotics. Nafcillin or oxacillin is

indicated for 1–2 weeks beyond initial clinical improvement, unually a 3-week duration. One study treated 19 patients for 18 days with full recovery, whereas 11 patients treated for 8 days all had relapses. The exquisite sensitivity of the organism to available antibiotics has made medical therapy alone adequate treatment even in some cases with mild to moderate empyema. Surgical drainage should be undertaken in patients with a tension pneumothorax, tracheal and mediastinal shift associated with considerable fluid, or extremely toxic infants who do not respond to adequate antibiotic therapy. Repeated needle thoracentesis was commonly used from 1950–1955 but was supplemented by closed tube drainage, which effects more complete removal of fluid. Decortication is not necessary, since fibrothorax and restrictive lung disease do not occur in children.

Roentgenographic resolution, primarily of pneumatoceles, has been reported to take as long as 14 months in the immunocompetent host and 5 years in immunocompromised patients. Pleural thickening may be evident for years. Follow-up studies at 5–15 years reveal no sequelae and normal pulmonary function tests in over 97 percent of cases; a rare patient develops bronchiectasis.

Table 13-7 *Culture Detection of* H. influenzae *Type b Pneumonia*

Site	Percentage (%)
Blood	87
Lung aspirate/tissue	86
Pleural fluid	75

OTHER BACTERIAL PNEUMONIAS

Group A streptococcal pneumonia is currently a rare disease. Most reviews of bacterial pneumonia in children contain only 1 or 2 cases, in contrast to 20 to 30 cases with *H. influenzae* or pneumococcal disease. Most often, the child is between 6 and 16 years of age and has the abrupt onset of fever, chills, respiratory distress, myalgia and pleuritic chest pain. In some series up to 50 percent of the cases occurred after varicella, rubeola, or occasionally rubella. The symptoms often progress rapidly in severity with cyanosis, hypotension, and often hemoptysis appearing shortly after admission. The most striking roentgenographic finding is massive, early pleural effusion. Thoracentesis yields a copious amount of serosanguineous fluid, which has rare organisms on gram stain, but invarialby yields the organisms on culture. In the majority of cases, the organism is cultured from the blood, but only one third are bacteria cultured from the throat. Other laboratory findings include evidence of disseminated intravascular coagulation, anemia, hypoproteinemia, and hyponatremia.

Penicillin G is the antibiotic of choice, administered intravenously at 50,000 μ/kg/day divided into 8–12 equal doses. Despite the uniform sensitivity of group A streptococci to the antibiotic, the clinical response to treatment is slow; most patients are febrile until 8–10 days of treatment have been completed. During the first few days of treatment, infectious complications are not uncommon. Pericarditis, osteomyelitis, or septic arthritis occur in one half of the patients. The pleural effusion should be drained to permit lung expansion. In certain patients, an empyema will develop despite early appropriate therapy.

A month of hospitalization may be necessary for treatment of the primary disease, as well as for the complications. Since the availability of penicillin G, fatalities have not been reported.

Long-term evaluation of lung function after treatment has not been reported.

Pneumonia due to gram-negative enteric bacilli is rare in children. These organisms, *K. pneumoniae, E. coli, P. aeruginosa,* and *Enterobacter* species produce pneumonia in immunosuppressed children (those receiving glucocorticoids or chemotherapy for neoplastic disease), those with burns, and those with intrinsic lung disease, such as cystic fibrosis. These predisposing factors are the only distinguishing features of the disease other than the tendency to have severe disease with extensive tissue necrosis. Appropriate antibiotic therapy and adequate drainage of the infected and necrotic tissue are the mainstays of therapy. The outcome depends on the underlying disease.

Unusual Causes of Pneumonia

A complete discussion of pneumonias due to less common pathogens is beyond the scope of this chapter. A summary of characteristic features of pneumonias due to certain less common bacterial, fungal, and protozoan pathogens is shown in Table 13-11. A more complete discussion of these entities and their treatment can be found in the general references.

CASE REPORTS

P.J. was a previously healthy 3-month-old infant who had the onset of rhinorrhea 2 days before evaluation. One day before evaluation, he developed a severe cough and anorexia, although he still took clear liquids well; on the day of evaluation tachypnea was noted. His temperature had not been greater than 38.2°C. Although his 6-year-old brother had had an upper respiratory tract infection the previous week, none of his other three siblings or parents had been ill. During the physical examination, he was alert and occasionally playful. His temperature was 37.8°C, his respiratory rate was 64 breaths/min, and he had mild intercostal retractions. Chest auscultation revealed scattered rhonchi, but there were no rales. The physical examination was otherwise normal. His peripheral white blood cell count was 12,500/mm^3 with 50 percent polymorphonuclear cells and 10 percent bands. A chest roentgenogram revealed flattened diaphragms with bilateral perihilar infiltrates.

Discussion. The mildness of this child's clinical course suggests nonbacterial pneumonia. The most likely agents in this age group would be RSV parainfluenza virus type 3, and *Chlamydia* organisms. The acute

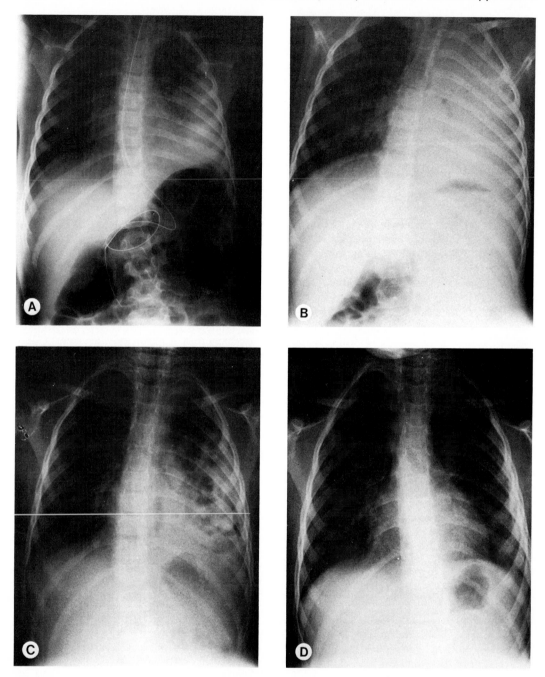

Figure 13-5. Staphylococcal pneumonia in a 4-year-old child. (**A**) Dense left lower lobe infiltration with effusion. (**B**) The effusion has increased 4 days later. Air bronchograms are evident. (**C**) Cavitation and pneumatocele formation occurred within 8 days after admission. (**D**) The process has nearly resolved 5 weeks after admission.

Table 13-8   *Characteristics of* S. aureus *Pneumonia*

Age	70% <12 months of age; median, <6 months of age
Sex	Male/female, 1.5:1
Season	Winter
Mean temperature	38.7°C
Mean WBC count	>25,000/mm^3
Mean fever duration	7 days
Mean hospital stay	28 days

Table 13-9   *Roentgenographic Features in* S. aureus *Pneumonia*

Findings	Percentage (%)
Empyema	70
Pneumothorax	30
Pneumatoceles	23
Abscess	6.3
Atelectasis	14
Right lung involvement	63
Left lung involvement	20
Bilateral involvement	17

onset of the illness and presence of sibling illness are against *Chlamydia* organisms as the etiology of the pneumonia. The occurrence in midwinter suggests that RSV is the most probable etiology. This child was admitted to the hospital for observation.

RSV was detected in nasal washings by, the fluorescent antibody test; P.J. was observed in the hospital, and was not treated with antibiotics. His coughing and tachypnea continued for 2 days and then improved; he had mild tachypnea for an additional 12 days, but was treated at home.

D.L. was a 15-year-old boy who was healthy until 4 days before evaluation. At the beginning of his illness, he had a fever of 38.4°C and a sore throat with nasal congestion. The next day he developed a cough, which worsened during the next 2 days. His physical examination was normal, except for his tired appearance and the presence of bibasilar rales. The peripheral white blood cell count was 8500/mm^3; 45 percent were polymorphonuclear cells and 5 percent were bands. His serum did not contain cold agglutinins, and a chest roentgenogram revealed bibasilar patchy consolidation.

Discussion.   The age of this child helps distinguish viral from *Mycoplasma* pneumonia. A likely viral agent at this age is parainfluenza type 1, but this virus is not a common cause of pneumonia during the summer. The season of the year and the roentgenographic pattern suggest *M. pneumoniae* as the etiology.

This patient was treated with erythromycin but continued to cough. The serum was again examined for cold agglutinins, which were present in a titer of 1:64. This further strengthens the diagnosis of *M. pneumoniae* pneumonia, but growth of the organism or a rise in complement-fixing antibodies would be necessary for confirmation.

The patient, a 27-month-old boy, presented to the emergency department in acute respiratory distress with a 7-day history of coughing and rhinorrhea and a 2-day history of fever. His vital signs included a temperature fo 39.7°C; pulse, 150 beats/min; respira-

tions, 60 breaths/min; and blood pressure, 100/60. His height and weight were in the tenth percentile. Examination revealed a seriously ill child with intercostal retractions, dullness to percussion at both bases, and diffuse bilateral rales. The liver was palpated 3 cm below the right costal margin. Assay of arterial blood gas showed the following results: pH, 7.41; Pao$_2$, 60mm Hg; and Pco$_2$, 32 mm Hg. He had a hemoglobin level of 10.2 g/L and a white blood cell count of 17,000/mm^3 with 36 percent segmented neutrophils, 33 percent band forms, 17 percent lymphocytes and 14 percent monocytes. A chest roentgenogram revealed right upper and left lower lobe infiltrates with bilateral pleural effusions.

Blood cultures and a cerebrospinal fluid examination were performed. Thoracentesis of the left chest yielded 5 ml of serosanguineous fluid, and the gram stain did not reveal bacteria. Ampicillin and chloramphenicol were administered. An intermediate strength purified protein derivative of tuberculin (PPD) was placed.

Discussion: He improved over the next 24 hours, and there was no increase in pleural fluid or respiratory distress. On the second hospital day, his blood cultures yielded *H. influenzae* type b. The next day the pleural fluid also grew *H. influenzae* type b. Chloramphenicol was discontinued, and ampicillin was administered at a dosage of 200 mg/kg/day, intravenously. The PPD skin

Table 13-10   *Culture Detection of* S. aureus *Pneumonia*

Site	Percentage (%)	
Pleural fluid	84	(131/158)
Lung aspirate	54	(185/354)
Blood	12	(19/158)

Table 13-11 *Unusual Causes of Pneumonia*

Disease	Environmental Exposure	Host Factors	Clinical Features	Roentgenographic Features	Diagnostic Tests	Treatment
Bacterial pathogens Tularemia (*Francisella tularensis*)	Exposure to infected mammals such as rabbits, foxes, cats, squirrels, ticks, deer flies, mosquitos	None	Abrupt onset of fever, chills; 10% have skin lesions or peripheral lymphadenopathy	Patchy parenchymal infiltrates ± effusion	Culture on special media; agglutinins-titers peak in 4–6 weeks	Streptomycin, 20–30 mg/kg/day for 10–14 days
Plague (*Yersinia pestis*)	Exposure to infected rodents, rabbits, fleas	None	Acute onset, peripheral lymphadenopathy common	Diffuse lobular or lobar infiltrates ± effusion	Culture	Streptomycin, 30 mg/kg/day for 10 days, or chloramphenicol, 50–75 mg/kg/day for 10 days
Brucellosis (*Brucella* sp.)	Exposure to infected cows, sheep, goats, pigs, dogs, raw milk, cheese	None	Insidious onset common; fever, malaise, weight loss	Hilar adenopathy, peribronchial and perihilar infiltrates ± effusion	Culture (may require weeks to grow); agglutinins; titers peak in 4–6 weeks	Streptomycin, 20–30 mg/kg/day for 14 days, and tetracycline, 25–50 mg/kg/day for 21 days, or trimethoprim-sulfamethoxazole with 10 mg/kg of trimethoprim for 21 days
Legionnaire's disease (*Legionella* sp.)	Cooling towers, other contaminated water sources	Immunosuppression, smoking	Subacute onset progressing to severe pulmonary disease in several days; diarrhea and neurologic symptoms common	Patchy alveolar infiltrates leading to consolidation	Direct fluorescent antibody staining of secretions, tissue; culture on special medium; acute and convalescent (>22 day) titers	Erythromycin, 50–60 mg/kg/day for 14 days
Anthrax (*Bacillus anthracis*)	Exposure to animal hair or hides	None	Mild prodrome of 3–5 days; sudden onset of respiratory distress and fever; edema of neck and chest	Mediastinal adenopathy, infiltrates, effusion	Characteristic gram stain; culture	Penicillin, mild, 30–50 mg/kg/day, severe, 150 mg/kg/day for 10–14 days; alternative, erythromycin

Disease	Epidemiology	Predisposing Factors	Clinical Features	Radiographic Findings	Diagnosis	Treatment
Nocardiosis (*Nocardia* sp.)	None	Steroids, immunosuppressive agents; alveolar proteinosis, chronic granulomatous disease	Acute to chronic onset of pulmonary and systemic symptoms; brain involved in ~30% of patients	Bronchopneumonia, cavitation, effusion, empyema, pulmonary nodule	Characteristic gram stain; modified acid fast stain; culture (may require up to 2–4 weeks to grow)	Sulfisoxazole, 100–150 mg/kg/day for ≥ 2 months, or trimethoprim-sulfamethoxazole with 10mg/kg of trimethoprim
Melioidosis (*Pseudomonas pseudomallei*)	Travel to S.E. Asia, W. Indies, Australia, Guam, S. and Central America	None	Latent infection for days to years leading to acute fulminant pneumonia or septicemia; mild to subclinical pneumonia	Pulmonary consolidation; cavitation; upper lobes commonly involved	Culture	Chloramphenicol, 50–75 mg/kg/day, plus sulfisoxazole, 100–150 mg/kg/day, or trimethoprim-sulfamethoxazole plus gentamicin, 6–7.5 mg/kg/day for 10–14 days, then one drug for 2–3 months
Leptospirosis (*Leptospira* sp.)	Exposure to dogs, rodents, cats, pigs, cattle, horses, or water contaminated with their urine	None	Pneumonia occurs in first phase of biphasic illness; associated with acute onset of systemic symptoms	Patchy infiltrates, particularly in periphery; diffuse consolidation	Clinical suspicion; agglutination titers that peak at 3–4 weeks; cultures take up to 6 weeks	Efficacy of therapy unproven; if diagnosed in the first weeks, tetracycline, 30/mg/kg/day, or penicillin, 200,000–300,000 units/kg may be given
Actinomycosis (*Actinomyces* sp.)	None	Dental or chronic pulmonary disease	History of aspiration or penetrating chest injury; minimal systemic response	Pulmonary infiltrate spreading across lobes or invading adjacent structures; small cavities	Presence of sulfur granules; characteristic gram stain; anaerobic culture of tissue or drainage	Penicillin, 50–100 mg/kg/day, for at least 6 months
Q fever (*Coxiella burnetti*)	Exposure to goats, cattle, sheep, raw milk, or cheese	None	Abrupt onset of fever, prostration, cough; occasionally enlarged liver or spleen	Discrete segmental infiltrates	Antibody titers	Tetracycline, 25–50 mg/kg/day, or chloramphenicol, 50 mg/kg/day

Table 13-11 *Continued*

Disease	Environmental Exposure	Host Factors	Clinical Features	Roentgenographic Features	Diagnostic Tests	Treatment
Psittacosis (*Chlamydia psittaci*)	Exposure to birds	None	Onset over 1–4 days, prominent systemic symptoms with headache, persistent cough; enlarged liver or spleen common	Patchy perihilar infiltrates; less commonly nodular or lobar pattern	Antibody titers	Tetracycline, 25–50 mg/kg/day, or chloramphenicol, 50 mg/kg/day
Fungal pathogens Coccidioidomycosis (*Coccidioides immitis*)	Travel to southwestern U.S.; northern Mexico; exposure during dust storm	None usually	Primary,—>50% asymptomatic, or acute onset of fever, malaise, cough, pleuritic pain, arthralgia, erythema nodosum; progressive or persistent pneumonia,—fever, weight loss, cough, chest pain, prostration	Primary,—infiltrates, nodules, transient cavities, pleural effusions and hilar adenopathy 10–20%; persistent infiltrates, cavities, miliary disease, nodules, abscesses	Isolation of organism; elevated precipitin titers in acute disease; elevated complement fixation titers in progressive disease	Primary, none; progressive, amphotericin B or ketoconazole
Histoplasmosis (*Histoplasma capsulatum*)	U.S. excluding far west; dust from soil enriched with bird or bat droppings	None usually; severe disease more common in infants	Primary,—>50% asymptomatic, commonly mild cough, variable fever, malaise; progressive primary,—progressive infiltrates, multisystem illness	Primary,—hilar adenopathy, patchy infiltrates; progressive,—same as coccidioidomycosis except scattered infiltrates more common	Isolation of organism; serologic tests occasionally useful	Primary, none; progressive, amphotericin B
Blastomycosis (*Blastomyces dermatitidis*)	Focal distribution in south, south central and Great Lakes regions of N. America	None usually	Resembles coccidioidomycosis and histoplasmosis	Resembles coccidioidomycosis and histoplasmosis	Isolation of organism	Primary, amphotericin B or none; progressive, amphotericin B

Disease	Source/Exposure	Host factors	Clinical features	Radiographic findings	Diagnosis	Treatment
Cryptococcosis (*Cryptococcus neoformans*)	Dust from soil enriched with pigeon droppings	~50% normal; ~50% diabetes, immunosuppression, or pulmonary alveolar proteionosis	>50% asymptomatic; mild cough, fever, malaise	Homogeneous infiltrates, nodules; hilar adenopathy < 10%	Isolation of cryptococcus neoformans from tissue or multiple sputum samples	Solitary lesion in normal host, surgery; complicated, amphotericin B and flucytosine
Aspergillosis (*Aspergillus* sp.)	None usually	Neutropenia, immunosuppression	Progressive pulmonary infiltrates, respiratory distress, fever	Bronchopneumonia, commonly necrotizing; mass lesion (Aspergilloma), commonly with cavitation	Lung biopsy; circulating antigen detection or rising antibody titers are less sensitive	Amphotericin B
		Chronic lung disease	Progression of primary lung disease, hemoptysis	Funga ball (aspergilloma)	Precipitins to *Aspergillus* organisms; immediate skin-test response to *Aspergillus*	None or surgery
		Allergy	Episodic wheezing, infiltrates, eosinophilia	Variable infiltrates, hilar widening, central bronchiectasis		Corticosteroids
Parasites Pneumocystis (*Pneumocystis carinii*)	None	Immunosuppression, prematurity, malnutrition	Progressive respiratory distress and fever	Diffuse interstitial disease; rarely infiltrates, nodules, pleural effusions	Demonstration of organism in lung tissue or respiratory secretions	Trimethoprim-sulfamethoxazole, 15–20 mg/kg/day of trimethoprim, or pentamidine, 4 mg/kg/day
Toxoplasmosis (*Toxoplasma gondii*)	Undercooked meat, cat feces, transplacental	Neonates, immunosuppression	Systemic symptoms predominate, variable respiratory disease	Interstitial infiltrates	Demonstration of trophozoites in tissue; diagnostic antibody studies	Pyrimethamine, 0.5–1 mg/kg/day (maximum 25 mg), and sulfadiazine, 100–150 mg/kg/day; may add folinic acid

test was less than 5 mm 48 and 72 hours after admission. His hospital course remained uneventful. He became afebrile on day 6, and oral ampicillin

therapy was started on day 7. He was discharged on day 19 with bilateral pleural thickening on the chest roentgenogram.

REFERENCES

1. Cherry JD: New respiratory viruses: their role in repiratory illnesses of children. *Adv Pediatr* 20:225–290, 1974.
2. Murphy TF, Henderson, FW, Clyde WA, Jr, et al: Pneumonia: an eleven-year study in a pediatric practice. *Am J Epidemiol* 113:12–21, 1981.
3. Loda FA, Clyde WA, Jr, Glezen WP, et al: Studies on the role of viruses, bacteria and *M. pneumoniae* as causes of lower respiratory tract infections in children. *J Pediatr* 72:161–176, 1968.
4. Foy HM, Cooney MK, McMahan R, et al: Viral and mycoplasmal pneumonia in a prepaid medical care group during an eight-year period. *Am J Epidemiol* 97:93–102, 1973.
5. Glezen WP, Denny FW: Epidemiology of acute lower respiratory disease in children. *N Engl J Med* 288:498–505, 1973.
6. Scanlon, Unger JD: The radiology of bacterial and viral pneumonias. *Radiol Clin North Am* 11:317–338, 1973.
7. Levine DP, Lerner AM: The clinical spectrum of *Mycoplasma pneumoniae* infections. *Med Clin North Am* 62:961–978, 1978.
8. Denny FW, Clyde WA, Glezen WP: *Mycoplasma pneumoniae* disease: Clinical spectrum, pathophysiology, epidemiology and control. *J Infect Dis* 123:74–91, 1971.
9. Todd JK: Pneumonia in children. *Postgrd Med* 1977; 61:251.
10. Schachter J, Grossman M: *Chlamydia* infections. *Ann Rev Med* 32:45–61, 1981.
11. Beem MO, Saxon EM: Respiratory-tract colonization and a distinctive pneumonia syndrome in infants infected with *Chlamydia Trachomatis*. *N Engl J Med* 296: 306–310, 1977.
12. Harrison HR, Phil D, English M, et al: *Chlamydia trachomatis* infant pneumonitis. *N Engl J Med* 298:701:708, 1978.
13. Schachter J, Holt J, Goodner E, et al: Prospective study of Chlamydia infection in neonates. *The Lancet* II:377–379, 1970.
14. Frommell GT, Rothenberg R, Wang S, et al: Chlamydial infection of mothers and their infants. *J Pediatr* 95:28–32, 1979.
15. The pneumococcus. *Rev Infect Dis* 1981; 3:183.
16. Assessment of the pneumococcal polysaccharide vaccine. *Rev Infect Dis* 3 (suppl):1, 1981.
17. Ginsburg CM, Howard JB, Nelson JD: Report of 65 cases of *H. influenzae* b pneumonia. *Pediatrics* 64:283–286, 1979.
18. Asmar BI, Slovis TL, Reed JO, Dajani AS: *H. influenzae* type b pneumonia in 43 children. *J. Pediatr.* 93(3):389–393, 1978.
19. Jacobs NM, Harris VJ: Acute *H. influenzae* type b pneumonia in childhood. *Amer. J. Dis. Chld.* 133:603–605, 1979.
20. Wald ER, Levine MM: *H. influenzae* type b pneumonia. *Arch. Dis. Chld.* 53:316–318, 1978.
21. Rebhan AW, Edwards HE: Staphylococcal pneumonia: a review of 329 cases. *Can Med Assoc J* 82:513–517, 1960.
22. Koch R, Carson MJ, Donnell G: Staphylococcal pneumonia in children: a review of 83 cases. *J Pediatr* 55:473–480, 1959.

SUGGESTED READINGS

Feigin RD, Cherry JO (eds:) *Pediatric Infectious Diseases.* Philadelphia, 1981. WB Saunders Co.
Mandell GL, Douglas RC, Bennett JE (eds): *Princi-* *ples and Practice of Infectious Diseases.* New York, 1979. John Wiley and Sons, Inc.

14

Tuberculosis

Richard F. Jacobs
Jack Levy
Christopher B. Wilson
Arnold L. Smith

Tuberculosis is a systemic disease caused by *Mycobacterium tuberculosis*. Although the lungs are the primary site of infection, up to 15 percent of the patients have involvement of other organs. This chapter will deal primarily with pulmonary manifestations of tuberculosis.

EPIDEMIOLOGY

Tuberculosis was a disease of limited importance in American Indians. The arrival of the European immigrants started an epidemic cycle. Successive peaks in the incidence of the disease were observed until the end of the nineteenth century in areas where urbanization with new immigrants occurred. The morbidity and mortality of tuberculosis began to decrease throughout the United States in the early part of the twentieth century; this decline was accelerated by the introduction of specific antituberculous chemotherapy in the late 1940s. In 1953 the annual new case and mortality rates were respectively 53 and 12.4/100,000 population. By 1979 these numbers were reduced to 12.6 and 0.9/100,000. The prevalence of tuberculin skin-test reactors in children entering school is now estimated to be 0.2 percent and in adolescents it is 0.7 percent.

Age, race, socioeconomic status, and geographic location influence the distribution of the disease. The incidence in the elderly has decreased more slowly than in younger age groups, causing a gradual rise in the average age of the patient with tuberculosis. From 1953 to 1978, the percentage of new cases in children less than 15 years of age decreased slightly from 6.2 percent

to 5.2 percent. The lowest incidence is observed in the 5–15 age group. During the same period, the population of patients who were older than 65 years increased from 13.8 percent to 28.6 percent. The incidence is five times higher in nonwhites than whites and two times higher among men than women. Differences between races are apparent in childhood; the incidence of differences between sexes is not apparent until the age of 25 years. The prevalence of the disease is higher in the southern half of the United States and in cities with 500,000 or more residents. In these cities, socioeconomic factors such as poor living conditions, crowding, and malnutrition are associated with the highest case rates.

Since 1973 the overall downward trend of tuberculosis has leveled off, particularly in the younger age groups. This observation has been attributed to the influx of Indochinese refugees with a high prevalence of the disease. In contrast to what is observed in the rest of the population, 17 percent of the cases reported in 1979 in Indochinese refugees were children younger than 15 years old. About one third of the isolates of tubercle bacilli recovered from these patients are resistant to at least one antituberculous drug; this phenomenon may have considerable impact on the treatment and epidemiology of tuberculosis in the United States.

BASIC MECHANISMS

Mycobacteria are acid-fast, alcohol-fast, nonmotile, nonspore-forming, aerobic rods. Various species can be isolated from humans. Some are

157

saprophytes, and two are responsible for tuberculosis (*M. tuberculosis* and *M. bovis*); others, although less pathogenic for humans, can cause diseases other than tuberculosis.

M. tuberculosis bacilli are identified by their slowly developing, rough, nonpigmented, corded colonies on oleic acid—albumin agar. Recognizable growth may require incubation for 4–6 weeks. Biochemical characteristics used to identify *M. tuberculosis* include a positive niacin test, the ability to reduce nitrates, and weak catalase activity that is lost by heating at 68°C.

In 2114 autopsies on children, tuberculosis was found to have a primary pulmonary focus in 95.9 percent of the cases. It is possible that this value actually underestimates the frequency of primary lung involvement, since the study[1] was performed at a time when bovine tuberculosis was prevalent. Other forms of acquiring tubercle bacilli that result in primary nonpulmonary tuberculosis include ingestion, contact with the skin or mucous membranes, inoculation with a contaminated syringe, and congenital acquisition. Respiratory tract infection occurs when coughing or expectoration by an infected individual results in formation of airborne droplet nuclei of 1- to 10-$\mu\mu$ diameter containing *M. tuberculosis*. Such droplets are small enough to be kept aloft by air currents normally present in any room and to reach distal airways and alveoli when inhaled. If such nuclei pass beyond the mucociliary blanket, which acts as a primary defense against distal disease, they may implant in the terminal bronchioles and alveoli (Fig. 14-1). At these sites bacilli are engulfed by resident pulmonary phagocytes (alveolar macrophages) in which they survive and multiply. After local replication bacilli spread through the lymphatics to regional, hilar, and mediastinal lymph nodes. Hematogenous spread to distal organs also may occur; the most common organs involved are the lung, bone marrow, liver, and spleen. Other organs are relatively resistant to infection by the tubercle bacillus. Regional lymph nodes in particular may contain large numbers of organisms. Organisms can multiple (before the establishment of immunity) in upper portions of the lung, epiphyseal lines of bones, regional lymph nodes, renal parenchyma, and cerebral cortex. Pleural effusion may occur at any time after the initial infection; it is most commonly, but not invariably, found on the same side as the primary pulmonary focus. The etiology of this effusion

seems to be the release of caseous material into the pleural space, which causes an inflammatory response and exudation of a clear, protein-rich fluid; a direct hematogenous seeding of the subpleural space also has been proposed. Undiagnosed or untreated primary tuberculosis with pleural effusion can organize and progress over several weeks to months into tuberculous empyema; this is a rare complication in children.

Lurie[2] in 1964 concluded that a favorable host response to invasion by tubercle bacilli depends on augmentation of the antimicrobial activity of the host's mononuclear phagocytes (macrophages). The incubation period from the time the tubercle bacillus enters the body until an acquired cellular immune response develops, as indicated by cutaneous sensitivity to tuberculoprotein, is 2–10 weeks. With the development of delayed hypersensitivity (acquired immunity), lymphocytes release products (lymphokines) that attract, localize, and activate macrophages; activated macrophages are able to destroy intracellular organisms. The development of specific immunity results in tissue inflammation, and this response rather than products of the tubercle bacillus results in the clinical symptoms and signs of primary tuberculosis. Acquired immunity does not depend on serum antibodies, but is exclusively cellular. Acquired immunity, in more than 90 percent of instances, is adequate to limit the initial multiplication of organisms, and the host remains asymptomatic or minimally symptomatic, with healing of the initial infectious focus. In a small percentage of persons who are initially infected, limitation of organism replication is inadequate, and clinical disease results. Natural resistance to tuberculous infection varies among ethnic groups and is affected by genetic factors, sex, age (women appear highly susceptible during adolescence or pregnancy), other disease processes (such as diabetes, measles, influenza, silicosis, malnourishment, immunosuppression), corticosteroid administration, and after a gastrectomy. In individuals with clinical disease, the causative organisms are almost always the persistent progeny of the original inhaled bacilli; they are not newly acquired bacteria. Over a period of weeks to years, a broad spectrum of disease can be produced by these organisms, with dissemination to organs that favor their persistence.

In children the first 5 years after the initial infection, and especially the first year, are the times when complications most commonly occur.

Figure 14-1. Pathogenesis of tuberculosis.

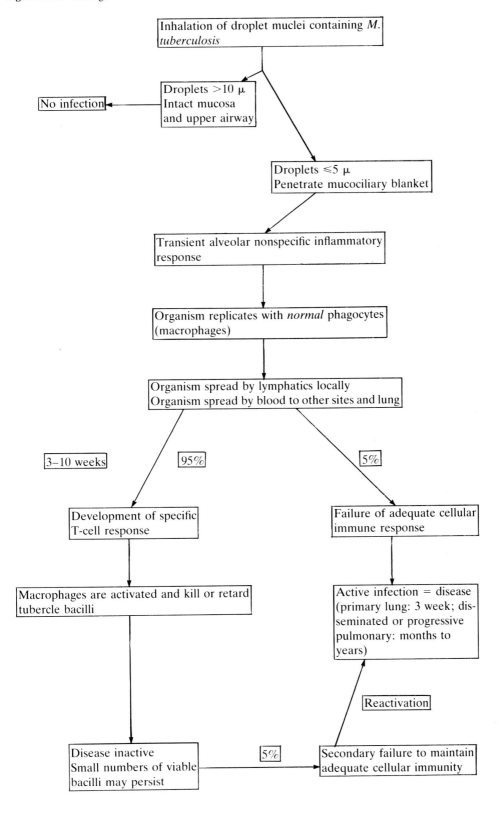

Walgren's timetable concept[3] is a useful approach for the clinician. It allows anticipation of complications and permits a realistic prognosis to be made. According to Walgren, there are three basic forms of pulmonary tuberculosis in children: (1) lymphohematogenous dissemination, (2) endobronchial tuberculosis, and (3) chronic pulmonary tuberculosis. Symptomatic lymphohematogenous spread, which results in manifestations such as miliary tuberculosis or tuberculous meningitis, occurs in only 0.5–3 percent of infected children; such infections usually occur within 3–6 months after the initial infection. Endobronchial tuberculosis (segmental pulmonary lesions due to infected regional lymph nodes) develops at a slightly later time. Metastatic bone and joint lesions, seen in 5–10 percent of infected children, appear about 1 year after the initial infection. Renal lesions appear only after 5–25 years. The appearance of chronic pulmonary tuberculosis is extremely variable, depending on the age when initial infection occurs; adolescents tend to have a short interval, whereas infants have a longer interval.

CLINICAL MANIFESTATIONS

Asymptomatic infection, defined as a reactive tuberculin test but no clinical or roentgenographic evidence of disease, is a frequent occurrence in children. However, children with a reactive tuberculin test and exposure to a patient with active tuberculosis should be suspected of having disease. Asymptomatic initial infection occurs more frequently in school-age children (elementary school) than in infants or adolescents; 40–50 percent of infants under 1 year of age and 80–90 percent of older children with newly reactive tuberculin tests have no recognizable symptoms. Physical findings are nonspecific and may or may not be present. Although a few patients have an acute onset of coughing, fever, chills, myalgias, and diaphoresis, a cough is rarely associated with pulmonary tuberculosis in children. Hemoptysis, dyspnea, acute or recurrent pleuritic pain, and erythema nodosum may be present but are seldom the initial complaint. Some older children and adolescents are first aware of anorexia, weight loss, fatigue, low-grade fevers, and irregular menses that do not resolve over weeks to months. A careful history and contact investigation should be undertaken.

As described in more detail later, chemotherapy for these children is mandatory along with close follow-up.

The endothoracic primary complex, as described by Ghon[4] in 1916, usually includes the primary pulmonary parenchymal focus, lymphangitis, and regional lymphadenitis with a heavy inoculum of tubercle bacilli in these nodes. The location of the primary pulmonary focus is subpleural in over 70 percent of patients. Tuberculosis may involve any lymph node; hilar or mediastinal involvement or both are frequently seen soon after the initial pulmonary infection. Although cervical and supraclavicular nodes are frequently involved in tuberculosis, young children with cervical adenitis due to mycobacteria are more likely to be infected with atypical mycobacteria.

Histopathologic evolution is characterized by the influx of acute inflammatory cells into the alveolus, producing localized consolidation. This is followed by the influx of alveolar macrophages with the formation of tubercles (granulomas). Granulomas organize and resolve or central caseation may develop; lesions that caseate contain large numbers of multiplying tubercle bacilli, which can then produce lymphangitis and regional lymphadenitis. All lobes of the lung are at equal relative risk of being infected with tubercle bacilli in children. Of the primary pulmonary infections 70–85 percent are initiated by one focus; Ghon[4] described 170 cases in which two foci were found in 15 percent, three foci in 7 percent, four foci in 3 percent, and five foci in 2 percent. When the cellular infiltrate reaches its maximal level 3–10 weeks after the initial infection, lymph node enlargement is usually much more striking than pulmonary parenchymal disease. Also at this time, infection may spread along adjacent lymphatics to distant lymph nodes. Spread occurs from left to right in most cases, and the right upper paratracheal nodes are most commonly involved. Cervical nodes may become infected after lymphatic spread to the apical pleura from subpleural sites; deep cervical and abdominal nodes may become infected by communication with the paratracheal nodes.

Localized or generalized pleural effusions (unilateral or bilateral) are seen so frequently with primary pulmonary infection that some investigators consider it to be part of the nonsegmental primary complex. Pleural seeding from an adjacent subpleural pulmonary or lymph node focus may produce no clinical symptoms or may produce localized pleuritis within 3–6 months of primary infection. Tuberculous pleural effusion is uncommon in children less than 2 years of age; it is more common in boys, almost never seen in segmental lesions, and only rarely seen in miliary infections. Symptoms, if present, are abrupt in onset (fever, pleuritic chest pain, dyspnea). The diagnostic procedure of choice in cases with pleural effusion is thoracentesis with a concomitant pleural biopsy. Up to 30 ml of fluid may be aspirated for chemistry, cytologic examinations, stains, and culture without complications. The characteristic findings in tuberculous pleural effusions are a greenish yellow color, often blood tinged, a specific gravity of 1.011 to 1.022, a pH level of 7.1 to 7.3, an increased protein level, and a low glucose (less than 30 mg/dL) concentration with inflammatory cells (polymorphonuclear leukocytes or lymphocytes, depending on the age of the effusion). Pleural fluid contains few bacilli; acid-fast stains and cultures are usually not rewarding. A pleural biopsy specimen more often reveals acid-fast bacilli and glanulomas on histologic staining and more often yields *M. tuberculosis* on culture.

Endobronchial tuberculosis, a complication, results from bronchial obstruction secondary to compression by enlarged, infected peribronchial nodes. This produces segmental pulmonary lesions on roentgenograms. In a study of children with endobronchial tuberculosis by Daley,[5] enlarged nodes were responsible for bronchial obstruction in more than one half of the cases. Damage to bronchial cartilage with gradual perforation and occlusion of the bronchus by caseous plugs or granulomatous tubercles were the other causes of bronchial obstruction. Potential clinical or roentgenographic manifestations can vary from sudden death by asphyxia (rare) to obstructive hyperaeration or a segmental lesion. Obstructive hyperaeration is not commonly seen; 7 of 538 cases with primary pulmonary infection were found in the study by Walker.[6] It occurs most often in children less than 2 years of age. These children are brought to medical attention with wheezing; the diagnosis is made using expiratory roentgenography. A segmental lesion is mainly due to atelectasis. It occurs in the segment involved in the primary infection and is fan shaped on the chest roentgenogram. Segmental lesions are more common in younger children and usually occur in the first 3–6 months after

infection. Focal physical findings in children with segmental lesions are usually absent.

In endothoracic primary complex disease, other less common complications resulting from impingement or erosion by infected nodes are dysphagia, tracheoesophageal fistulas, peripheral edema secondary to venous obstruction, erosion into major vessels, rupture into the mediastinum, phrenic nerve compression (with diaphragm paralysis), and pericarditis. Late manifestations of endothoracic primary complex disease are complete reexpansion of segmental lesions with residual calcifications, and, less frequently, scarring and segment contraction leading to bronchiectasis. Calcification of segmental caseous lesions occurs in 75–80 percent of children and usually involves the regional lymph nodes with or without pulmonary parenchymal calcification. Although most sequelae are asymptomatic and not visible on chest roentgenograms, permanent anatomic sequelae occur in up to 60 percent of segmental lesions.

Progressive primary pulmonary tuberculosis (cavitary disease) is a serious complication of primary pulmonary disease. It occurs when the primary focus does not resolve, but undergoes central caseation necrosis and enlarges. The caseous center is associated with large numbers of infectious bacilli that can empty into an adjacent bronchus, creating a cavity at the primary focus. This allows contiguous dissemination of tubercle bacilli to other lung areas or adjacent structures in the chest. The lesion occurs in adolescents and is associated with dramatic clinical symptoms and findings: spiking fever, malaise, coughing, weight loss, occasional hemoptysis, and physical signs of consolidation. Compared to the prechemotherapy era when up to 60–70 percent of children with progressive primary lesions died, the prognosis now is very good.

Endogenous reinfection in a localized dormant focus of previous tuberculous disease causes chronic pulmonary tuberculosis in up to 5 percent of patients. These sites are believed to be initially infected by a hematogenous route from the primary focus, remain small and quiescent for variable periods of time, and, if untreated, progress to the lesions of chronic pulmonary tuberculosis. The clinical manifestations of chronic pulmonary tuberculosis include coughing, chest pain, fever of unknown origin, cervical and supraclavicular lymphadenitis, and occasion-

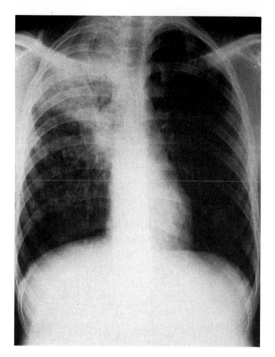

Figure 14-2. Active tuberculosis in a 16-year-old child. There is a dense infiltrate principally involving the posterior segment of the right upper lobe with early cavitation. This probably represents reactivation.

ally hemoptysis. This entity is rare in children and was uncommon even in the prechemotherapy era. Posterior apical involvement is most common (Fig. 14-2).

Extrapulmonary foci are inoculated with infectious bacilli by lymphohematogenous dissemination from the primary complex. Hematogenous spread is required for bacilli to reach distal organs; the spleen, liver, skin, meninges, and bone marrow are common sites of dissemination. The extent of disease is probably determined by host susceptibility at the time of primary infection, which determines the number of bacilli that disseminate. This initial spread may be occult, with symptoms subsequently occurring months to years later (renal tuberculosis), or protracted periods of symptomatic hematogenous focal or miliary dissemination may occur. The clinical picture of miliary tuberculosis varies greatly and probably depends on the quantity of tubercle bacilli in the bloodstream at any one time. The diagnosis is usually established by the combination of a compatible clinical picture with a reactive tuberculin skin test or evidence of an

infectious contact and a typical chest roentgenogram (Fig. 14-3). In miliary disease, tuberculin skin tests are commonly unreactive (25–30 percent). In such patients the diagnosis may be confirmed by a liver or bone marrow biopsy; occasionally, culturing the organism from urine confirms the diagnosis. Antituberculous therapy is usually successful in children with disseminated tuberculosis.

In newborns with suspected congenital or neonatal tuberculosis, the primary sites of infection are the liver and the lung. Hematogenous spread of bacilli through the placenta to the portal vein results in primary liver involvement; hematogenous spread or aspiration of infected amniotic fluid results in pulmonary involvement. In patients with congenital pulmonary tuberculosis, the mediastinal nodes are enlarged and caseous. Symptoms usually appear during the second week of life and include nasal discharge, bronchopneumonia, jaundice, hepatosplenomegaly, anorexia, and failure to gain weight. Congenitally and neonatally acquired tuberculosis cannot always be differentiated. Disease acquired during the neonatal period is predominantly pulmonary and may have a fulminant course, resembling an overwhelming bacterial infection. Although the diagnosis of congenital or neonatal tuberculosis has been made at autopsy on several occasions, a history of recent active tuberculous disease in the mother and increased clinical awareness have led to earlier diagnosis in recent years. Because the tuberculin test is very rarely reactive in infants, a higher index of suspicion, careful investigation of contacts, and confirmation of tubercle bacilli in endotracheal or bone marrow aspirates, gastric washings, or liver or lymph node biopsy specimens is essential. Although the clinical response is usually slow, successful treatment of congenital and neonatal tuberculosis has been reported.

DIFFERENTIAL DIAGNOSIS

In children tuberculosis may simulate many other diseases. Especially in the newborn and young infant, bacterial infections, including sepsis, pneumonia, or meningitis, may be difficult to differentiate. It may mimic or occur concurrently with pneumonia, sarcoidosis, lung abscess, or fungal infection. Mediastinal, axillary, cervical, or supraclavicular lymphadenopathy due to *M. tu-*

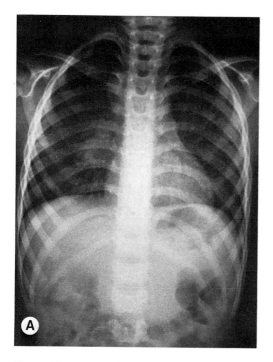
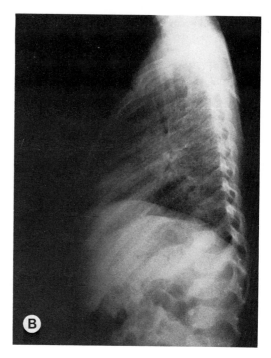

Figure 14-3. Tuberculosis in a 2½-year-old child. Diffuse miliary involvement is evident. A primary complex involving the right perihilar area and the perihilar nodes is present (**A**) Postero-anterior view. (**B**) Lateral view.

berculosis should be differentiated from atypical mycobacteria, bacterial and fungal lymphadenitis, tularemia, cat-scratch disease, and neoplasms.

DIAGNOSTIC TESTS AND CRITERIA

The diagnostic approach should include a careful history of the present illness, family history and history of contacts, tuberculin skin testing (with appropriate controls to rule out an anergic state), chest roentgenograms, and acid-fast stain and culture of body fluids and biopsy material. The importance of extensive and accurate historical information cannot be overemphasized in the pediatric age group. A history of exposure, the skin-test status of contacts, thereby, and the duration of therapy of tuberculous contacts should be elicited. This is especially important in newborns and young infants in whom skin testing is less accurate and the diagnosis more difficult.

In children, tuberculin reactivity usually develops 3–6 weeks (the range is a few days to 3 months) after the initial infection. Reactivity thus is usually present at the time symptoms are apparent; delayed development of reactivity is more common in newborn infants than in older children.

Purified protein derivative tuberculin, stabilized with Tween 80 (PPD-S) and standardized by biologic assay to 5 tuberculin units (TU) is the recommended antigen. The standard technique (Mantoux test) is the intracutaneous injection of 0.1 ml of PPD-S tuberculin (5 TU standard) into the skin. Multiple-prong (tine) tests should not be used for testing individuals suspected of having tuberculosis, since their sensitivity and specificity are inadequate for this purpose. The volar surface of the forearm is the usual injection site; the injection is made with a short, bluntly beveled 26- or 27-gauge needle. The injection should be made just beneath the surface of the skin with the needle bevel upward so as to create a discrete, pale 6- to 10-mm wheal. Tuberculin should never be transferred from one container to another, and skin tests should be performed immediately after the syringe is filled. The vial should be kept refrigerated and in the dark.

Tuberculin skin tests should be read 48–72 hours after injection when induration, if present, is most evident. Interpretation of the skin test is based on the presence or absence of induration, which should be judged both by inspection and by palpation. The diameter of induration should always be measured transversely to the long axis. Erythema without induration is not considered evidence of tuberculous infection. The skin test must be recorded as the "millimeter of induration" and the interpretation recorded; this avoids the simplistic and often misleading record of "positive" or "negative." Available data indicate that induration of 10 mm (or more) to a 5 TU PPD is significant. This test identifies at least 90 percent of those children infected with *M. tuberculosis* and identifies the lowest number of noninfected children as positive. When evaluating close contacts of infected persons, however, a reaction of 5 mm or more may be significant. In this situation, the goal is to identify as many individuals as possible who could be infected with *M. tuberculosis;* thus the reaction of 5 mm is appropriate. This interpretation may lead to the inclusion of a higher percentage of children infected with nontuberculous mycobacteria. Control skin testing to exclude anergy in children is important in proper interpretation of a PPD skin test having 0- to 5-mm induration (negative). Commonly used control skin-test antigens contain materials that most children have come into contact with or have been immunized with: *Candida, Trichophyton,* streptokinase-streptodornase, tetanus toxoid, or mumps antigens. The control skin test is applied and interpreted in the same manner as the PPD tuberculin. Control skin-test antigens must be standardized and routinely checked for reactivity in order to be used as indicators of anergy. Possible immunologic mechanisms of anergy include the presence of serum inhibitors, antigen-antibody complexes, a faulty inflammatory response, chemotaxis inhibitors, compartmentalization of sensitized lymphocytes, and adherent, immune suppressor cells. Compromised immune function in patients with localized, pulmonary tuberculosis tends to improve with treatment and recovery. This supports the view that immunologic abnormalities may be the result of, and not the cause of, tuberculous disease. There is evidence that immunologic response to mycobacteria may be linked to certain HLA phenotypes, suggesting that the presence of anergy may have a genetic component.

Delayed hypersensitivity to tuberculin, once present after mycobacterial infection or vaccination, may gradually wane over years. These individuals may have an insignificant initial skin test, but have a notable response to a subsequent test. This booster effect can be seen with a second test done as soon as 1 week after the initial test and can persist for up to 1 year. The booster phenomenon is present in all age groups, increases with age, and is prevalent in endemic areas for nontuberculous mycobacteria. Repeated skin testing of uninfected children does not sensitize them to tuberculin. Skin-test reactivity may temporarily decrease or disappear during any severe or febrile illness, rubella or other viral exanthemas, influenza, measles, live virus vaccinations, Hodgkin's disease, sarcoidosis, overwhelming miliary or pulmonary tuberculosis, and administration of adrenal corticosteroids or immunosuppressive drugs. Breast feeding or multiple transfusions from sensitized individuals rarely may result in passive transfer of delayed hypersensitivity and transient reaction to PPD tuberculin in a recipient who is not infected with *M. tuberculosis.*

Since the strength and duration of tuberculin reaction after the bacillus Calmette Guerin (BCG) vaccination is quite variable and cannot be distinguished from a reaction due to atypical or typical tuberculous infection, it has been suggested that the history of vaccination not alter the guidelines for interpretation of reactions.

Some authors consider the 250-TU skin test helpful in excluding tuberculosis with a negative reaction. When there is no reaction to 250 TU in a person with intact immunity, the presence of tuberculosis is unlikely. Precise guidelines for interpretation of reaction size are not available, however, and cross-reactivity with other mycobacteria is greater due to the high concentration of tuberculin.

Smith and Marquis[7] have described a combination of criteria for making the diagnosis of tuberculous disease in children. A combination of any two of the following six criteria is diagnostic for infection with *M. tuberculosis:*

1. A positive tuberculin skin test (PPD, 5 TU).
2. Clinical findings compatible with tuberculosis.
3. A history of close contact with an individual with active tuberculosis.
4. The presence of hilar or mediastinal lym-

phadenitis with or without a pulmonary lesion on a chest roentgenogram (posteroanterior and lateral view).

5. The presence of acid-fast bacilli on histologic examination of lymph nodes, bone, bone marrow, skin lesions, or pleura.

6. The most crucial single procedure for proving the diagnosis of tuberculosis is isolation of *M. tuberculosis;* this also allows for drug-susceptibility testing. The frequency of false-negative cultures and slow recovery time make reliance on the other criteria important.

If the diagnostic criteria suggest a tuberculous infection, but skin tests are unreactive (less than 5 mm) and cultures are pending, it is often worthwhile to repeat the skin test after 1–2 weeks. Tuberculin sensitivity may be developing or depressed; alternatively, the skin test may not have been satisfactorily performed. Other nonspecific laboratory findings are not helpful in diagnosing tuberculous infection in children. Among the laboratory values commonly associated with tuberculosis in children are an elevated erythrocyte sedimentation rate, anemia, and relative monocytosis.

The earliest manifestation of tuberculous involvement of the lung, whether in the young infant or child, is usually a parenchymal lymph node complex seen on chest roentgenography. A parenchymal lesion may appear at any stage of development and in any portion of the lung. If the lesion is large enough to be seen, unilateral involvement of the hilar or paratracheal mediastinal nodes are present (Fig. 14-3). Lymph node changes tend to persist longer than the parenchymal lesions, and calcification generally occurs within several years of the infection.

For optimal recovery of tubercle bacilli, clinical specimens should be transported to the laboratory promptly and processed immediately. Since disease may involve multiple sites, collection of samples for culture should be based on suspected sites of infection as shown in Table 14-1. In younger children sputum collection may not be feasible; in older children and adolescents who can cooperate, a series of at least three single, early-morning specimens should be collected on separate days. Early-morning gastric aspiration (approximately 50 ml) after an 8- to 10-hour fast permits the culture of swallowed sputum on 3 successive days. In patients with active pulmonary tuberculosis, the yield of positive cultures from three expectorated sputa is approximately 80 percent, three induced sputa is approximately 50 percent, and three optimally collected gastric aspirates is approximately 30 percent.

The time from receipt of the clinical specimen to confirmed culture with a report averages 3–6 weeks. All clinical specimens, once in the laboratory, should be inoculated directly into culture media to maximize the change of recovering the etiologic organism; culture media are sensitive enough to detect as few as 10 organisms for each milliliter of concentrated material. Mycobacterial culture media are of two basic categories: egg-potato–base media (Lowenstein-Jensen or American Trudeau Society media) and agar-base media (Middlebrook 7H10 and 7H11 media and Dubos media). Incubation of cultures at 5–10 percent carbon dioxide is optimal for growth.

THERAPY

Chemotherapy is highly effective in tuberculosis and is the major factor in the current decrease in the communicability of tuberculosis. Antituberculous chemotherapy is used to treat patients with clinical disease; it is used in asymptomatic individuals with a positive tuberculin skin test to prevent development of active disease and in certain tuberculin-negative patients to prevent infection after exposure to tuberculosis.

Of the 10 drugs currently used in the United States, isoniazid, rifampin, streptomycin, and ethambutol are the most effective and the least toxic. Second-line drugs, which may be used because of microbial resistance to first-line drugs, are pyrazinamide, ethionamide, para-aminosalicylic acid, kanamycin, capreomycin and cycloserine. Only the first-line drugs will be reviewed in this text.

Isoniazid, the hydrazide of isonicotinic acid, is the primary drug used for prophylaxis and treatment of disease caused by sensitive strains of *M. tuberculosis*. The drug is bacteriostatic at concentrations of 0.025–0.05 μg/ml; it is bactericidal if the bacilli are in an actively growing phase. Approximately 1 in 10^5 organisms is spontaneously resistant to isoniazid. The usual dosage in children is 10–20 mg/kg/day to a maximum of 300 mg in one daily dose. The drug is well absorbed orally, and peak plasma concen-

Table 14-1   *Diagnostic Methods of Choice in Childhood Tuberculosis*

Site	Diagnostic Procedure
Lungs	Smear and culture of spontaneous or induced sputum or three early morning gastric aspirates
Pleural Cavity	Culture and histologic examination of pleural biopsy specimens
Pericardium	Culture and histologic examination of pericardial biopsy specimens
Lymph nodes	Culture and histologic examination of excised node
Genitourinary tract	Culture of concentrated urine specimens
Skeletal system	Histologic examination and culture of bone
Peritoneum	Histologic examination and culture of peritoneal biopsy specimens
Meninges	Smear and culture of spinal fluid
Miliary	Culture and histologic examination of hepatic biopsy specimens; bone marrow biopsy has a somewhat lower yield

trations of 3–5 μg/ml are reached within 2 hours after ingestion. Isoniazid diffuses readily into pleural and peritoneal fluids and into cells. Concentrations in the cerebrospinal fluid are about 20 percent of those measured in the serum. The drug is metabolized in the liver by enzymatic acetylation and hydrolysis. The rate of acetylation of isoniazid is genetically determined. Rapid acetylators are more frequent in Eskimos and the Japanese. The incidence of slow acetylators among the various races in the United States is 50 percent. The rate of acetylation determines the pharmacokinetics of the drug; fast acetylators have lower serum levels and shorter half-lives. With the recommended dosage in children, however, there is no evidence that the acetylator phenotype interferes with the effectiveness of the drug. The half-life of the drug is prolonged in the presence of hepatic insufficiency.

Rifampin is a semisynthetic derivative of rifamycin B, a macrocyclic antibiotic with a broad spectrum of antimicrobial activity. Minimal inhibitory concentrations for *M. tuberculosis* range from 0.005 to 0.2 μ/ml. One of every 10^7 or 10^8 organisms in a population of *M. tuberculosis* bacilli is resistant to rifampin. Rifampin is readily absorbed after oral administration, if given on an empty stomach. The usual dosage is 20 mg/kg/day up to a maximum of 600 mg. Serum concentrations of about 10μg/ml are measured in adults 2 hours after an oral dose of 10 mg/kg. In infants, the same dose results in serum concentrations of about one third of those measured in adults. Rifampin undergoes deacetylation in the

liver, is excreted in the bile in the deacetylated form, and enterohepatic circulation follows. The deacetylated metabolite is fully active. The half life of the drug is increased in the presence of hepatic dysfunction. About 30 percent of the drug is excreted in the urine. There is no need to adjust the dosage in patients with impaired renal function. After usual doses, rifampin is present in significant concentrations in various tissues or body fluids such as sputum or cerebrospinal fluid. Concentrations of about 4μg/ml have been measured in tuberculous cavitary lesions. Both isoniazid and rifampin are active against intracellular, as well as extracellular, organisms.

Streptomycin is an aminoglycoside antibiotic. It is a bactericidal drug active against gram-negative bacilli, some strains of staphylococci, and mycobacteria. The minimal inhibitory concentration for *M. tuberculosis* may be as low as 0.5 μg/ml, and most of the strains are inhibited by 10μg/ml. One organism in a population of 10^6 tubercle bacilli is resistant. Streptomycin is not significantly absorbed from the gastrointestinal tract and must be administered intramuscularly. The usual dosage is 15–20 mg/kg/day in one injection. The drug diffuses readily in pleural or peritoneal fluid and in tuberculous cavities but does not penetrate adequately into the cerebrospinal fluid. Streptomycin is excreted in the urine, and the dosage must be adjusted in patients with impaired renal function. It is only active against extracellular organisms.

Ethambutol is a tuberculostatic agent. The usual dosage is 15 mg/kg/day orally in one dose, and 75–80 percent of the dose is absorbed from the gastrointestinal tract. Sixty-five percent of an ingested dose is excreted in the urine. Ethambutol accumulates in patients with impaired renal function, and the dosage must be adjusted.

Isoniazid, rifampin, streptomycin, and ethambutol, although safe in the majority of patients when administered at the recommended dosage, may produce untoward effects varying in severity. Isoniazid has been associated with peripheral neuritis and hepatitis and rarely with hypersensitivity reactions. Peripheral neuritis, which is manifested by paresthesia in the hands and feet, is due to competitive inhibition of pyridoxine utilization. This adverse reaction is very rarely observed in children with adequate dietary sources of pyridoxine; patients who are receiving isoniazid therapy and whose nutrition may be inadequate should also take 5–50 mg of pyridoxine each day. Of more concern is the liver disease that has been associated with isoniazid. The clinical features of isoniazid liver toxicity may vary from isolated biochemical signs of hepatocellular necrosis to a syndrome resembling typical viral hepatitis. Significant elevation of transaminases precedes the clinical symptoms, and promp cessation of therapy generally causes a rapid improvement in liver function tests. The incidence of hepatitis probably due to isoniazid is very low in children, but increases with age. In a large cooperative surveillance study performed by the Public Health Service, no cases of hepatotoxicity were detected in individuals younger than 20 years. In contrast, in the 35- to 43-year-old age group, the incidence of progressive liver damage from isoniazid was 1.2 percent. Isolated biochemical signs of hepatocellular necrosis occur more frequently; in a series of 363 children receiving isoniazid at a single daily dose of 10 mg/kg, 6.8 percent had an increase in serum transaminases during the course of therapy. Overt clinical manifestations did not develop in any of these patients. Slow acetylator phenotypes have been believed to be associated with an increased risk of isoniazid hepatotoxicity, but this remains controversial. Monitoring for toxicity should be performed by questioning and examining the patient for prodromal signs of liver dysfunction at monthly intervals. Routine monitoring of liver function tests is not necessary in children. Isoniazid has been demonstrated to interfere with the pharmacokinetics of diphenylhydantoin, resulting in toxicity. During therapy, the dosage of diphenylhydantoin should be reduced and the serum concentration monitored. Hypersensitivity reactions to isoniazid are manifested by a fever, skin rash, and lupuslike appearance.

Adverse effects of rifampin can be divided into three categories: (1) those associated with an immunologic reaction to the drug, (2) direct tissue toxicity, and (3) interactions with other drugs. A flulike syndrome, possibly associated with renal function impairment, thrombocytopenia, and rarely hemolysis, has been associated with the presence of circulation antibodies that react with rifampin. This group of manifestations appears to occur more frequently in patients who have taken the drug at irregular intervals and only infrequently when this drug is taken daily without interruption. Severe reactions respond generally to supportive therapy and discontinuation of the drug; moderate reactions respond to reinstitution of regular administration of the drug. Hepatitis is due to direct toxicity of the drug. Clinical and biochemical manifestations are comparable to isoniazid hepatitis. Although the incidence of mild liver toxicity is higher in patients receiving the combination of isoniazid and rifampin than in patients receiving either drug alone, it appears from the very low rate reported in children that the combination of these drugs is probably safe. Being a hepatic mixed-function oxidase inducer, rifampin has adverse interactions with drugs that depend on the oxidase enzyme system for clearance. Warfarins, para-aminosalicylic acid, methadone, corticoids, and oral contraceptives are among the drugs whose metabolism is accelerated by rifampin.

Streptomycin, as all aminoglycosides, is nephrotoxic and can cause eighth cranial nerve damage. The dosage should be modified in the presence of renal insufficiency. Renal and auditory function should be monitored during therapy.

Ethambutol produces very few toxic reactions when a dose of 15 mg/kg is used. If higher doses are administered, the major toxicity is retrobulbar neuritis. This involves generally the central fibers of the optic nerves and results in blurred vision, a decrease in visual acuity, central scotoma, and sometimes loss of the ability to perceive the color green. Baseline visual acuity and red–green color discrimination tests are required; this prohibits the use of ethambutol in very young children.

MODALITIES OF TREATMENT

The observation that natural resistance to each of the major antituberculous drugs occurs in a significant proportion of organisms precludes monotherapy of the disease. Treating patients with combinations of two or more drugs lowers the chance of selecting a resistant organism during treatment. For example, in a patient with cavitary lesions containing up to 10^9 organisms, 10^5 organisms will be naturally resistant to isoniazid and 10^7 to rifampin. Only 1 out of 10^5 times 10^7 (1 out of 10^{12}) organisms will be resistant to both drugs, that is, there is only 1 chance in 1000 that a single bacterium which harbors this pattern of resistance is present. The usual regimen for therapy of pulmonary tuberculosis consists of isonizaid at 10 mg/kg (maximum 300 mg/day) and rifampin at 20 mg/kg (maximum 600 mg/day) or, in children older than 13 years, ethambutol at 15 mg/kg. If the possibility of drug resistance is suspected, for example, when the infecting source is known to harbor a resistant organism or in children of Indochinese refugees, three drugs should be used to assure that the organism is at least sensitive to two antibiotics, the third agent may be either streptomycin, ethambutol, or kanamycin. The standard duration of therapy was previously 18 months to 2 years, depending on the bacteriologic status of the patient at the time of diagnosis. The major obstacle to the success of therapy is patient compliance. In recent years, increasing efforts have been made to shorten the duration of therapy and to administer drugs intermittently.[8] It has been demonstrated that 9 months of treatment are as effective as the longer courses, provided that both isoniazid and rifampin are used. Moreover, in underdeveloped countries, after an initial daily phase of therapy ranging from 2 weeks to 2 months, which results in a substantial decrease in the number of infecting organisms, treatment may be given on a twice-weekly basis with acceptable results. This regimen can be fully supervised, if necessary, to ensure compliance.

The recommendation that patients with active tuberculosis be isolated has also been reconsidered. Patients can be admitted to community hospitals rather than to sanitariums, provided that effective isolation measures are applied while therapy reduces the infectiousness. Patients with non cavitary disease may not require hospitalization. It has been shown that patients with a sputum culture growing *M. tuberculosis* are quickly rendered noninfectious by effective chemotherapy.[9] Return of the patients to their families soon after initiation of chemotherapy therefore has been advocated. Monitoring of the outpatient should be directed toward observing the regression of the disease with therapy, compliance, and evidence of drug toxicity. Clinical improvement should be present after 2 weeks of treatment. If the disease has been bacteriologically proven by sputum or gastric fluid culture, the smears and culture should be repeated. The cultures should be repeated 3–6 weeks after the beginning of the treatment to verify the appropriateness of the therapy. Chest roentgenograms should be repeated after 1 month of treatment. Patients and their families must be educated on the reasons and modalities of prolonged, regular therapeutic regimens, including multiple drug use and the early signs of drug toxicity. A monthly clinic visit should be recommended. After a successful course of chemotherapy, supervision of the patient can be discontinued.

PREVENTION OF TUBERCULOSIS

The opportunity to prevent tuberculosis exists at two stages. Vaccination or chemoprophylaxis can be used before the acquisition of infection in individuals at high risk, and chemoprophylaxis can prevent active disease in asymptomatic tuberculin reactors.

Chemoprophylaxis

The administration of isoniazid for 3 months after a household exposure to a person with active disease is highly effective in reducing the rate of tuberculin conversion. The skin test should be repeated at the end of that period. If it becomes positive (greater than 10-mm induration) the patient should be evaluated for tuberculosis infection, and treatment is indicated.

It also has been convincingly demonstrated that isoniazid prevents patients with tuberculosis infection from developing active disease. A 19-year follow-up study[10] has shown that this protective effect persists. All individuals who recently have had a change in skin test from negative to positive should receive prophylaxis. Other groups of patients in whom the benefit of chemoprophylaxis outweighs the risk of isoniazid hepatotoxicity are tuberculin reactors with medical conditions such as immunosuppressive therapy, diabetes, or a gastrectomy or skin-test reactors with a chest roentgenogram suggestive of inactive disease. With non-recent tuberculin reactors, the risk of developing active tuberculosis is lower than the risk of hepatic toxicity after the age of 35 years. Isoniazid prophylaxis is therefore not recommended after the age of 35 years in patients whose skin test reactivity is not from recent acquisition.

BCG

Vaccine-induced protection against tuberculosis depends on establishment of a specific cell-mediated immune response. BCG was produced early in this century by attenuation of a virulent strain of *M. bovis*. Since vaccines are produced in different countries using different BCG "daughter" strains, notable differences in their immunizing potency exist. There are still questions about the efficacy of the vaccine; controlled trials[11] have shown discordant results, ranging from 0 to 80 percent protection. The World Health Organization recommends administration of the vaccine by intradermal injection. A local reaction usually develops within 6 weeks and consists of a papule at the site of injection. This is generally followed by a small ulceration and results in a scar. In 1–10 percent of vaccinees, ulceration may be more severe and prolonged, with purulent drainage and enlargement of the regional lymph nodes. BCG osteomyelitis has been reported in one out of a million vaccines. A tuberculin skin test should be performed 2 or 3 months after vaccination. If the skin test remains unreactive, a second dose should be given. After BCG vaccination, it is generally not possible to distinguish a reactive skin test resulting from post vaccination sensitivity from a reactive skin test caused by infection.

Because of the questions about its efficacy and the success of tuberculosis control in the United States by case identification, treatment, and prophylaxis with isoniazid, the use of BCG vaccine in this country is restricted to specific circumstances. The advisory committee on immunization practices of the Public Health Service recommends its use in individuals, particularly infants in a household, who have repeated exposure to untreated patients with pulmonary tuberculosis whose sputum grows the organism or in groups with an excessive rate of new infection and in which the other measures of control have failed.

DRUG SUSCEPTIBILITY TESTING

Patients with newly diagnosed tuberculosis and no previous treatment should begin receiving chemotherapy before isolation of the organism and susceptibility testing. Less than 30 percent of the tuberculosis cases occurring in children under 15 years old are confirmed bacteriologically. If the organism is recovered, however, sensitivity testing allows the physician to adapt the chemotherapy specifically; testing also helps by providing epidemiologic data on the general pattern of drug resistance in the country. Susceptibility tests are based on the growth of the organism on a solid medium. The amount of growth on antibiotic containing media is compared with the growth on drug-free controls. Because mycobacteria are slow-growing organisms, sensitivity testing requires 4–6 weeks of incubation, although more rapid methods are now being evaluated. Control organisms with known drug sensitivity should be included in every testing to check the activity of drug-containing media. The drug susceptibility test can be performed by using a clinical specimen, if acid-fast bacilli can be demonstrated on the smear (direct drug susceptibility test), or a subculture from the primary isolation medium as the inoculum (indirect sensitivity test). Resistance occuring in isolates from patients with no previous exposure to antituberculous drugs is called primary drug resistance. A recent survey[12] of primary resistance in the United States indicated rates varying from 3.3 to 15.1 percent (mean 8.5 percent) among the various geographic areas. Resistance rates were higher in younger patients than older ones and varied among various racial groups; it was highest in southeast Asians and Mexican-Americans. Resistance to more than one drug was present in one third of these organisms. About 3.9 percent of the organisms were resistant to streptomycin, 4.1 percent to isoniazid, 0.2 percent to rifampin, and 0.3 percent to ethambutol.

Patients who relapse after having been treated for tuberculosis are particularly likely to be infected by drug-resistant organisms. (secondary drug resistance). In these patients, susceptibility testing of the isolate is mandatory. Before the results are available, therapy should be started with a regimen including at least two drugs to which the patient has never been exposed.

CASE REPORTS

A 30-year-old nurse working in a community hospital was found to have pulmonary tuberculosis. A tuberculin test performed 8 months earlier was negative. She complained of coughing and fatigue for 2 months and had lost 12 pounds. Her chest roentgenogram showed an infiltrate in the left apex with multiple small cavities. Her two children, 5 and 7 years of age, had normal physical examinations but had positive (greater than 10-mm induration) intermediate-strength PPD skin tests. The eldest child had a normal chest roentgenogram and was considered to have asymptomatic tuberculous infection. Chemoprophylaxis was started with isoniazid and was continued for 1 year; at that time clinical examination indicated a normal child, as did a chest roentgenogram performed after 1 month of treatment. The youngest had right hilar lymphadenopathy with a small infiltrate in the right lower lobe on the chest roentgenogram. He was diagnosed as having primary pulmonary tuberculosis and was treated with isoniazid and rifampin for 1 year. He remained clinically asymptomatic, and the chest infiltrate disappeared after 2 months of treatment. None of the children had signs of drug toxicity. A culture of the mother's sputum yielded *M. tuberculosis* resistant to streptomycin but sensitive to isoniazid and rifampin. Culture of the gastric fluid and urine of the children did not yield the organism.

A 7-year-old boy of Laotian origin was brought to medical attention with a 10-day history of fever and progressive respiratory distress. On admission his temperature was 40°C, and he had chills and tachypnea. The physical examination revealed diminished breath sounds and thin rales in the left lung base. The neurologic examination was normal. A chest roentgenogram showed left hilar adenopathy and a dense left lower lobe infiltrate. Antibiotic treatment was started with penicillin G. A tuberculin test placed the day of admission was positive (35-mm induration with a blister). Two antituberculous drugs, isoniazid and rifampin, were added to the treatment. On the fifth hospital day, the child had a persistant high fever, and right third cranial nerve palsy developed. A spinal tap was performed. Cerebrospinal fluid examination was consistent with the diagnosis of tuberculous meningitis (a white blood cell count of 150/mm^3 with 70 percent lymphocytes and 30 percent neutrophils; the protein level was 150 mg/dl, and the glucose level was 32 mg/dL with a blood glucose level of 88 mg/dL). Two other antituberculous drugs were started (ethambutol and streptomycin), as well as corticosteroids. The clinical course was uneventful. The child was afebrile on the eighth hospital day. Pulmonary signs improved greatly in the first 2 weeks of treatment, and the child gradually recovered full range of motion of his eyes. Cultures of the gastric fluid and cerebrospinal fluid grew *M. tuberculosis* sensitive to the four antituberculous drugs. Corticosteroids were tapered and stopped in 3 months. Streptomycin was discontinued after 1 month, and ethambutol was discontinued after the sensitivity of the isolate was known. Therapy with isoniazid and rifampin was continued for 18 months.

REFERENCES

1. Ghon A, Kuedlich H: Die Eintrittspforten der Infektion. In Engel, S., and Pirquet, C. (eds): *Handbuch der Kindertuberkulose.* Stuttgart, Georg Thieme Verlag, 1930.
2. Lurie MB: *Resistance to Tuberculosis: Experimental Studies in Native and Acquired Defense Mechanisms.* Cambridge, Mass, Harvard University Press, 1964.
3. Walgren A: The timetable of tuberculosis. *Tubercle* 29: 245–251, 1948.
4. Ghon A: *The Primary Lung Focus of Tuberculosis in Children.* London, JA Churchill Ltd, 1916.
5. Daley JF, Brown DS, Lincoln EM, et al. Endobronchial tuberculosis in children. *Dis. Chest* 22:380–398, 1952.
6. Walker CHM. Pulmonary primary tuberculosis in childhood. *Lancet* 1: 218–223, 1955.
7. Smith MHD, Marquis JR. Tuberculosis and other mycobacterial infections, in Feigin RD, Cherry JD (eds). *Pediatric Infectious Diseases.* Philadelphia,

WB Saunders Co, 1981, p 1016.
8. Guidelines for short-course tuberculosis chemotheraphy. *MMWR* 29:97, 1980.
9. Gunnels JJ, Bates JH, Swindol H. Infectivity of sputum positive tuberculosis patients on chemotherapy. *Am Rev Respir Dis* 109: 323–330, 1973.
10. Comstock GW, Baum C, Snider DE Jr. Isoniazid prophylaxis among Alaskan Eskimos: a final report of the Bethel isoniazid studies. *Am Rev Respir Dis* 119:827–830, 1973.
11. Eickhoff TC. The current status of BCG immunization against tuberculosis. *Annu Rev Med* 28:411, 1977.
12. Kopanoff DE, Kilburn JO, Glassroth JF, et al. A continuing survey of tuberculosis primary drug resistance in the United States: March 1975 to November 1977: A United States Public Health Service cooperative study. *Am Rev Respir Dis* 118:835–842, 1978.

SUGGESTED READINGS

American Thoracic Society. Diagnostic standards and classification of tuberculosis and other mycobacterial diseases. *Am Rev Respir Dis* 1981; 123:343.

BCG Vaccines. Recommendations of the Public Health Service advisory committee on Immunization practices. *MMWR* 28, 21:241, 1979.

Glassroth JG, Robins AG, Snider DE. Tuberculosis in the 1980's. *N Engl J Med 3*302:1441–1460, 1980.

Kopanoff DEC, Snider DE, Jr, Caras GJ. Isonazid related hepatitis: A U.S. Public Health Service cooperative surveillance study. *Am Rev Respir Dis.* 117:991–1001, 1978.

Lincoln EM, Sewell EM. *Tuberculosis in children.* New York, McGraw-Hill Book Co, 1963.

Mandall GL, Sande MA. Antimicrobial agents: drugs used in the chemotherapy of tuberculosis and leprosy, in Goodman L, Gilman A (eds). *The Pharmacological basis of therapeutics.* Macmillan Publishing Co, Inc, New York, p 1200–1221. 1975.

Primary resistance to antituberculosis drugs–United States. *MMWB* 29:345, 1980.

Rich AR. *The Pathogenesis of Tuberculosos.* Springfield, Ill, Charles C Thomas Publisher, 1944.

Tuberculosis Statistics: States and Cities, 1979. Atlanta, Center for Disease Control, Tuberculosis Control Division, 1980.

15

Respiratory Failure in Children

Eliezer Nussbaum

Respiratory failure is defined as the inability of the lungs to adequately deliver oxygen to the pulmonary circulation and/or remove carbon dioxide. The partial pressure of arterial oxygen (Pao_2) is therefore below the predicted normal range for the patient's age at the prevalent barometric pressure, or the partial pressure of arterial carbon dioxide ($Paco_2$) is elevated above the upper normal range. It has been accepted that in respiratory failure the Pao_2 is below 60 mm Hg in room air, and the $Paco_2$ is above 50 mm Hg.

An elevated $Paco_2$ can occur in patients with chronic obstructive pulmonary disease who manifest chronic carbon dioxide retention.

This chapter is limited to Pulmonary diseases of children beyond the perinatal period, thus excluding infants with hyaline membrane disease, congenital diaphragmatic hernias, and other diseases unique to the perinatal period. Some of these diseases will be discussed in detail in other chapters.

INCIDENCE

The precise incidence of respiratory failure in the pediatric age group is difficult to assess, since its clinical manifestations overlap a broad spectrum of syndromes and diseases.

The incidence of respiratory failure in asthmatic children in two major children's hospitals has been estimated to range from 1 to 5.3 percent. This represents only one example. In the majority of cases, the term respiratory failure is frequently substituted for its underlying disease entity, such as cystic fibrosis, acute epiglottitis, and muscular dystrophy (Table 15-1), resulting in a low and probably underestimated incidence.

CAUSES OF RESPIRATORY FAILURE

In the majority of cases, respiratory failure can be linked to an underlying disease. But recent studies of unexplained respiratory failure have demonstrated an association with depressed ventilatory responses to hypoxia or hypercapnia or both. Decreased chemosensitivity to the hypoxic ventilatory drive or an attenuated response to hypercapnia has been recently demonstrated in children with bronchial asthma.

For a systematic approach we have divided the causes of respiratory failure in children into five major groups (Table 15-1): (1) central nervous system and neuromuscular disorders, (2) upper airway obstruction, (3) lower airway obstruction, (4) cardiovascular diseases, and (5) hematology/oncology causes.

PATHOPHYSIOLOGIC MECHANISMS

Respiratory failure is invariably associated with hypoxemia. If one excludes the presence of an intracardiac shunt or low barometric pressure (such as found in high altitudes), a low Pao_2 is the result of any or a combination of the following:

1. Poor ventilation
2. Abnormal diffusion
3. Imbalance between alveolar ventilation and pulmonary perfusion
4. Intrapulmonary shunting

The concentration of inspired oxygen (Fio_2) should be taken into account so that alveolar oxygen tension (P_Ao_2) can be calculated to derive the alveolar-arterial oxygen gradient. Since the

173

Table 15-1 *Causes of Respiratory Failure*

Central Nervous System and Neuromuscular Disorders	Upper Airway Obstruction	Lower Airway Obstruction	Cardiovascular Diseases	Hematology/Oncology Causes
Head trauma	Aspiration of a foreign body	Acute bronchial asthma	Congenital heart diseases with pump failure	Severe anemia
Spinal cord injury	Congenital anomalies (e.g., Pierre Robin syndrome)	Pneumothorax	Vascular ring or enlarged heart with secondary compression of large airways	Tumors compressing major bronchi (e.g., Hodgkins disease, bronchogenic cysts, and tumors with massive metastases to the lung)
Sedative overdose		Severe pneumonia (such as that caused by *Pneumocystic carinii*, staphylococcal organism, or adenoviruses)		
Guillain-Barré syndrome	Choanal atresia		Severe pulmonary hypertension with ventilatory decompensation secondary to prolonged massive left-to-right shunting	
Intracranial tumors	Acute epiglottitis	Massive pleural effusion or severe empyema (also includes chylothorax, hemothorax, and hydrothorax)		
Myasthenia gravis	Severe laryngotracheitis			
Meningoencephalitis	Severe subglottic stenosis			
Muscular dystrophy	Vocal cord paraylsis	Pulmonary contusion		
Poliomyelitis	Vascular ring	"Shock lung" or adult type respiratory distress syndrome (ARDS)		
Intracranial hemorrhage	Tumors in upper airways (e.g., papillomas or hemangiomas)	Hyaline membrane disease		
Central apnea or primary alveolar hypoventilation (e.g., obesity-hypoventilation syndrome)		Massive atelectasis		
		Bronchiolitis		
		Cystic fibrosis		
		Pulmonary edema		
		Pulmonary emboli		
		Aspiration of foreign material		
		Diaphragmatic hernia		

normal alveolar-arterial oxygen gradient is below 15 mm Hg, a significant increase may suggest hypoxemia resulting either from ventilation/perfusion imbalance, intrapulmonary (or intracardiac) shunting, or poor diffusion. When hypoxemia results from hypoventilation, however, both Pao_2 and P_AO_2 will be low, thereby giving minimal or no change in the alveolar-arterial oxygen gradient. The P_AO_2 can be calculated as follows:

$$P_AO_2 = PIO_2 - \frac{P_ACO_2}{R} + F$$

$$PIO_2 = FIO_2(PB - PH_2O)$$

PIO_2 is the partial pressure of inspired oxygen, P_ACO_2 is the partial pressure of alveolar carbon dioxide, and R (respiratory exchange ratio) represents the ratio of carbon dioxide production to oxygen consumption. FIO_2 represents the percentage of inspired oxygen, PB is the barometric pressure, and PH_2O is the pressure of water vapor at body temperature (47 mm Hg). For simple calculation R is considered to be 0.8 and the P_ACO_2 equals the $Paco_2$.

The difference between the P_AO_2 and Pao_2 represents the alveolar-arterial oxygen gradient as follows:

$$P(A - aDO_2) = P_AO_2 - Pao_2$$

Calculation of $P(A - aDO_2)$ allows approximation of intrapulmonary shunting.

$Paco_2$ is the arterial representation of alveolar ventilation, and when increased it signifies hypoventilation. A relationship between timed alveolar ventilation (V_A) and P_ACO_2 is expressed by the following formula:

$$P_ACO_2 = \frac{0.863 \times \dot{V}CO_2}{\dot{V}A}$$

This formula shows the inverse relationship between V_A and P_ACO_2. In practical terms, a disease causing hypoventilation, such as acute bronchial asthma or severe pneumonia, will result in an elevated level of $Paco_2$, poorly ventilated alveoli, and a low ratio of ventilation/pulmonary perfusion.

Keeping the above introduction in mind, respiratory failure has been divided into two major groups: types I and II.

Type I Respiratory Failure

Type I respiratory failure represents poor oxygenation but relatively adequate ventilation. Patients in this group have a low Pao_2 and a normal or low $Paco_2$. This type has been also termed *nonventilatory*, or *normal ventilatory*, respiratory failure. Type I is manifested by an increase in $P(A - aDO_2)$ usually due to any pathologic condition affecting alveolar or distal airways such as found in bronchial asthma or cystic fibrosis. This results in ventilation/perfusion ($\dot{V}A/\dot{Q}$) imbalance, shunting, and failure of oxygenation without failure of ventilation. Since poor compliance with a low tidal volume (V_T) may accompany this situation, the human body will attempt to compensate for minute ventilation ($\dot{V}E = V_T \times f$) by increasing the respiratory frequency (f). The majority of patients with status asthmaticus will fall into this category. They have tachypnea and a low Pao_2, but also normal or a low $Paco_2$ due to hyperventilation. Decompensated carbon dioxide retention results in progression to type II respiratory failure.

Type II Respiratory Failure

Type II respiratory failure represents a ventilatory defect with a low Pao_2, rising $Paco_2$, and an imbalance in $V_A/\dot{Q}$. Patients can manifest both types of respiratory failure during the course of one disease. For example, patients with status asthmaticus with a low Pao_2 and a low or normal $Paco_2$ may progress to type II respiratory failure with rising $Paco_2$. Other examples include hypoxic patients with cystic fibrosis, "shock lung," severe pneumonia, or acute epiglottitis who may progress from type I to type II respiratory failure. On the other hand, some patients will manifest type II respiratory failure during the initial course of the disease and later shift into type I respiratory failure, for example, a child who aspirates gastric contents after an accidental barbiturate overdose. Initially, the respiratory drive will be depressed, leading to hypoventilation with rising $Paco_2$ and concomitant hypoxemia due to aspiration (a combination of types I and II respiratory failure). Later, on awakening and regaining the respiratory drive, the child will hyperventilate and blow carbon dioxide but remain hypoxic, thus representing a shift to type I respiratory failure. In bronchial asthma arterial

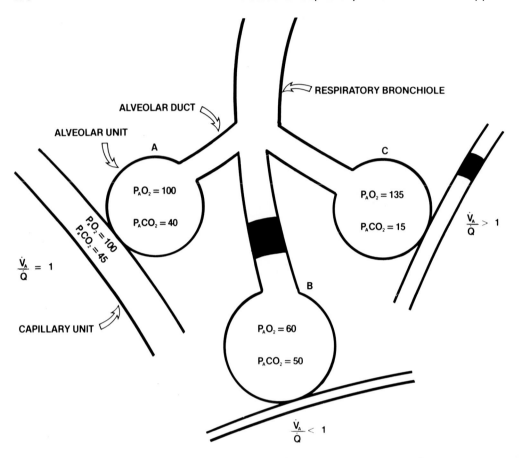

Figure 15-1. Relationships between alveolar ventilation ($\dot{V}A$) and capillary perfusion ($\dot{Q}$). (*A*) Normal relationship when ventilation and perfusion are perfectly matched ($\dot{V}A/\dot{Q} = 1$). (*B*) Alveolus is underventilated with respect to capillary perfusion ($\dot{V}A/\dot{Q} < 1$). (*C*) Alveolus is relatively hyperventilated with respect to poor capillary perfusion ($\dot{V}A/\dot{Q} > 1$).

blood gas studies may combine both types I and II respiratory failure, representing areas of the lung with an abnormal relationship between ventilation and perfusion (Fig. 15-1). Arterial blood gas studies therefore should be interpreted as the sum of alveolar-capillary units with a low, normal, and high ratio between $\dot{V}A$ and capillary perfusion (Fig. 15-1).

Hypoxia and hypoxemia are the common denominators for any type or combination of respiratory failure and can potentially result in pulmonary hypertension and increased pulmonary vascular resistance (PVR). Hemodynamic assessments of PVR will be discussed later.

Although the importance of arterial blood gases in the objective assessment of either type I or II respiratory failure has been emphasized,

they should be interpreted in view of the clinical picture. Type II is considered more critical than type I respiratory failure, although this may be sometimes misleading. For example, patients can die from hypoxia alone (type I), such as in adult respiratory distress syndrome, without having carbon dioxide retention, whereas some individuals with chronic carbon dioxide retention, such as cystic fibrosis patients, may live. Also, serial samples of arterial blood gases should be obtained in order to evaluate dynamic changes in the acid-base status of these patients.

The most common cause of hypoxemia or an increase in the $P(A - aDO_2)$ is a $\dot{V}A/\dot{Q}$ imbalance in which the $\dot{V}A$ is not proportional to capillary perfusion. During such an imbalance, hypoxemia can be accompanied by hypercapnia, although hyperventilation may actually lower the $Paco_2$. Since hypoxemia may persist, the resulting P(A − aDO_2) indicates either $\dot{V}_A/\dot{Q}$ mismatching, a diffusion abnormality, or shunting.

The mechanisms of hypoventilation are somewhat different. The following formula shows the basic process associated with hypoventilation:

$$\dot{V}_A = \dot{V}_E - \dot{V}_D$$

Minute alveolar ventilation $\dot{V}_A$ is proportionally related to the total amount of air moved each minute ($\dot{V}_E$) and is inversely related to total dead space ventilated each minute ($\dot{V}_D$). Based on this formula the following three basic mechanisms, separate or in combination, may be responsible for hypoventilation:

1. Increased $\dot{V}_D$, for example, children with bronchial asthma or cystic fibrosis with segmental atelectasis secondary to a mucous plug
2. Decreased $\dot{V}_E$, for example, central nervous system depression secondary to drug overdose, chest wall paralysis, poliomyelitis, or any disease involving central nervous system output
3. Poor elimination of progressive carbon dioxide production, which can be found in patients with cystic fibrosis, end-state muscular dystrophy, or severe bronchial asthma

Acute respiratory failure may result in respiratory acidosis (a pH level below 7.35) that can be corrected if the primary defect has been resolved, namely, the poor ventilatory status of the child. Attempts to restore the acid-base balance by giving sodium bicarbonate (HCO_3^- therefore are futile. For clarification, the Henderson-Hasselbalch equation can be expressed as a physiologic relationship between the respiratory and renal systems as follows:

$$pH = PK + \log \frac{HCO_3^-}{0.03 \times Paco_2}$$

$$\approx \frac{HCO_3^-}{Paco_2} = \frac{Kidney}{Lungs}$$

Since the $Paco_2$ is increased in acute respiratory failure, the pH level will be lowered; therefore this imbalance will be corrected only after correcting the ventilatory status of the patient. In chronic situations the kidneys will preserve HCO_3^-, thus maintaining a normal pH level. It is recognized that therapy for this condition should be aimed at improving $\dot{V}_A$ rather than correcting the chemical-metabolic imbalance. In patients with cardiovascular failure or prolonged hypoxemia, this process can be complicated by metabolic acidosis due to lactic acid accumulation. A combination of respiratory and lactic acidosis will require ventilatory support and Na/HCO_3 I.V. therapy.

Arterial blood gas studies (mainly the $Paco_2$ level) should confirm the diagnosis, since clinical evaluation in most situations is unreliable.

CLINICAL MANIFESTATIONS

Respiratory failure is associated with a variety of entities as described in Table 15-1. Since it is unrealistic to comprehend the entire spectrum of respiratory failure, it may be more productive to focus on limited, but recognized, disorders and also introduce modern concepts in monitoring and therapy.

General Considerations

The criteria for respiratory failure combine clinical assessments with arterial blood gas studies. It is emphasized that since clinical evaluation may be unreliable, arterial blood gas studies are mandatory. An example is a patient with severe respiratory failure who is anemic and therefore does not have peripheral cyanosis. In general, children in respiratory failure will have tachypnea, dyspenia with chest retractions and flaring of the ala nasi, tachycardia, and occasionally cyanosis. They may be exhausted, irritable, and even comatose due to carbon dioxide retention. Breath sounds are usually decreased, and pulsus paradoxus may be present. Any patient who is lethargic, dyspneic, restless, or confused should have arterial blood gases drawn. Rising of the $Paco_2$ may be indicative of a primary ventilatory defect. In critical situations where patients are exhausted, cyanotic, or have notably decreased breath sounds, it is imperative to provide adequate ventilation and intervene promptly rather than postpone critical care due to the unavailability of arterial blood gas studies. Although arterial blood gas studies are of paramount importance in establishing the diagnosis of respiratory failure, in critical situations prompt intervention is mandatory. A Pao_2 below 60 mm Hg (excluding congenital heart disease with intracardiac shunting) and a $Paco_2$ above 50 mm Hg constitute the diagnosis. Patients with an elevated $Paco_2$ are confused, lose their judgment, and may be wrongly considered as having a psychologic disturbance. The importance of serial arterial blood gas studies cannot be overemphasized. A child with status asthmaticus who progresses to respiratory failure may manifest absence of wheezing on physical examination and dangerously may be considered as one whose condition is improving. In certain situations, such as in acute asthmatic attack or acute epiglottitis, continued deterioration toward respiratory failure may occur, whereas in other conditions, such as cystic fibrosis, muscular dystrophy, or even shock lung, progression toward respiratory failure is more gradual.

General Approach to Therapy and Monitoring

All children in respiratory failure are hypoxic, and therefore acute hypoxia (or hypoxemia) should be corrected promptly regardless of the level of $Paco_2$. If the need for Fio_2 exceeds 60 percent one should not withhold therapy for fear of pulmonary oxygen toxicity. Correcting hypoxia is by far more critical than oxygen lung toxicity, and the benefit of oxygen therapy in hypoxic patients outweighs the risk of potential oxygen toxicity. Children die from hypoxia, and the following are only some of the deleterious results of hypoxia or hypoxemia:

1. Anaeorbic metabolism and lactic acidosis
2. Cytotoxic cerebral edema with a rise in intracranial pressure and subsequent demise
3. Pulmonary hypertension, an increase in PVR, right ventricular failure, and death (Fig. 15-2).
4. Impairment of myocardial contractility.

Prolonged hypoxemia may result in cerebral edema and subsequent brain damage. It is therefore critical to assess the adequacy of oxygenation and ventilation by serial arterial blood gas studies.

Oxygen can be given by a mask, nasal cannula, hood, or tent. Monitoring in critical situations may be accomplished with an indwelling percutaneous arterial catheter. Capillary blood gas studies are not reliable. Noninvasive means include ear oximetry for continuous oxygen saturation monitoring and transcutaneous measurement of Po_2, and Pco_2 in those children without circulatory failure. In critical conditions such as "shock lung" (ARDS) (which will be discussed later), the Po_2 in mixed venous blood ($P\bar{v}o_2$) should be monitored by a Swan-Ganz flow-directed catheter and maintained above 35 mm Hg. Pvo_2 reflects tissue oxygenation and in certain situations provides useful information for therapy. A Swan-Ganz catheter also can assist in evaluating the degree of intrapulmonary shunting ($\dot{q}s/\dot{q}t$), pulmonary artery pressure, and cardiac output. The following can be computed with the Swan-Ganz catheter:

$$PVR = \frac{\begin{array}{c}\text{Mean pulmonary artery pressure}\\ -\text{Pulmonary capillary wedge pressure}\end{array}}{\text{Cardiac output}}$$

$$SVR = \frac{\begin{array}{c}\text{Systemic blood pressure}\\ -\text{Central venous pressure}\end{array}}{\text{Cardiac output}}$$

where PVR = Pulmonary Vascular Resistance
SVR = Systemic Vascular Resistance

Systemic oxygen transport
(or oxygen tissue availability)
= Cardiac output $\times Cao_2$

where Cao_2 (Arterial oxygen content)
= Hemoglobin concentration $\times 1.36$
$\times$ Oxygen saturation (Sao_2)
$+ 0.0031 \times Pao_2$

Sao_2 represents oxygen saturation of hemoglobin in arterial blood, 1.36 is millimeters of oxygen bound to 1 g of fully saturated hemoglobin, and 0.0031 is the amount of dissolved oxygen. It is therefore possible to calculate the optimal positive end expiratory pressure (PEEP), which is defined as the best PEEP at which cardiac output and therefore oxygen delivery are optimal.

Caution should be exercised when oxygen is being administered to patients with chronic obstructive pulmonary disease such as cystic fibrosis. In this situation 28 percent Fio_2 is given in order to minimize depression of the patient's hypoxic drive, which may inadvertently cause carbon dioxide retention. Oxygen therapy is aimed at keeping the Pao_2 above 60 mm Hg so that the risk of pulmonary hypertension is minimized (Fig. 15-2).

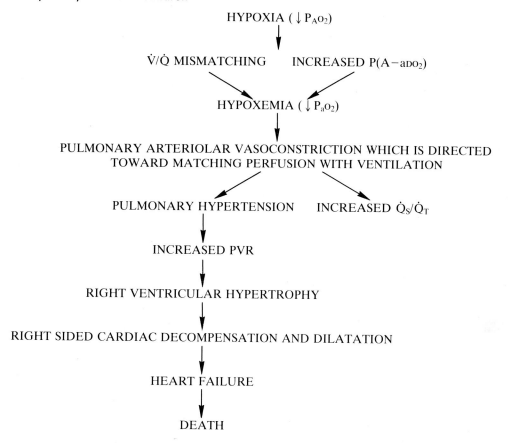

Figure 15-2. Basic pathophysiologic mechanism of hypoxia.

Children who are unresponsive to oxygen or pharmacologic therapy (e.g., patients with status asthmaticus and respiratory failure who are unresponsive to an intravenous isoproterenol drip) with a rising $Paco_2$ may require intubation and ventilatory support. This approach does not apply to cystic fibrosis patients with chronic carbon dioxide retention, since mechanical ventilation carries a very poor prognosis and invariably is associated with death. Every patient in acute respiratory failure should be mechanically ventilated if other measures have failed, however. Also, children who are exhausted, have a changing mental status, and have shallow respirations are decompensated and must be ventilated regardless of the arterial blood gas studies. Failure of adequate oxygenation may lead to cerebral edema with a subsequent rise in intracranial pressure, low cerebral perfusion pressure, and possible irreversible brain damage or even death.

Generally, indications for intubation and mechanical ventilation are listed in Tables 15-2 and 15-3. Indications for weaning from the respirator are listed in Table 15-4.

Guidelines for Extubation

Children will be considered ready for extubation if they can breathe spontaneously and maintain a $Paco_2$ below 50 mm Hg, a Pao_2 above 80 mm Hg and pH level between 7.35 and 7.45 with 40 percent inspired oxygen. They should have adequate gag and cough reflexes and not be dyspneic.

Extubation will be possible if the child is fully alert and does not have upper airway obstruction. Ten minutes before extubation elevation of the patient's head and administration of 100 percent inspired oxygen are recommended as a precautionary measure. Atropine, 0.01 mg/kg, is given either intravenously or intramuscularly (a

Table 15-2 *Indications for Intubation and Mechanical Ventilation*

1. $Paco_2$ rise of greater than 10 mm Hg/hr (e.g., a rise from 40 to 50 mm Hg) in a child who is exhausted, restless, or has a change in mental status

2. A $Paco_2$ above 50 mm Hg unresponsive to other modes of therapy

3. Poor oxygenation with a falling Pao_2 despite oxygen administration (e.g., a Pao_2 below 60 mm Hg that is unresponsive to high demands of oxygen supplementation)

Table 15-4 *Indications for Weaning a Child from the Respirator*

1. A $Paco_2$ below 50 mm Hg and a Pao_2 above 80 mm Hg with 40 percent inspired oxygen

2. Negative peak inspiratory pressure greater than -20 cm H_2O

3. Tidal volume more than 5 cc/kg of body weight

4. Forced vital capacity more than 15 cc/kg of body weight in a child who can perform the test

5. $P(A - aDo_2)$ less than 300 mm Hg with 100 percent oxygen

6. Shunt fraction ($\dot{Q}s/\dot{Q}t$ less than 15 percent with 100 percent oxygen

7. Ratio of dead space to tidal volume (VD/VT) less than 0.55

minimal total dose of 0.1 mg and a maximal total dose of 0.5 mg) to prevent a vagal reflex during extubation and minimize secretions. If vital signs are stable, the child is extubated during peak inspiration (or the beginning of expiration) to facilitate removal of potential mucous plug. Since stridor is present in any child who has been intubated for more then 2 hours, racemic epinephrine aerosol should be given as needed.

In extreme cases of acute respiratory failure extracorporeal membrane oxygenation (ECMO) was advocated with varying results. Extracorporeal circulation with a membrane oxygenator is currently under intensive research and should be used only in selected cases of acute respiratory failure.

SPECIFIC CLINICAL CONDITIONS ASSOCIATED WITH RESPIRATORY FAILURE

Status Asthmaticus

Children who have status asthmaticus can progress rapidly from type I to type II respiratory failure. This group of children will be in extreme respiratory distress, with little wheezing due to poor airflow and grossly diminished breath

Table 15-3 *Indications for Intubation Without Mechanical Ventilation*

1. Life-threatening upper airway obstruction (e.g., acute epiglottitis)

2. Comatose children with inadequate pulmonary toilet

3. Central nervous system depression accompanied by fatigue and potential life-threatening aspiration

sounds. In some, a change in level of consciousness will be evident. The $Paco_2$ will exceed 50 mm Hg or will rise at a rate greater than 10 mm Hg/hr. The Pao_2 will be invariably below 70 mm Hg with 40 percent inspired oxygen. Since therapy with intravenous aminophylline in conjunction with steroids, oxygen and adrenergic agents has failed to restore adequate ventilation, the use of isoproterenol in an intravenous drip is indicated. Table 15-5 outlines the use of isoproterenal in respiratory failure.

When adequate ventilation is restored patients may shift into type I respiratory failure.

Case 1: Status Asthmaticus and Type II Respiratory Failure.

E.N., an 8-year-old boy with asthma, was admitted with status asthmaticus after three subcutaneous injections of epinephrine. On arrival the Pao_2 with room air was 56 mm Hg and the $Paco_2$ 37 mm Hg. An hour later the $Paco_2$ was 45 mm Hg, and 2 hours after admission the $Paco_2$ had risen to 55 mm Hg. E.N. was in severe respiratory distress with maximal chest retractions, poor breath sounds, and minimal audible wheezing.

He had type II respiratory failure and despite oxygen therapy with 40 percent inspired oxygen, Pao_2 could not be maintained above 60 mm Hg and $Paco_2$ was rising. In this situation, an intravenous isoproterenol drip as described in Table 15-5 was clearly indicated.

Case 2: Status Asthmaticus and Type I Respiratory Failure with Hypoxia, Hypoxemia, and Intrapulmonary Shunting

T.J., a 9½-year-old boy with asthma, was admitted with status asthmaticus after three unsuccessful subcutaneous injections of epinephrine. On arrival the $Paco_2$

was recorded as 33 mm Hg and the Pao_2 was 55 mm Hg with 40 percent inspired oxygen. A chest roentgenogram disclosed right middle lobe and right lower lobe atelectasis secondary to mucous plugging. The P_Ao_2 was calculated as described earlier and subsequently the $P(A - aDo_2)$ is derived as follows:

$$P_Ao_2 = 0.40(757 - 47) - \frac{40}{0.8} = 284 - 50 = 234 \text{ mm Hg}$$
$$P(A - aDo_2) = 234 - 55 = 179 \text{ mm Hg}$$

This child was in type I respiratory failure with hypoxemia but did not have hypercapnia. His level of oxygenation was very poor, taking into account that he was provided with 40 percent inspired oxygen.

His $P(A - aDo_2)$ was significantly increased, which may be consistent with intrapulmonary shunting secondary to atelectasis with or without diffusion defect.

"Shock Lung" or Adult Type Respiratory Distress Syndrome (ARDS).

The term *"shock lung,"* or *adult respiratory distress syndrome* (ARDS), gained recent recognition in the pediatric age group. Although it does not have a defined etiology, it has been associated with many disorders and a complex of factors. A prerequisite for shock lung is the exclusion of its relationship to previous pneumonia, atelectasis, pulmonary edema, and cardiovascular disease. It has been associated with sepsis, pulmonary infection, microemboli, blood clotting abnormalities, pulmonary and nonpulmonary trauma, head injury, cardiovascular insufficiency, fractures, near drowning, smoke inhalation, cerebral edema, oxygen toxicity, aspiration, and barbiturate and narcotic overdose. The etiology of "shock lung" has not been well defined, which results in confusing terminology. Some of them include adult respiratory distress syndrome, adult hyaline membrane disease, adult insufficiency syndrome, wet lung, hemorrhagic atelectasis, stiff lung syndrome, post-traumatic pulmonary insufficiency, progressive respiratory distress, and progressive pulmonary consolidation. The basic defect involves injury to the alveolar-capillary membrane, resulting in $\dot{V}_A/\dot{Q}$ mismatching, increased intrapulmonary shunting, and hypoxemia. This is complicated by increased pulmonary microvascular permeability with subsequent pulmonary edema and poor lung compliance.

It is characterized by respiratory distress and severe hypoxemia in a patient who has had no history of previous cardiopulmonary disease. Within 72 hours after trauma or life-threatening

Table 15-5 *Intravenous Isoproterenol (Isuprel) for Respiratory Failure Associated with Status Asthmaticus*

1. Medical therapy remains unchanged. Aminophylline should be given at an optimal dose as determined by theophylline serum levels. Aerosolized isoproterenol and other β-adrenergic agents must be discontinued.

2. An additional intravenous site should be established for the use of isoproterenol.

3. Begin isoproterenol infusion at 0.1 μg/kg/min.

4. Increase the dosage by 0.1 μg/kg/min increments every 15 minutes based on close monitoring of arterial blood gases obtained through an arterial line. The $Paco_2$ is the most important factor in evaluating arterial blood gases in respiratory failure.

5. When a response is achieved as indicated by a decreasing $Paco_2$, the higher level should be maintained for 3 hours and then tapered off for the next 30–36 hours.

6. Rarely this mode of therapy fails. Failure of intravenous isoproterenol therapy is indicated by clinical deterioration, a rise in the level of $Paco_2$, a heart rate above 200, arrhythmias or relatively low heart rate.

7. Myocardial ischemia, arrhythmias, a heart rate above 200 beats/min, or chest pain are indicators to discontinue the isoproterenol drip.

8. Intubation is indicated after failure of isoproterenol therapy.

disease, children manifest severe respiratory distress, poor oxygenation, and progressive pulmonary insufficiency. Chest roentgenograms are characterized by diffuse reticular infiltrates, pulmonary edema, and progression from patchy infiltrates to dense consolidation. In some cases interstitial emphysema, a pneumomediastinum, and a pneumothorax develop.

Differential Diagnosis

This syndrome should be differentiated from aspiration, atelectasis, pneumonia, pulmonary emboli, a pneumothorax, and fat emboli.

Therapy

In treating children with "shock lung," maximal attention should be focused on ventilatory support with optimal PEEP in order to improve oxygenation, expand functional residual capacity, and increase compliance. Adequate therapy will result in diminution of intrapulmonary shunting. The SaO_2 is kept above 90 percent, the PaO_2 above 60 mm Hg, the $PaCO_2$ below 50 mm Hg. A Swan-Ganz flow-directed catheter plays an important role in the objective assessment of the cardiac output, $P\bar{v}O_2$, PVR, and oxygen tissue availability as previously described. Dynamic compliance will help determine the best PEEP, and the V_D/V_T is helpful in evaluating the relative perfusion of the pulmonary capillary bed. When PaO_2 cannot be maintained above 60 mm Hg with 60 percent inspired oxygen, and the $PaCO_2$ is greater than 50 mm Hg, artificial ventilation is inevitable.

"Shock lung" represents a severe form of acute respiratory failure with an estimated mortality between 60 and 95 percent in the pediatric age group. This form of respiratory failure represents a progressive shift from type I to type II respiratory failure with reversal back to type I after ventilatory support.

Case 3: ARDS in a Child Following Trauma

S.G., a 5-year-old boy, was admitted to the pediatric intensive care unit after an auto accident that resulted in multiple rib fractures, severe pulmonary contusion, and a lacerated liver. His past medical history was unremarkable in that he had never suffered from cardiac or pulmonary disease. His admitting chest roentgenogram (Fig. 15-3) showed pulmonary contusion, rib fractures, and pulmonary edema. His condition necessitated intubation, ventilatory support, administration of furosemide, 1 mg/kg, intravenously. Arterial blood gas studies during the first 24 hours after admission revealed a pH level of 7.36, a PaO_2 of 100 mm Hg, and a $PaCO_2$ of 35 mm Hg. Seventy-two hours after admission his condition had deteriorated. He required 100 percent inspired oxygen and a PEEP of 16 cm H_2O, a pH level of 7.50, a PaO_2 ranging from 60 to 74 mm Hg, and had a $PaCO_2$ from 35 to 42 mm Hg. His $P(A - aDO_2)$ was in excess of 500 mm Hg, and the $\dot{Q}s/\dot{Q}t$ was 48 percent. The pulmonary artery pressure was 65/40, and $P\bar{v}O_2$ was maintained above 35 mm Hg to ensure adequate tissue oxygenation. The low cardiac output necessitated an intravenous dopamine drip at a rate ranging from 10 to 15 μg/kg/min. Figure 15-4 shows the chest roentgenogram 4 days after admission.

After 10 days of ventilatory support, including 2 days of therapy with intravenous nitroprusside at a rate ranging from 2 to 6 μg/kg/min, his condition had improved remarkably with subsequent extubation and normalizing of the arterial blood gases.

Although type II respiratory failure is considered to be worse then type I, this case illustrates the clinical aspects of type I respiratory failure. This child suffered mainly from poor oxygenation, which resulted in an increased $P(A - aDO_2)$ and severe intrapulmonary shunting.

Upper Airway Obstruction Secondary To Acute Epiglottitis

Case 4: A Girl with Acute Epiglottitis

C.N., a 4-year-old girl, presented to the emergency room with a sore throat, hoarseness, a fever of 40°C, mild shortness of breath, and drooling. She was a frightened girl, preferred a sitting position, and was slightly dyspneic. There was no evidence of peripheral desaturation on physical examination. She was febrile and slightly stridorous. Roentgenograms of the soft tissues of the neck disclosed an enlarged epiglottis.

This case represents a severe form of acute upper airway obstruction that may be associated with mortality or high morbidity if prompt medical attention is not rendered. This child should not be stressed for arterial blood gas studies or extensive physical examination, but rather taken promptly to the operating room where intubation should be attempted by a highly trained anesthesiologist. An ear, nose, and throat or pediatric surgeon should be standing by in the operating room, and, if intubation fails (which is very rare), a tracheostomy can be performed. After relief of upper airway obstruction either by intubation or a tracheostomy, the child should receive intravenous ampicillin, 200 mg/kg/day, in combination with chloramphenicol, 100 mg/kg/day while awaiting the culture and sensitivity report from blood and throat specimens. This type of respiratory failure is invariably associated with *Haemophilus influenzae* type b and rarely is complicated by meningitis or pneumonia.

If unattended, this child can rapidly progress into combined type I and type II respiratory failure with subsequent brain damage and in some cases death.

Cystic Fibrosis (CF)

Cystic fibrosis is the most frequent lethal genetic syndrome among white children and adolescents causing chronic progressive pulmonary disease. The majority of patients have mucoid *Pseudomonas aeruginosa* or *Staphylococcus aureus* infections in the bronchial tree that are difficult to eradicate. These organisms can cause chronic pulmonary infection and subsequent irreversible saccular bronchiectasis. The diagnosis is confirmed by an elevated sweat chloride test (above 60 mEq/L). The disease is complicated by hypoxemia, pulmonary hypertension, increased PVR, and right ventricular hypertrophy and can lead to cardiac decompensation

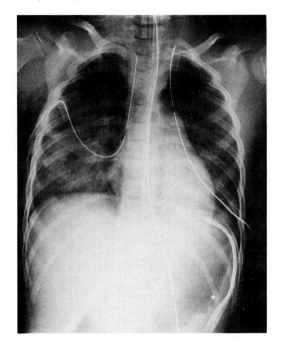

Figure 15-3. Chest roentgenogram on admission demonstrating multiple rib fractures and pulmonary contusion.

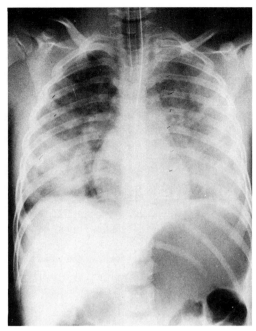

Figure 15-4. Chest roentgenogram 4 days after admission showing more consolidation and diffuse bilateral reticular pattern.

and death (Fig. 15-2). Although relative hypoxia is present in the majority of those with progressive pulmonary disease, in its late stages carbon dioxide retention develops, leading to type II respiratory failure.

Early pulmonary lesions include dilation and hypertrophy of bronchial glands and goblet cell metaplasia of the bronchiolar epithelium followed by mucous plugging of peripheral airways, segmental atelectasis, intrapulmonary shunting, and hypoxemia (type I respiratory failure). As the disease progresses, chronic infection leads to accelerated mucous production and vice versa. This result in saccular bronchiectasis and finally progression to type II respiratory failure.

Treatment of cor pulmonale is directed toward improvement of hypoxemia and airway obstruction with agressive antibiotic therapy, postural drainage, aerosols, oxygen for a Pao_2 below 60 mm Hg, vitamin supplementation, and enzyme replacement.

Previous studies have shown that in chronic carbon dioxide retention, mechanical ventilation is of little benefit, since the majority of patients die. In acute respiratory failure with a sudden rise of $Paco_2$ or acute hypoxemia secondary to mucous plugging of major airways, mechanical ventilation has been partially successful.

Case 5: CF and Acute Respiratory Failure due to Pneumothorax

B.J., a 14-year-old girl with a confirmed diagnosis of cystic fibrosis, was seen in the pediatric pulmonary center complaining of shortness of breath and left-sided chest pain. Physical examination disclosed tachypnea and a respiratory rate of 48/min accompanied by chest retractions and peripheral desaturation. Breath sounds over the left side of the chest were diminished. Previous arterial blood gas with room air revealed a pH level of 7.44, a Pao_2 of 48, and a $Paco_2$ of 44 mm Hg.

The chest roentgenogram on admission revealed a left-sided pneumothorax, and arterial blood gas studies showed a Pao_2 of 34 mm Hg and a $Paco_2$ of 52 mm Hg. Fifty percent oxygen by mask and placement of a left-sided chest tube resulted in resolution of the symptoms, an increase of the Pao_2 to 90 mm Hg and a lowering of the $Paco_2$ to 44 mm Hg.

This patient initially represented progression to type II respiratory failure. Despite therapy with oxygen and alleviation of the pneumthorax with a chest tube, the

P(A $-$ aDO$_2$) remains significant. The level of inspired oxygen should be taken into account, since the otherwise "excellent" PaO$_2$ may be misleading. It should be noted that in this patient mucous plugging and segmental atelectasis will promote intrapulmonary shunting and further aggravate hypoxemia.

Depression of the Central Nervous System

Depression of the central nervous system can be caused by barbiturate or narcotic overdose, anesthesia, head trauma, meningitis, cerebral edema secondary to near drowning, or intracranial hermorrhage. Primary or central alveolar hypoventilation can be found in obese children and is known as the *obesity-hypoventilation syndrome*.

The hallmark of this group is type II respiratory failure, although a shift to type I respiratory failure has been reported.

Case 6: Combined Types I and II Respiratory Failure Due to CNS Depression

J.C., a 1½-year-old girl, was admitted to a pediatric intensive care unit after a barbiturate overdose. She presented with shallow respirations, was depressed, and had right lower lobe and left lower lobe atelactasis on the chest roentgenogram. Arterial blood gas studies with 40 percent inspired oxygen revealed a PaO$_2$ of 55 mm Hg and a PaCO$_2$ of 60 mm Hg. She was treated with intravenous fluids, intubation and mechanical ventilation. A few hours later she became alert, gained her own respirations, and was successfully extubated. At that time arterial blood gas studies with 35 percent inspired oxygen revealed a PaO$_2$ of 100 and a PaCO$_2$ of 38 mm Hg.

This girl originally had type II respiratory failure with hypoxemia and hypercapnia. The PaCO$_2$ was elevated due to central hypoventilation, and the PaO$_2$ was decreased due to the same process but was also a result of atelectasis, probably from aspiration of gastric content, leading to $\dot{V}_A/\dot{Q}$ imbalance and intrapulmonary shunting.

After regaining consciousness, she began to hyperventilate, thus blowing carbon dioxide and normalizing the PaCO$_2$. The PaO$_2$ remained relatively low (taking into account her inspired oxygen). The degree of atelectasis accounts for the significant P(A $-$ aDO$_2$).

This case illustrates a change from type II to type I respiratory failure.

NEW DEVELOPMENTS IN THE FIELD

The trend in pediatrics is toward noninvasive measurements of ventilatory function. It is also believed that continuous assessment of pulmonary function provides, by far, more valuable information than sporadic isolated determinations.

New developments in the field have included continuous measurement of PO$_2$ and PCO$_2$ with transcutaneous electrodes, continuous measurements of SaO$_2$ with ear oximetry, measurement of tissue pH levels with special electrodes, and noninvasive measurements of end-tidal PCO$_2$.

Better assessment of the bronchial tree is possible by using a small pediatric flexible fiberoptic bronchoscope, CT and NMR scanners, and measurements of ventilation/perfusion relationships with sophisticated nuclear scanners.

New development in ventilatory support has included high jet frequency ventilators and computerized life-support systems.

REFERENCES

Anderson RR, Holliday RL, Driedger AA, et al: Documentation of pulmonary capillary permeability in the adult respiratory distress syndrome accompanying human sepsis. *Am Rev. Respir Dis* 119:869, 1979.

Ashbaugh DG, Bigelow DB, Petty TL, et al: Acute respiratory distress in adults. *Lancet* 2:319, 1967.

Ashbaugh DG, Petty TL, Bigelow DB, et al: Continuous positive-pressure breathing (CPPB) in adult respiratory distress syndrome. *J Thorac Cardiovasc Surg* 57:31, 1969.

Bartlett RH, Gazzaniga AB, Fong SW, et al: Extracorporeal membrane oxygenator support for cardiopulmonary failure: experience in 28 cases. *J Thorac Cardiovasc Surg* 73:375, 1977.

Bartlett RH, Gazzaniga AB, Huxtable RF, et al: Extracorporeal circulation (ECMO) in neonatal respiratory failure. *J Thorac Cardiovasc Surg* 74:826, 1977.

Battaglia JD, Lockhart CH: Management of acute epiglottitis by nasotracheal intubation. *Am J Dis Child* 129:334, 1975.

Baxter JC, Pashley NR: Acute epiglottitis—25 years' experience in management, the Montreal Children's Hospital. *J Otolaryngol* 6:473, 1977.

Bone RC: Treatment of adult respiratory distress syndrome with diuretics, dialysis, and positive end-expiratory pressure. *Crit Care Med* 6:136, 178;

Bone RC, Pierce AK, Johnson RL: Controlled oxygen administration in acute respiratory failure in chronic obstructive pulmonary disease. *Am J Med* 65:896, 1978.

Davison FW: Acute laryngeal obstruction in children: a fifty-year review. *Ann Otol Rhinol Laryngol* 87:606, 1978.

Esrig BC, Fulton RL: Sepsis, resuscitated hemorrhagic shock and "shock lung." *Ann Surg* 182:218, 1975.

Gallagher TJ, Civetta JM, Kirby RR: Terminology update: optimal PEEP. *Crit Care Med* 6:323, 1978.

Geelhoed GW, Adkins PC, Corso PJ, et al: Clinical effects of membrane lung support for acute respiratory failure. *Ann Thorac Surg* 20:177, 1975.

German JC, Gazzaniga AB, Amlie R, et al: Management of pulmonary insufficiency in diaphragmatic hernia using extracorporeal circulation with a membrane oxygenator (ECMO). *J Pediatr Surg* 12:905, 1977.

Goulon M, Raphael JC, Gajdos P, et al: Membrane oxygenators for acute respiratory insufficiency. *Intensive Care Med* 4:173, 1978.

Heinemann HO: Right-sided heart failure and the use of diuretics. *Am J Med* 64:367, 1978.

Hicks RE, Kinney TR, Raphaely RC, et al. Successful treatment of varicella pneumonia with prolonged extracorporeal membrane oxygenation in a child with leukemia. *J Thorac Cardiovasc Surg* 73:297, 1977.

Hodgkin JE, Bowser MA, Burton GG: Respirator weaning. *Crit Care Med* 2:96, 1974.

Holbrook PR, Taylor G, Pollack MM, et al: Adult respiratory distress syndrome in children. *Pediatr Clin North Am* 27:677, 1980.

Hopewell PC, Murray JF: The adult respiratory distress syndrome. *Ann Rev Med* 27:343, 1976.

Hudgel DW, Weil JV: Depression of hypoxic and hypercapnic ventilatory drives in severe asthma. *Chest* 68:493, 1975.

Hunt, CE, Matalon SV, Thompson TR, et al: Central hypoventilation syndrome: experience with bilateral phrenic nerve pacing in 3 neonates. *Am Rev Respir Dis* 118:23, 1978.

Kirby RR, Downs JB, Civetta JM, et al: High level positive and expiratory pressure (PEEP) in acute respiratory insufficiency. *Chest* 67:156, 1975.

Kolobow T, Stool E, Sacks K, et al: Acute respiratory failure: Survival following ten days' support with a membrane lung. *J Thorac Cardiovasc Surg* 69:947, 1975.

Lamy M, Fallat RJ, Koeniger E, et al: Pathologic features and mechanisms of hypoxemia in adult respiratory distress syndrome. *Am Rev Respir Dis* 114:267, 1976.

Lyrene RK, Truog WE: Adult respiratory distress syndrome in a pediatric intensive care unit: predisposing conditions, clinical course, and outcome. *Pediatrics* 67:790, 1981.

Martin L: Respiratory failure. *Med Clin North Am* 61:1369, 1977.

Newth CJL: Recognition and management of respiratory failure. *Pediatr Clin North Am* 26:617, 1979.

McFadden ER, Feldman NT: Asthma pathophysiology and clinical correlates. *Med Clin North Am* 61:1229. 1977.

Moore GC, Zwillich CW, Battaglia JD, et al: Respiratory failure associated with familial depression of ventilatory response to hypoxia and hypercapnia. *N Engl J Med* 295:861, 1976.

Parry WH, Martorano F, Cotton EK: Management of life-threatening asthma with intravenous isoporterenol infusions. *Am J Dis Child* 130:39, 1976.

Peters, RM: Lifesaving measures in acute respiratory distress syndrome. *Am J Surg* 138:368, 1979.

Petty TL, Reiss OK, Paul GW, et al: Characteristics of pulmonary surfactant in adult respiratory distress syndrome associated with trauma and shock. *Am Rev Respir Dis* 115:531, 1977.

Pontoppidan H, Geffin B, Lowenstein E: Acute respiratory failure in the adult. *N Engl J Med* 287:690, 743, 799, 1972.

Schwartz AL, Lipton JM, Warburton D, et al: Management of acute asthma in childhood *Am J Dis Child* 134:474, 1980.

Shuller DE, Birck HG: The safety of intubation in croup and epiglottitis: an eight-year follow-up. *Laryngoscope* 85:33, 1975.

Simons FER, Pierson WE, Bierman CW: Respiratory failure in childhood status asthmaticus. *Am J Dis Child* 131:1097, 1977.

Simpson H, Mitchell I, Inglis JM, et al: Severe ventilatory failure in asthma in children: experience of 13 episodes over 6 years. *Arch Dis Child* 53:714, 1978.

Soloway HB, Castillo Y, Martin AM: Adult hyaline membrane disease: relationship to oxygen therapy. *Ann Surg* 168:937, 1968.

Tumalewicz WE: Assessment of arterial blood oxygenation in various states of acute respiratory failure. *Anaesth Resusc Intensive Ther* 3:25, 1975.

Wanner A: Conservative management of acute respiratory failure. *Prac Cardio* 5:32, 1979.

Wood DW, Downes JJ, Scheinkopf H, et al: Intravenous isoproterenol in the management of respiratory failure in childhood status asthmaticus. *J Allergy Clin Immuno* 50:75, 1972.

Wood RE, Boat TF, Doershuk CF: State of the art: cystic fibrosis. *Am Rev Respir Dis* 113:833, 1976.

Zapol WM, Snider MT: Pulmonary hypertension in severe acute respiratory failure. *N Engl J Med* 296:476, 1977.

16

Pharmacotherapy of Respiratory Disease

Miles Weinberger
Elliot Ellis

Diseases of the respiratory tract are related to the unique exposure of this system to insults from the outside world. The mucosa is exposed repeatedly to various pollutants and noxious substances of the atmosphere, extremes of temperature, and infectious agents. The upper respiratory tract is heavily colonized with a wide range of microbiologic flora with varying degrees of virulence. The contiguous lower respiratory tract maintains its sterility through the constant action of mucociliary clearance aided by secretory antibodies. In addition, immunologic reactions to airborne antigens can result in the release of endogenous substances that cause acute and sustained inflammatory responses of both the upper and lower respiratory tract.

The responses of the respiratory tract are more limited than the variety of insults to it. Infection results in inflammation that is manifested by vascular engorgement and mucosal edema, causing obstruction at the site of the inflammation. Rhinitis, otitis media, laryngitis, tracheitis, and bronchitis are terms that describe such inflammatory responses at various sites in the airway. At all of these sites, however, inflammation can also occur on a noninfectious basis. Vascular congestion and mucosal edema, whatever the cause, results in similar symptoms. Except when specific antimicrobial therapy is indicated for susceptible bacterial infections, therapy of respiratory tract disease is directed at preventing the release of mediators of inflammation, treating the vascular engorgement and edema of the mucous membrane, or relaxing the smooth muscle of the lower respiratory tract when bronchospasm contributes to the airway obstruction.

Because of the similarity of symptoms and the various types of insults, specific diagnosis is essential for the choice of therapy. Antibiotics will be effective in the presence of infection with susceptible bacteria but not with a viral infection or noninfectious inflammation. Airway obstruction can occur by both anatomic and physiologic processes. Even when the airway obstruction is physiologic, inflammation of the respiratory tract mucosa must be distinguished from bronchospasm in the lungs or vascular congestion in the nose. An understanding of the pathophysiologic process of airway disease and the specificity of the pharmacologic agents available allows a rational approach to therapy. Unfortunately, the similarity of symptoms that results from the limited nature of responses of the airways to various insults often causes confusion and consequent ineffective treatment.

RHINITIS

Rhinitis, inflammation of the nasal mucosa, occurs most commonly in response to common viral respiratory tract infection such as the common cold. Symptoms of the usual viral upper respiratory tract infection are generally mild and self-limited, and medical treatment is not commonly needed. Except under unusual circumstances, such as a retained foreign body in the nose, bacterial rhinitis generally is not recognized as a clinical entity.

Chronic noninfectious rhinitis includes a spectrum of nasal disorders that can best be characterized as hyperreactivity of the nasal mucosa to a variety of stimuli. At least 10 percent of the population suffer from chronic or recurrent

Table 16-1   *Response of Rhinitis to Treatment**

Therapy	Diagnostic Category			
	AR!	AR?	NARWES	NARES
Antihistamine-decongestant therapy	(19)68%	(12)50%	(30)63%	(6)83%
Inhaled corticosteroid therapy	(29)66%	(9)56%	(22)45%	(15)93%

*Modified from Mullarkey MF, Hill JS, Webb DR: *J Allergy Clin Immunol* 1980; 65:122. With permission.[176]

†Parenthetical values indicate the number of patients treated; the percentage indicates those responding; AR!, definite allergic rhinitis; AR?, possible allergic rhinitis; NARWES, nonallergic rhinitis without eosinophilia; NARES, nonallergic rhinitis with eosinophilia.

sneezing, rhinorrhea, nasal congestion, and sometimes a discharge into the posterior pharynx that is commonly called postnasal drip.[1]

Often identified by the lay public as "sinus problems," the medical literature classifies this disorder variably as seasonal or perennial allergic rhinitis when specific antigens can be identified and as vasomotor or nonallergic rhinitis when antigens are not identifiable. Chronic nonallergic rhinitis has been further subdivided into nonallergic rhinitis with eosinophilia (NARES) and nonallergic rhinitis without eosinophilia. A higher degree of clinical response to treatment with antihistamines and topical steroids has been reported with NARES, although the distinction is not sufficiently reliable to predict unresponsiveness to therapy in patients without eosinophils in their nasal secretions (Table 16-1).

Symptoms of chronic rhinitis are often sufficiently mild that little or no medical treatment is indicated. Frequent or continuous rhinorrhea or nasal congestion, however, may require treatment with one or more pharmacologic agents.

Clinical Pharmacology of Drugs Used for Rhinitis

Antihistamines (H₁ Blockers)

The classic antihistamines inhibit the physiologic effects of histamine at H_1 receptors; they do not block H_2 receptors that stimulate gastric acid secretion. In addition, they often possess anticholinergic properties. Traditionally antihistamines have been classified into one of six groups according to chemical structure (Fig. 16-1). These categories, however, do not relate to efficacy or side effects. For example, diphenhydramine (Benadryl), which is strongly sedating, is

in the ethanolamine group along with carbinoxamine (in Rondec) and clemastine (Tavist), which are reported to rarely produce sedation.[2] The comparative efficacy of the antihistamines has been screened by examining the extent and duration to which the wheal and flare response to an intradermal injection of allergic extract can be suppressed. Cook et al.,[3] in a double-blind cross-over study, compared the efficacy of five structurally distinct antihistamines and showed that hydroxyzine suppressed the wheal size initially to the greatest extent (60 percent) and for the longest duration (4 days). In that study, diphenhydramine produced side effects as frequently as hydroxyzine but suppressed the wheal size to a significantly lesser extent and for a shorter duration. These findings suggest that drowsiness is a poor indicator of potency.

In a subsequent well-designed study, patients receiving hydroxyzine required 750 times the minimal histamine dose needed to induce pruritis compared to only a tenfold increase in histamine tolerance for diphenhydramine and a fivefold increase for both cyproheptadine (Periactin) and a placebo.[4]

In a double-blind study of patients with seasonal allergic rhinitis, hydroxyzine effectively decreased the severity and frequency of nasal pruritis, sneezing, rhinorrhea, and conjuctivitis when it was administered on a constant daily basis.[5] Persistent side effects, particularly drowsiness and dry mouth, were uncommon when therapy was initiated with a small amount of drug at bedtime and the dose increased progressively over a 10-day period as tolerated. In a subsequent double-blind placebo-controlled study, the authors found that hydroxyzine suppressed disabling symptoms of ragweed allergic rhinitis to a somewhat greater extent than chlorpheniramine,[6]

HISTAMINE

$$HC = C - CH_2 - CH_2 - NH_2$$

$$X - CH_2 - CH_2 - N \big< \begin{matrix} R_1 \\ R_2 \end{matrix}$$

CHEMICAL GROUP	GENERIC NAME	BRAND NAME	H₁ BLOCKERS	T½ PLASMA (HRS)	WHEAL SUPPRESSION EXTENT (%)	DURATION (DAYS)	COMMENT
Ethanolamine	Diphenhydramine	Benadryl		3-4	31	1.9	Therapeutic range (25–50 ng/ml) Marked anticholinergic effect
	Carbinoxamine	(in Rondec)		14			Sedation infrequent
	Clemastine	(Tavist)					Sedation infrequent
Ethylenediamine	Tripelenamine	(Pyribenzamine)		2-3	44	2.8	
	Methapyriline	Histadyl					In non-prescription sleep aids
Alkylamine	Chlorpheniramine	Chlortrimeton		12-15	34	2.4	In many OTC products
	Brompheniramine	Dimetane		36			
	Triprolidine	(in Actifed)		5			
Piprazine	Hydroxyzine	Atarax		3	63	4.3	
Piperidine	Cyproheptadine	Periactin					Less effective than hydroxyzine in itch suppression. Uniquely effective in some cases of cold urticaria.
Phenothiazine	Promethazine	Phenergan		51	2.8		
	Trimeprazine	Temaril					
	Methdilazine	Tacaryl					

Figure 16-1. Classification of antihistamines according to chemical structure.[75] This classification, however, does not necessarily predict effect. Except for diphenhydramine,[13] chlorpheniramine,[174] and hydroxyzine.[175] half-life data are unpublished but on file with the manufacturer. From Weinberger M. Hendeles, L. Pharmacologic management of asthma, rhinitis, anaphylaxis, and urticana. In Bierman. CW and Pearlman, PS [Eds.]: *Allergic Diseases in Infancy*. Philadelphia, WB Saunders Co., p. 328. (With permission.)

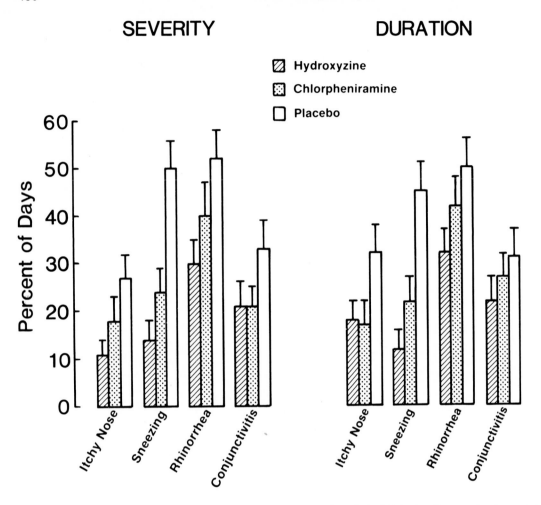

Figure 16-2. The frequency of days during weeks 3–6, the 3-week period of highest pollen counts when symptoms are annoying or disabling or lasted more than 2 hr/day. Both antihistamine regimens differed significantly from the placebo for severity and duration of sneezing and itchy nose, but only hydroxyzine differed significantly from the placebo for rhinorrhea (p is less than 0.05). Placebo-controlled evaluation of hydroxyzine and chlorpheniramine for seasonal allergic rhinitis. From Wong L, Hendeles L, Weinberger M: Placebo-controlled evaluation of hydroxyzine and chlorpheniramine for seasonal allergic rhinitis. *J. Allergy Clin Immunol* 63:203, 1979.[6]

although chlorpheniramine was clearly more effective than the placebo (Fig. 16-2).

In contrast to other symptoms of seasonal allergic rhinitis, nasal stuffiness does not appear to be suppressed by continuous antihistamine therapy.[5-7] This suggests that stuffiness may not be mediated by histamine, but possibly by another chemical factor such as slow-reacting substance of anaphylaxis (SRS-A). For this reason, benefit from antihistamines in patients with perennial allergic rhinitis is often not apparent in the presence of substantial nasal stuffiness.

There is no evidence that combining two or more antihistamines minimizes side effects or increases efficacy. On the other hand, a combination of antihistamine and decongestant may offer at least additive benefit for the symptoms of seasonal allergic rhinitis.[5-7] Adverse effects from antihistamine therapy include drowsiness, dry mouth, irritability, and occasionally a complaint of dizziness. These side-effects, although annoying to some patients, are rarely serious and are generally transient. A large overdose may result in atropine-like toxicity with delirium, hallucinations, ataxia, muscular twitching, fever, convulsions, and even cardiorespiratory collapse and death. Chronic toxicity with any of the antihistamines is relatively rare. Appetite stimulation has been reported with cyproheptadine.[9] Cyclizine has produced teratogenic effects in rats,[10] and brompheniramine has been implicated in congenital malformations in humans. Although the commonly used antihistamines such as chlorpheniramine are probably without effects on the fetus, there are little data to provide specific guidance. Antihistamines may increase the sedative effects of central nervous system depressants, including alcohol.[11]

Previous concern about the use of antihistamines in the presence of asthma was based on the potential for the anticholinergic properties of these drugs to increase the tenacity of the already viscous sputum of asthmatic patients. A controlled evaluation in children with chronic asthma did not support these concerns, however.[12] There is therefore no contraindication to using antihistamines in patients with asthma except perhaps during prolonged acute symptoms requiring hospitalization.

The therapeutic efficacy of diphenydramine appears to relate to serum concentrations in the range of 25–50 ng/ml, which can be achieved with a single 50-mg oral dose in most adults.[12,13] Toxicity commonly occurs when the serum concentration exceeds 50 ng/ml. As a result of the first-pass effect (i.e., the metabolic degradation following absorption into the portal system and subsequent first pass through the liver), oral bioavailability is poor, averaging 43 percent of the dose when compared to an intravenous reference.[13,14] The half-life of diphenhydramine in serum is about 3–4 hours, but suppression of the wheal and flare response to allergenic extracts may extend as long as 2 days.[3] This discordance between the duration of biologic effect and serum half-life suggests persistence of the antihistamine in tissues at histamine receptor sites for extended periods beyond substantial elimination from plasma. Thus, there is no rationale for prescribing diphenhydramine, and probably all other antihistamines, multiple times each day; two times a day should be quite sufficient.

Sympathomimetic Decongestants

Most oral decongestants constrict nasal mucous membranes by directly or indirectly stimulating α-adrenergic receptors. Although decreased nasal airway resistance after single doses of pseudoephedrine and phenylpropanolamine has been documented by rhinometry,[15,16] the efficacy of these drugs during chronic therapy has not been studied adequately.

Sympathomimetics are used conventionally for nasal decongestion with dosing intervals of 4–8 hours. Pseudoephedrine, however, has a relatively short half-life that averages only 4 hours.[15] When administered in the form of plain tablets, it produces a significant decrease in nasal airway resistance for at least 3 hours. Six hours after a dose, however, the effect is no different from that of a placebo. As a consequence, slow-release pseudoephedrine capsules have been introduced, and bioavailability equivalent to that of plain tablets has been demonstrated for two of the preparations, Novafed and Sudafed S.A. Such data are also available for combinations of pseudoephedrine and antihistamine in Novafed A and Isoclor.

Phenylephrine is included in many oral products in combination with an antihistamine (e.g., Dimetapp) for its decongestant effect. Oral bioavailability of this sympathomimetic, however, is poor, apparently as a result of rapid degradation in the gut or liver by the enzyme monoamine oxidase.[7,18] In one double-blind study of patients with chronic rhinitis, doses of 10, 20, or 40 mg of phenylephrine had no greater effect on nasal airway resistance than a placebo. In contrast, phenylpropanolamine, 40 mg, and pseudoephedrine, 60 mg, each produced a significant effect that persisted for 3 hours.[19] In the doses commonly recommended, phenylephrine is thus unlikely to be of benefit.

Oral decongestants frequently produce mild transient side effects, consisting of nervousness, insomnia, and irritability. These effects, however, are troublesome only to a minority of patients and are usually transient. Since ephedrine and theophylline have synergistic toxicity in asthmatic patients,[20,21] it is possible that pseudoephedrine, a stereoisomer of ephedrine, may interact similarly, although perhaps less frequently. In normotensive patients, pseudoephedrine and phenylpropanolamine do *not* produce an elevation of blood pressure.[5,6] The α-adrenergic stimulation from these drugs, however, may elevate diastolic blood pressure in patients with labile or overt hypertension or patients taking monoamine oxidase inhibitors.[18] Through a similar mechanism, men with symptomatic benign prostatic hypertrophy can experience urinary retention when taking oral decongestants.

Topical nasal decongestants such as phenylephrine (Neo-Synephrine) or oxymetazoline (Afrin) are transiently more potent than oral sympathomimetics but must be avoided in patients with allergic rhinitis because of the potential for overuse and the development of rhinitis medicamentosum,[22] whereby rebound congestion with often greater nasal stuffiness than before occurs despite persistence of the initial transient decongestant effect.

Corticosteroids

Repository corticosteroid injections and dexamethasone nasal aerosol have been used in the past to relieve the symptoms of allergic rhinitis, but they present the unnecessary and potentially hazardous risk of adrenal suppression and other systemic corticosteriod effects when used repeatedly or for prolonged periods.[23–25] On the other hand, beclomethasone dipropionate has about 100 times the topical activity of dexamethasone and has only a small degree of systemic effect when administered topically to respiratory tract mucous membranes.[27] Both are highly effective in the majority of patients, particularly when persistent nasal congestion is the dominant symptom.[28–30]

Because of its predominantly local effect, intranasal topical beclomethasone dipropionate does *not* provide benefit for accompanying allergic conjunctivitis. The only adverse effect associated with this therapy has been the rare occurrence of epistaxis.[29]

On occasion, poor effect may be a result of the aerosol failing to penetrate severe congestion with impatent nares. A short course of oral prednisone in dosages of 20–40 mg twice a day will generally provide sufficient clearing within 5 days to allow subsequent use of the inhaled beclomethasone dipropionate.

Anticholinergics

In selected patients in whom rhinorrhea is the primary manifestation of vasomotor rhinitis, an anticholinergic such as propantheline (Pro-Banthine) or belladonna alkaloids (Donnatal)

may provide symptomatic relief. The predominant side effects of anticholinergics are dry mouth, constipation, and urinary retention in patients with benign prostatic hypertrophy. These drugs should be avoided in patients with tachyarrhythmias, obstructive uropathies, and the rare narrow-angle glaucoma.

Cromolyn Sodium

Cromolyn sodium can prevent mast cell degranulation and thus inhibit release of histamine and other chemical mediators of the acute inflammatory response involved in allergic rhinitis. Clinical studies, however, have documented only a modest beneficial effect in suppressing allergic rhinitis[26] and conjunctivitis[31] in patients with high levels of antigen specific IgE. Therapy with this drug is inconvenient, since it must be instilled in both eyes and nose four to six times a day, and a therapeutic advantage over antihistamines has not been established.

Guide to Treatment

When rhinitis is predominantly caused by extrinsic factors, elimination of the offending agent is the most rational mode of therapy. Sensitivity to household pets, house dust, or other antigens (or irritants such as cigarette smoke) is best treated by removal of the pet or initiation of measures to minimize airborne dust or irritants. Complete avoidance of exogenous factors triggering rhinitis is often not practical, however, and much rhinitis may persist even in the absence of identifiable triggering factors.

Antihistamines have been used in the symptomatic treatment of noninfectious rhinitis for a few decades, but patients have experienced variable benefit and annoying side effects. Many patients prefer to tolerate discomfort from allergic rhinitis symptoms for a short time rather than experience drowsiness that impairs their ability to function. These limitations, however, appear in many cases to relate to the method of administration of the drug. Taking antihistamines only after symptoms have developed is inconsistent with the pharmacologic mechanism of these drugs. They must occupy histamine receptors in blood vessels, nerve endings, and mucous glands before release of histamine if they are to effectively act as competitive inhibitors and thus prevent the physiologic effects of histamine. If antihistamines are administered before antigen exposure, they are more likely to be effective, since they can occupy receptor sites before histamine is released and thereby block the effects of histamine.

Maximal suppression of symptoms of seasonal allergic rhinitis with minimal side effects therefore can be achieved by initiating therapy with a potent antihistamine such as hydroxyzine in low doses just before the season associated with exacerbations (e.g., early August for ragweed and hay fever) and increasing the dose as tolerated over a 10-day period. For hydroxyzine, the first dose of 25 mg in adults or 10 mg in children is given at bedtime so the patient can develop tolerance to the transient drowsiness at a time least likely to interfere with functioning. If the patient has no "antihistamine hangover" after 1 or 2 days, the same dose can then be given twice daily in equal amounts and progressively increased at 2- to 3-day intervals until a maximum of 150 mg/day for adults or a proportionately lower dosage for children is attained. The dose is always lowered to the highest tolerated if sedation persists. The maximal tolerated dosage, administered twice daily, is then continued for prophylaxis until the season is over (e.g., the end of September for ragweed hay fever).

For the patients with only mild symptoms of seasonal allergic rhinitis, chlorpheniramine can be used as an inexpensive over-the-counter prescription antihistamine that is only somewhat less potent than hydroxyzine. The same procedure is followed with an initial bedtime dosage of 4 mg for adults and 2 mg for children and progressive increases as tolerated to 24 mg for adults or proportionately lower dosages for children. Since all antihistamines have a long duration of biologic effect, slow-release formulations are needed only when a combination containing an oral decongestant is used. Such products are indicated when nasal congestion plays a dominant role in the symptoms, since antihistamines have little effect on this symptom despite their high degree of efficacy in suppressing sneezing, rhinorrhea, nasal pruritis, and conjunctivitis. The sympathomimetic decongestants such as pseudoephedrine or phenylpropanolamine, however, lack any effects on these symptoms but do have at least a modest effect on nasal congestion. They have short durations of action, however, thus benefiting from sustained release preparation. Doses of pseudoephedrine are 60–120 mg in adults and proportionately lower doses for chil-

dren; the dose of phenylpropanolamine is generally considered to be 50–100 mg in adults with proportionately less for children. Both of these drugs must be given at least four times a day if used as plain tablets or capsules. The duration of effect of slow-release pseudoephedrine is not well documented but proportionately larger doses administered at 8- or 12-hour intervals have been used empirically.

When maximal doses of oral sympathomimetics do not provide adequate medical benefit or are not tolerated well, intranasal administration of the newer generations of topical corticosteroids (beclomethasone dipropionate or flunisolide) may provide effective relief of nasal congestion. A twice daily dosage is sufficient, beginning with one or two sprays in each nostril. When symptoms are controlled, the dosage can often be reduced even to one inhalation in each nostril once daily. Many patients with chronic rhinitis find that discontinuation is possible after a few months even though subsequent exacerbations of the rhinitis may require reinitiation of therapy at a later time. An antihistamine may be needed in addition to the topical steroid to reduce conjunctivitis and other antihistamine-responsive symptoms. Mild eye symptoms may also be treated with an ophthalmic decongestant such as phenylephrine, 0.12 percent.

In rare circumstances, symptoms may be of sufficient severity to warrant a short course of systemic corticosteroids. This may be particularly indicated when severe allergic conjunctivitis leads to swelling of subconjunctival tissues. Prednisone is administered twice daily for 3–5 days in a dose of 20 mg for children 2–5 years old, 30 mg for those 6–10 years old, and 40 mg for adolescents and adults.

Although a full discussion of immunotherapy is beyond the intent of this chapter, it is primarily indicated when airborne allergens contribute substantially to symptoms, and adequate relief with acceptable medication has not been attained. Injections of increasing doses of extracts of those allergens contributing to troublesome symptoms are administered in a manner that increases the quantity of antigen as rapidly as tolerated on a once- or twice-weekly basis. When the maximal tolerated dose is achieved, the frequency of injections is decreased to 2-, 3-, and then 4-week intervals. Adverse effects from immunotherapy include systemic allergic reactions that are relatively common although usually mild. Localized discomfort is even more common even though this is usually only a nuisance-type side effect. The patient is maintained on the highest tolerated dose at monthly intervals for as long as efficacy is apparent. When clinical efficacy is not apparent or the clinical course suggests complete remission, the injections should be discontinued. Although often effective in ameliorating symptoms of allergic rhinitis, immunotherapy should not be considered a priori as a preferred or more specific therapy. It is more appropriately considered an alternative to pharmacologic management with its own benefits and risks that need to be weighed in making therapeutic decisions.

SINUSITIS

The criteria for the diagnosis of acute and, in particular, chronic sinusitis in children are a source of continuing controversy.[32] Roentgenologists differ widely in their opinions concerning what constitutes normal anatomy and which findings indicate disease.[33-35] For all practical purposes, except during early life when ethmoidal sinus disease may extend into the orbit to cause orbital cellulitis, a serious infection, the maxillary sinuses are those most often diseased during childhood. The embryology, anatomy, and physiology of the sinuses have been reviewed recently.[32] The most important event in the pathogenesis of sinusitis is obstruction of the sinus ostium. This occurs commonly as a result of viral upper respiratory tract infection or swelling of the nasal mucous membranes secondary to nasal allergy. The obstructed sinus becomes secondarily infected by bacteria that generally are part of the normal nasopharanygeal flora. Oxygen is absorbed from a poorly ventilated sinus and the relatively anaerobic environment facilitaties the growth of Streptococcus pneumoniae and Haemophilus influenzae (nontypable most often), the organisms most commonly recovered from infected maxillary sinuses.[36] A high prevalence of "abnormal" sinus roentgenograms has been reported in a population of children with rhinitis or asthma[37,38]; the clinical implications of this finding in regard to therapy are far from clear.

Diagnosis

Facial pain, headache, and fever are the more common signs and symptoms of maxillary sinusitis in older children, as in adults. In younger children, the symptoms may be more obscure; tenderness and swelling of the tissue over the maxillary sinuses is observed in acute sinusitis. A mucopurulent discharge draining from the region of the middle meatus or seen on the posterior pharyngeal wall suggests maxillary sinus disease. Transillumination of the sinuses, largely because the findings are not clean cut, has not been found to be a useful diagnostic aid.

Widely varying opinions exist among respectable roentgenologists concerning the validity of roentgenograms in the diagnosis of sinus disease in chidren. John Caffey, the father of pediatric roentgenology, cautioned that films of the sinuses as indictors of disease in children were unreliable because of the normal presence of redundant mucosa that caused opacity. A large longitudinal growth and development study in Denver that included periodic sinus roentgenograms, showed substantial variation in the size, shape, aeration, and development of the sinuses from birth to adulthood. In this study, it was observed that roentgenologic findings commonly attributed to sinus disease could be found in healthy children who were clinically well at the time of the examination.[39,40] Similar "abnormal" roentgenogram findings have been observed in our institution in children who have had computed tomography (CT) scans of the skull for head injury, but no other disease save a mild upper respiratory infection (URI). Ultrasound has been reported to be of value in confirming the presence of fluid in the antra of children with abnormal maxillary sinus roentgenograms,[41] but the relationship of this finding to clinical symptoms must still be established. In view of the lack of validation of roentgenograms in the diagnosis of maxillary sinusitis in children, one wonders about the cost-effectiveness of obtaining sinus roentgenograms before institution of treatment when clinical signs of disease are suggestive.

Treatment

In the majority of children with the clinical signs of acute purulent sinusitis, antimicrobial treatment with either ampicillin, 100 mg/kg/day, or amoxicillin, 50 mg/kg/day, in three divided doses is the agent of choice. Since there is a poor correlation between bacteria recovered from cultures of the nasopharynx and those aspirated from the sinuses, selection of antimicrobials based on nasopharyngeal culture results is of no value. Although commonly prescribed (and perhaps they should be tried because of the low risk of adverse reactions), antihistamines and decongestants have not been adequately studied for efficacy in the treatment of acute or chronic sinusitis. If sinus pain results from IgE-mediated allergy that causes obstruction of the maxillary ostia along with the response of the nasal mucosa, then one might anticipate that allergy therapy directed either at avoidance of allergens or immunotherapy to those allergens not easily avoidable would be of benefit. No well-designed studies have addressed this question, however. When medical treatment fails and symptoms from chronic maxillary sinus disease persist, nasoantral irrigation or provision of a nasoantral window may be useful. Such treatment is not indicated, however, simply for rhinitis, that is, nasal congestion with or without rhinorrhea, even if sinus roentgenograms are abnormal.

OTITIS MEDIA

Aside from the common cold, acute otitis media is the most common respiratory tract disorder of childhood. In acute otitis media, the middle ear fluid is suppurative, whereas in chronic otitis media with effusion (OME), the effusion may be serous, mucoid, and occasionally purulent. For this reason, the commonly used term serous otitis media should be abandoned in favor of the term OME. The epidemiologic pattern of the disease has been well studied, as has its bacteriologic process. The highest attack rate for acute otitis media occurs between 6–36 months of age; about one third of the infants in one large study suffered at least one episode and another third had three or more episodes.[42] The attack rates diminish sharply after 6 years of age.

The studies of Bluestone and associates[43] have clearly shown that the pathogenesis of otitis media is related to eustachian tube dysfunction. Equilibration of air pressure in the middle ear with atmospheric pressure and clearance of middle ear secretions into the nasopharynx are two essential functions necessary for middle ear integrity. When disturbed by congenital (cleft palate and ciliary dyskinesia syndrome) or acquired (upper respiratory tract infection, enlargement of the adenoids, and in some cases allergy) abnormalities, otitis media may occur.

Chronic OME is a major pediatric problem, and much controversy exists concerning its pathogenesis, particularly in regard to the role of IgE-mediated allergy. In a study recently conducted at the Children's Hosptial of Buffalo,[44] IgE-mediated allergy was shown to play an etiologic role in only a minority of randomly selected children with recurrent OME. When allergy is involved, OME appears to be secondary to nasal obstruction and pressure changes associated with swallowing known as the "Toynbee phenomenon". There is no good evidence that allergy is a cause of intrinsic mechanical obstruction of the eustachian tube. Since bacteria are commonly present in aspirates of fluid from children with chronic OME, antimicrobial therapy is recommended if the child has not been previously treated.[45]

Diagnosis

The bacteriologic process of acute otitis media has been well studied. The organisms most commonly found are those normally resident in the nasopharynx of young children, namely, *S. pneumoniae* and *H. influenzae*. In the neonate, enteric bacteria are frequently encountered. Even in chronic OME about 50 percent of ears aspirated contain bacteria, but a much lesser percentage are clearly of the pathogenic variety. The typical patient with acute otitis media who has a history of an acute upper respiratory tract infection for a few days suddenly followed by earache, fever, and loss of hearing is easily diagnosed. Examination of the tympanic membrane reveals a red, bulging eardrum with obliteration of the normal landmarks. The tympanic membrane moves little when negative or positive pressure is applied to the canal with the pneumatic otoscope. In chronic OME the tympanic membrane is either retracted, with prominence of the short process of the malleus, or convex in appearance. The membrane is generally opaque in chronic OME, but if it is translucent, air bubbles or an air-fluid level may be seen. The patient, if old enough to complain, may be aware of the presence of fluid in the ear, and hearing may be reduced significantly. Audiometry can be performed to assess hearing loss. Tympanometry is the most reliable indicator of the mobility of the membrane and the presence of effusion. Reliable and relatively inexpensive tympanometers are available commercially, and many pediatricians find the instrument to be a good investment.

Treatment

Treatment of the usual case of acute otitis media is quite straightforward, since the bacteriologic process is predictable. Ampicillin, 50–100 mg/kg/24 hours, or amoxacillin, 25–50 mg/kg/24 hours in three divided doses, has been most frequently recommended. A combination of erythromycin, 50 mg/kg/24 hours, and sulfisoxazole, 150 mg/kg/24 hours, in four divided doses is an effective alternative for the penicillin-allergic child. Trimethoprim-sulfamethoxazole, 10–40 mg/kg/24 hours of the trimethoprim in two divided doses, is another alternative. Although a more expensive choice, cefaclor, 40 mg/kg/24 hours, in three divided doses can be used. Ampicillin-resistant strains of H. influenzae are being encountered on a regular basis. The occasional patient who continues to have a fever and persistent earache after 24–48 hours of optimal therapy should have a myringotomy with middle ear aspiration for bacteriologic culture and relief of pain. The traditional use of antihistamines appears not to alter the outcome.[46] A well-publicized study[47] purporting to show that antibiotics were not essential for acute otitis media was seriously flawed, however, and appropriate antibiotic therapy is routinely indicated for acute otitis media even though many patients would recover spontaneously without treatment.[48] Frequently the patient with recurrent acute otitis media may benefit from maintenance antimicrobial therapy to prevent recurrences; both sulfa and ampicillin administered twice daily have been used for this purpose.[49,50]

After adequate treatment, the middle ear may have persistent effusion that may clear spontaneously, without treatment beyond an initial 10-day antibiotic course, after as long as 3 months.[51] Thus "tincture of time" rather than rigorous therapy is indicated when effusion does not clear rapidly after treatment of acute otitis media, as long as symptoms have cleared and hearing is not compromised to a clinically important degree. A course of an oral decongestant combination has frequently been tried in an attempt to restore eustachian tube function, but a controlled clinical trial did not support the efficacy of such treatment.[52] Oral (but not inhaled) corticosteroids may influence the course of the disease. At least two controlled trials appear to have shown an increased frequency of resolution of OME when prednisone, 1 mg/kg/day, was used for up to 10 days.[53,54] Although further study is indicated before this becomes routine therapy, some surgical intervention might be prevented from this form of therapy.

For effusions that persist beyond 2–3 months, audiometric evaluation is indicated. Further investigation should consider extrinsic mechanical obstruction of the eustachian tubes such as enlarged adenoids, congenital abnormalities, or tumors. A myringotomy with insertion of a ventilation tube is indicated if medical management fails and hearing is impaired to a clinically important degree. Sometimes the problem resolves after one procedure. In other cases, reinsertion of the tube is performed if it falls out or becomes nonfunctional. In a long-term evaluation of 55 children with bilateral persistent OME treated with insertion of a ventilation tube in only one ear, with the other left as a control, improved hearing was associated with tube insertion within the first 6 months but not beyond. When the ears were examined after 5 years, there was a 42-percent incidence of tympanosclerosis and a 13-percent incidence of thin scars in the treated ears, although these abnormalities were not seen in the untreated ear, which averaged slightly (but not significantly) better hearing.[55] Thus chronic OME seems to be a developmental disease due to a combination of anatomic, infectious, and perhaps other factors affecting mostly young children. As such, the disorders resolves with "tincture of time" with or despite treatment, which therefore is primarily indicated when a dysfunctional hearing deficit results.

ASTHMA

Asthma is a disease characterized by abnormal physiology of the airways. Smooth muscle contraction, mucosal edema, and mucous secretions constitute the pathophysiologic mechanisms of the airway obstruction that results in the troublesome symptoms. Pharmacologic management is directed at reversing these abnormalities during acute symptoms and preventing their return with continuous therapy when symptoms are chronic. Since airway obstruction is uniquely reversible, appropriate use of available pharmacologic measures offers the potential to control the disease process with a high degree of efficacy and safety. The use of these medications without an understanding of their pharmacokinetic and pharmacodynamic properties, however, is likely to result in suboptimal clinical effect and increased risk of toxicity.

Clinical Pharmacology of Drugs Used for Asthma

Sympathomimetic Bronchodilators

The multiple drugs in this class include some of the oldest antiasthmatic agents still used, epinephrine and ephedrine, as well as many of the newest medications, some not yet on the American market. Parenterally and by inhalation these drugs relieve acute symptoms resulting from bronchospasm. The newest drugs in this class also offer the clinical advantage of greater specificity, longer duration, and efficacy by the oral route as compared with older drugs.

All of the currently available sympathomimetic amines have the phenylethylamine structure as their nucleus (Fig. 16-3). Alterations of this structure have been effective in increasing the β_2-specificity, oral bioavailability, and duration of action. The newer agents such as terbutaline, albuterol, and fenoterol thus can be given systemically with less cardiac and peripheral vascular effect than with the older drugs; they can be given orally with less degradation by gut and hepatic enzymes before entering the systemic circulation, and their duration of effect will be longer.

The sympathomimetic bronchodilators are administered by inhalation, parenterally, and orally. The rapid onset of action, potent bronchodilation, and patient acceptability of the aerosol route make it well-suited for treatment of intermittent symptoms or during acute exacerbations of chronic disease. The newer longer acting aerosal β_2-agonists also may have some usefulness in the treatment of chronic asthma, although the rapid falloff of effect of even the longest acting agents limits the practicality of the aerosols for around-the-clock therapy.

Concern over abuse has made some physicians very cautious in prescribing the aerosols. Deaths from asthma were reported to have increased approximately three-fold in England and Wales between 1959 and 1966 and about 50% in Australia from 1964–1967 in association with the increased use of potent sympathomimetic inhalers sold without prescription.[56,56a,56b,56c] Although speculation related to the apparent toxicity of the isoproterenol metered dose inhalers

ranged from cardiotoxicity from overdose of the drug[57] or fluorocarbon propellant,[58] the more likely explanation was failure of the critically ill patient to seek medical care in the presence of decreasing effect from the drug.[59]

Terbutaline, albuterol, and fenoterol are currently the drugs of choice in this class because of their β_2-selectivity and duration of action. They can be effectively administered via metered dose inhalers or through compressed air–driven nebulizers. The latter are particularly useful for young children who cannot effectively use the metered dose inhalers.

Oral use of these agents does not provide nearly the efficacy and freedom from adverse effects as is seen with aerosol use. Moreover, they are still plagued by the short duration of action with elimination half-lives from plasma in adults of less than 4 hours.[60] Systemic side effects, primarily tremor, correlate well with the degree of bronchodilation, thereby limiting the administration of optimally effective doses.[61] Metaproterenol, one of the more popular oral β_2-agonists used in children in the United States is considerably less effective than theophylline in a double-blind crossover comparative study.[62] Fewer symptoms, better exercise tolerance, and less need for additional oral corticosteroids were documented with theophylline as compared with the metaproterenol. The study concluded that oral metaproterenol was primarily indicated for patients with mild symptoms who rarely have emergency care requirements and cannot effectively use the medication by metered dose inhaler. This very restricted indication probably applies to all of the oral β-agonists. Even the most popular of these agents worldwide, albuterol (salbutamol), has been associated with considerably less effect orally than by inhalation,[63] and tolerance has been documented with continued therapy for various of these agents by both the oral and inhaled route.[64–66]

Theophylline

Theophylline is an old drug that has undergone a recent transformation in usage. Long recognized as a potent bronchodilator for relief of acute asthmatic symptoms, this drug has now become a major "prophylactic" agent for controlling symptoms and signs of chronic asthma. This has resulted largely from the application of new knowledge related to the pharmacodynamic and pharmacokinetic characteristics of the drug,

PHENYLETHYLAMINE

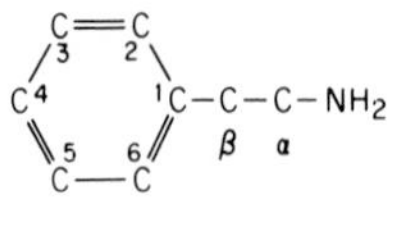

CATECHOLAMINE

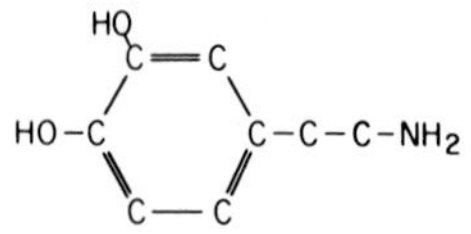

Drug Name	Structure	Major Receptor Activity	Oral Bioavailability In Conventional Doses	Approximate Duration Of Effect
NOREPINEPHRINE	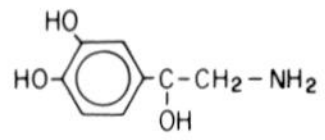	α	NO	<1 HOUR
PHENYLEPHRINE	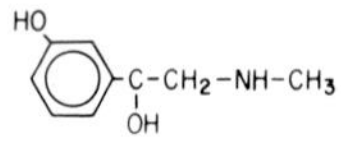	α	NO	<1 HOUR
EPINEPHRINE	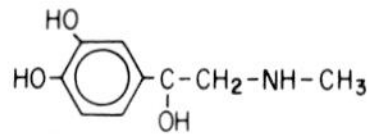	α, β_1, β_2	NO	<1 HOUR
EPHEDRINE	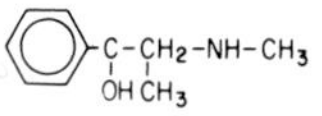	α, β_1, β_2 CNS	YES	4 HOURS
ISOPROTERENOL	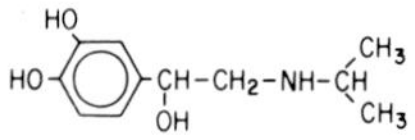	β_1, β_2	NO	<1 HOUR
ISOETHARINE	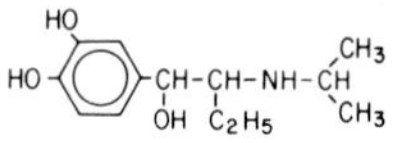	β_2	SOME	1 HOUR
METAPROTERENOL	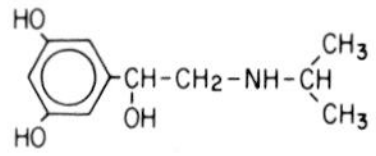	β_2	YES	4 HOURS
TERBUTALINE	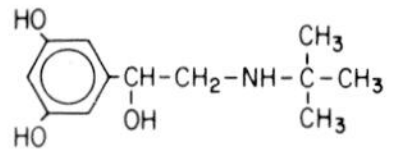	β_2	YES	6 HOURS
ALBUTEROL	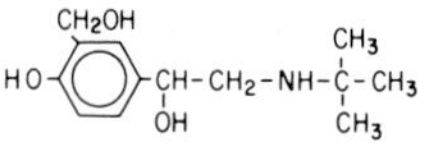	β_2	YES	6 HOURS
FENOTEROL	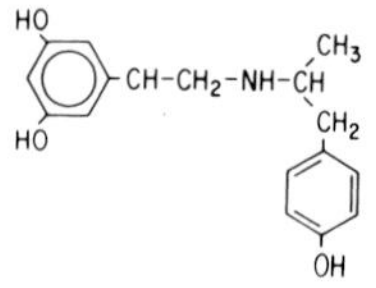	β_2	YES	6 HOURS

Figure 16-3. Structure and function of selected sympathomimetic amines. Numbers are used to identify the positions on the benzene ring and identify the carbon atoms of the basic phenylethylamine structure and the positions of the ethanol moiety. Adrenergic receptor activity is indicated by α, β_1, and β_2. From Weinberger M, Hendeles L: *Am J Hosp Pharm* 1976; 33:1071. With permission.[183]

the development of readily available rapid and specific assays, and the development of new controlled-release formulations for oral use.

Theophylline relaxes bronchial smooth muscle through mechanisms that are not well defined. Older speculation regarding the inhibition of phosphodiesterase with consequently delayed degradation of intracellular cyclic AMP has not been supported by more recent data. Concentrations in vitro required to inhibit phosphodiesterase exceed safe concentrations used clinically and other phosphodiesterase inhibitors are not bronchodilators. Others[67] have suggested that theophylline acts as a prostaglandin antagonist, and effects on intracellular calcium flux have been described.[68]

Theophylline also is a diuretic and central nervous system stimulant. Most patients, however, rapidly become tolerant to these effects. When theophylline and ephedrine are used in combination, the adverse effects on the central nervous system of the two drugs are synergistic, whereas the bronchodilator effect is, at most, additive.[69]

The bronchodilator effect of theophylline has been shown to be approximately proportional to the logarithm of serum concentrations within the range of 5–20 μg/ml[70,71] The relationship between serum theophylline concentration and therapeutic response also has been demonstrated for exercise-induced bronchospasm, a nearly universal manifestation of asthma.[72] Serum concentrations above 10 μg/ml are much more effective at inhibiting bronchospasm in response to a standardized treadmill exercise stress than lower levels, although some further increase in inhibitory effect was apparent at serum concentrations above 15 μg/ml. Furthermore, this effect of theophylline is maintained with continuous dosing.[73] Of greatest importance for the treatment of chronic asthma, the frequency and severity of symptoms are reduced to the greatest extent when serum theophylline concentrations are maintained on a continuous around-the-clock basis at levels ranging from 10 to 20 μg/ml (Fig. 16-4).

Theophylline has minor caffeinelike side effects that appear to have little direct relationship to serum concentration and are associated with rapidly acquired tolerance during long-term therapy. Adverse effects associated with serum concentrations above 20 μg/ml, however, generally are persistent and include nausea, vomiting, headache, diarrhea, irritability, insomnia, and, at higher serum levels (e.g., > 40 μg/ml), cardiac arrhythmias, seizures, and death (Fig. 16-5).

Deaths resulting from theophylline toxicity have been most frequently reported among small children who received multiple adult-size doses.[74] The common clinical course is characterized by irritability, vomiting of coffee ground–like material, and seizures, after which some patients fail to regain consciousness. Brain damage is common among survivors. Unfortunately, serious toxicity, including seizures and death, are not reliably preceded by less severe adverse effects. Charcoal hemoperfusion is recommended for levels over 60 μg/ml, preferably begun before the onset of seizures.[187]

Theophylline is rapidly, consistently, and completely absorbed when administered as an oral liquid, plain uncoated tablet,[76] or rectal solution.[77] Once absorbed, theophylline appears to distribute rapidly throughout extracellular and, to a lesser extent, intracellular body water.[70] The apparent volume of distribution (V_D) ranges from 0.3 to 0.7 L/kg and averages about 0.45 L/kg among adults and children[78,79] and about 0.6 L/kg in neonates.[80] Protein binding for theophylline is about 40 percent. Theophylline freely crosses the placenta[81] and also passes freely into breast milk.[82] Salivary levels are approximately 60 percent of serum concentrations.[83] No serious consequences have been reported as a result of either transplacental passage of therapeutic levels or ingestion of the amounts occurring in breast milk.

Theophylline is eliminated from the body at variable rates through multiple parallel pathways, some of which are saturable or capacity limited.[84] Approximately 10 percent is eliminated by the kidneys unchanged, whereas the remainder is metabolized, apparently in the liver, to 1,3-dimethyluric acid, 1-methyluric acid, and 3-methylxanthine. The proportion eliminated as 3-methylxanthine is variable and appears to be lower in patients who metabolize theophylline slowly.[85] Variability of dosage requirements among individuals occurs as a result of the variable rates of elimination.[84] Individual clearance rates and dose requirements remain relatively stable over time, however.

Variability in clearance appears to be a function of the rate of hepatic biotransformation which, on the average, changes with age (Table 16-2). Patients with hepatic cirrhosis generally have much lower theophylline plasma clearance rates and dose requirements than individuals with normal liver function.[86] Elimination of theophylline is also prolonged in patients with cardiac decompensation,[87] including those with cor pulmonale,[88] newborn infants,[80] and patients receiving macrolide antibiotics such as troleandomycin and erythromycin.[89–91] Cimetidine, an inhibitor of hepatic microtubular function,[92] has similar effects.[93–96]

There is no rationale for formulations that include added substances to form so-called salts or pharmacologically active solubilizers such as alcohol.[97] Even for an aminophylline injection the addition of ethylenediamine only serves to increase the pH level sufficiently to dissolve theophylline at the packaged concentration.

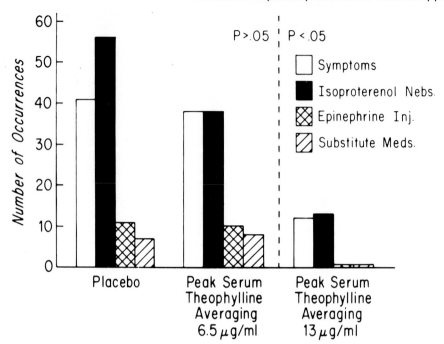

Figure 16-4. Frequency and severity of asthmatic symptoms during 1 week of treatment with a placebo, an ephedrine-theophylline combination in conventional doses that resulted in serum theophylline concentrations averaging 6.5 μg/ml, and individualized theophylline doses that resulted in serum theophylline concentrations averaging 13 μg/ml. Asthmatic symptoms during each 1-week period were treated when necessary with inhaled isoproterenol; if symptoms were not promptly relieved, epinephrine was administered subcutaneously. If the patient was unresponsive to these measures, known medications were substituted for the double-blind medications. From data in Weinberger M: Theophylline for treatment of asthma. *J Pediatr* 92:1–7, 1978.[69]

Consequently, all dosages and labeling of theophylline formulations should be in terms of the anhydrous theophylline content, for example, aminophylline injection, 25 mg/ml, would more appropriately be labeled as theophylline injection, 21 mg/ml.

The parenteral theophylline preparation is given only intravenously; it is painful and absorbed more slowly when given intramuscularly. [98] Although rectal suppositories are incompletely and erractically absorbed, this is a function of the formulation, since the rectal route allows rapid and complete absorption from a solution.[77]

Because of the decreased fluctuations in serum concentration, particularly in patients with rapid elimination, slow-release preparations have become the formulations of choice for management of chronic asthma. Of those products which are completely absorbed, Theo-Dur and Slobid have the slowest absorption that is relatively constant over approximately 12 hours.[76,99,99a] A 12-hour

dosage interval is therefore reasonable with this product, except in patients with very high dose requirements in whom 8-hour dosages may provide more stable blood levels. Furthermore, only products that allow dosage adjustment in 50-mg increments or less should be used routinely so that doses can be adequately individualized. Bead-filled capsules can be administered to small children by sprinkling the beaded contents on a spoonful of soft food, followed by a tasty beverage to wash down the beads unchewed.

Cromolyn

Cromolyn sodium (sodium cromoglycate) is a structurally and pharmacologically unique drug that inhibits, but does not reverse, bronchospasm. Limited clinical testing was begun in England in 1965, and it was introduced into that market in 1968 and in the United States in 1975.

Cromolyn blocks the release of chemical mediators of IgE-mediated hypersensitivity reac-

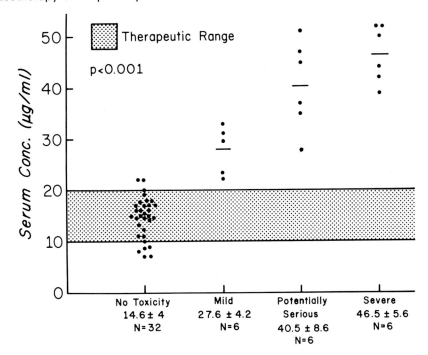

Figure 16-5. Serum theophylline concentrations resulting from intravenous theophylline administered to adults in the medical intensive care unit of the University of Iowa Hospital. Dosages were no greater than 0.7 mg/kg/hr of theophylline (0.9 mg/kg/hr of aminophylline). Using these previously recommended infusion rates, 17 of 49 patients experienced varying degrees of theophylline toxicity as a result of elevated serum concentrations. Mild toxicity included nausea, vomiting, headache, insomnia, and nervousness. Potentially serious adverse effects included sinus tachycardia with or without symptoms of mild toxicity. Severe toxicity included cardiac arrhythmias and seizures. Thus the relationship between the degree of toxicity and serum theophylline concentration was supported by these data. From Hendeles L, Bighley L, Richardson RH, et al: Frequent toxicity from IV aminophylline infusions in critically ill patients. *Drug Intell Clin Pharm* 11:12–18, 1977. With permission.[184]

tions. It appears to do this through direct activity at the mast cell surface. It does not interfere with the antigen-antibody interaction, nor does it oppose the action of the mediators once they are released. The effect of cromolyn is nonspecific and exerted regardless of the antigen involved. In addition, it blocks nonimmunologic stimulation of mediator release from rat mast cells that results from exposure in vitro to such compounds as phospholipase A, dextran, and polymyxin B.[100]

The mechanism of action is unclear. Some evidence suggests an alteration in membrane permeability to calcium, which may be an early step in the sequence of cellular events leading to degranulation.[101] Others have suggested that cromolyn acts on irritant receptors in the airways,[102,103] which could reduce vagal reflex pathways for bronchospasm. This theory would help to explain the clinical efficacy of cromolyn in

modifying asthmatic symptoms triggered by nonimmunologic factors such as exercise or cold air.

Less than 1 percent of a cromolyn dose is absorbed after oral administration. When administered by inhalation using a turboinhaler device for powder insufflation, only about 75 percent of the dose is delivered. Of that only 10 percent reaches the peripheral airways where it is rapidly removed by systemic absorption. The remainder is deposited in the mouth and pharynx, swallowed, and passed through the stool intact. The fraction that is absorbed is rapidly eliminated in bile and urine with a biologic half-life of 46–99 minutes.[104] Biotransformation into metabolites does not occur.

When administered before exposure to antigen, cromolyn can decrease or even completely block the resulting bronchospasm, both immediate and delayed.[105] Although the effect of cromo-

Table 16-2 *Relationship Between Age and Theophylline Elimination**

Age	Age (Years)[†]	Number of Patients	Clearance (ml/kg/min)	Half-Life (Hours)
Premature neonates with apnea	7.5 ± 4.4 days	6	0.29 ± 0.1	30 ± 6.5
	41 ± 12 days	8	0.64 ± 0.3	20 ± 5.3
Infants				
4–24 weeks	14 ± 5 weeks	10	—	13 ± 4.7
24–48 weeks	31 ± 8 weeks	9	—	6.8 ± 2.2
Young children, 1–4 years	2.5 ± 0.9	10	1.7 ± 0.6	3.4 ± 1.1
Older children				
4–12 years	9.4 ± 3	17	1.5 ± 0.4	—
6–17 years	10.7 ± 2.6	30	1.4 ± 0.6	3.7 † 1.1
13–15 years	14 ± 0.8	6	0.8 ± 0.2	—
Adults, otherwise healthy				
nonsmoking asthmatics	31 ± 10	16	0.65 ± 0.19	8.7 ± 2.2

*From Weinberger M, Hendeles L, Ahrens R: *Pediatr Clin North Am.* 28:47, 1981. With permission.[177]
†The statistics for age, clearance, and half-life are the mean ± the standard deviation.

lyn in blocking antigen blocking antigen-induced bronchospasm may be only partial when it is administered in conventional doses through a turboinhaler, near total protection has been reported using nebulization of a 5 percent solution.[106] The effect of a conventional dose in blocking antigen-induced bronchospasm begins to decline rapidly 2 hours after administration and is substantially gone by 5 hours.[107]

It is interesting that repeated challenge with the *same* antigen at 2 and 5 hours after a cromolyn dose is associated with continued blocking effect, but if different antigens are used at the two times, there is little suppression of bronchospasm at 5 hours. This indicates that the effect observed at 5 hours when the same antigen is used for both challenges is not due to the cromolyn but is a result of transient desensitization by continued occupation of the antibody receptor itself after the prior antigen exposure.[107]

Cromolyn appears also to affect nonimmunologically mediated bronchospasm such as that induced by aspirin[108] and some alcoholic beverages.[109] Cromolyn may also decrease bronchospasm induced by voluntary hyperventilation[110] and inhalation of histamine[111] or methacholine,[112] although others have failed to demonstrate a protective effect for bronchospasm induced by intravenous histamine,[113] inhaled histamine, or inhaled methacholine.[114]

The effectiveness of this drug for exercise-induced asthma has been reported.[115] The blocking effect is variable, however, and in most cases inferior to that which can be obtained with optimal bronchodilator therapy with theophylline or inhaled sympathomimetic bronchodilators.

In the treatment of chronic asthma, regular use of cromolyn prevents symptoms in many patients, but not to the degree seen with theophylline (Fig. 16-6). Interestingly, its efficacy appears not to relate to the presence of inhalant allergy, exercise-induced bronchospasm, or other identifiable clinical factors.[116,117]

Cromolyn has been the least toxic of all medications used for the treatment of asthma. Even when administered intravenously in doses far exceeding the amount normally absorbed in the human by inhalation, no adverse effects were consistently observed.[118] No clinically important adverse effects of cromolyn were detected in a multicenter study of long-term safety.[119]

The most common adverse responses to cromolyn are transient brochospasm, coughing, and dryness of the throat. The former is rarely more than a minor nuisance and may be prevented by prior use of an inhaled bronchodilator. The latter can generally be avoided by drinking water after its use. Adverse reactions consisting of generalized or facial dermatitis, myositis, or gastroenteritis were observed and found to be reproducible upon challenge in 8 of 375 patients receiving cromolyn.[120] Immunologic hyperreactivity to cromolyn was not demonstrated in these patients but has been reported elsewhere.[121]

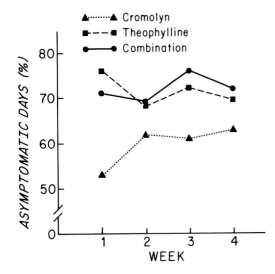

▲········▲ Cromolyn
■----■ Theophylline
●——● Combination

Figure 16-6. Frequency of asymptomatic days in 28 asthmatic children treated in a double-blind study for 4 weeks each with theophylline, cromolyn, and the combination. Although significant differences between cromolyn and theophylline were observed (*p* less than 0.025), differences between weeks during the same regimen were not significant for any of the three drug regimens (*p* greater than 0.1). From Hambleton G, Weinberger M, Taylor J, et al: *Lancet* 1:381, 1977. With permission.[185]

Corticosteroids

Corticosteroids are the only antiasthmatic agents that can effectively reverse airway obstruction of asthma that has become poorly responsive to bronchodilators. Since this is a major reason for hospitalization and for continuing morbidity in the patient with severe disease, these drugs are exceedingly important and should not be withheld when needed. When used inappropriately, however, they have the potential for serious adverse effects.

The anti-inflammatory effects of glucocorticoids include suppression of the redness, heat, pain, and swelling of the acute inflammatory reaction. They appear to do this by increasing the resistance of the capillary wall to extravasation of fluid, with subsequent reduction in the accumulation of leukocytes at the site of inflammation or injury. They also affect the distribution of various pools of leukocytes in the body. Neutrophils, which are normally marginated on the capillary endothelium of various tissues, reenter the circulation. Eosinophils, monocytes, and lymphocytes

(particularly thymus-derived lymphocytes) disappear from the peripheral circulation. Impairment of bactericidal activity has been observed in vitro for neutrophils and monocytes after exposure to corticosteroids, perhaps as a result of the stabilization of lysozymes.[122] Either the synthesis or release of vasoactive kinins[123] and prostaglandins[124] is inhibited, and it appears that corticosteroids potentiate the catecholamine stimulation of cyclic AMP synthesis.[125]

Glucocorticoids also have the potential for a profound influence on carbohydrate metabolism, response to stress, and function of the hypothalamic-pituitary-adrenal (HPA) axis. Suppression of growth, lymph node and thymus involution, eosinopenia, lymphocytopenia, and various other metabolic effects also may occur.[126] At an intracellular level, corticosteroids act by stimulating a protein receptor in the cytoplasm of the cell, which ultimately results in the formation of specific messenger ribonucleic acid (mRNA). The translation of mRNA leads to the formation of proteins that mediate the effects of the steroid hormone. Although the relevance of this to effectiveness in asthma has not been established, the time course of these events in vitro is consistent with the delayed onset of therapeutic effect that is generally observed.

Corticosteroids may be administered orally, topically, or parenterally. Phosphate and hemisuccinate conjugates suitable for both intravenous and intramuscular administration are absorbed rapidly and reach plasma concentrations similar to those following administration of the unconjugated steroids. Acetate derivatives, on the other hand, are very slowly absorbed over a long period of time and are thus useful as depot injections for intraarticular or intralesional therapy of dermatologic problems. They have no place in the treatment of asthma because their slow rate of onset would delay the relief of symptoms, and their duration may be longer than is needed. The absorption of oral prednisone *can* be quite rapid, but is influenced by tablet disintegration and dissolution; recent studies have demonstrated that the rate of absorption of prednisone may vary considerably among generic brands.[127]

Betamethasone and dexamethasone, used by inhalation in doses effective for asthma, appear to be efficiently absorbed and capable of clinically important systemic effects.[128,129] In contrast, triamcinolone acetonide, beclomethasone dipropionate, flunisolide, and others are topically active with relatively poor absorption in active form.[130]

Most of the corticosteroids, other than cortisone and prednisone, do not require biotransformation to become active. Although the hydroxylation required for these two compounds to become active may be delayed or decreased in some patients,[131] this rarely, if ever, is a clinical problem. Phenobarbital and rifampin increase the clearance of dexamethasone and methylprednisolone, and these interactions have been associated with apparent decreases in clinical effect.[132,133] Similarly, phenytoin increases the rate of elimination of prednisone, thus decreasing its effect.[134]

Circulating corticosteroids can be inactivated in the liver by conjugation to glucuronides, which are then excreted in the urine. This constitutes a major pathway of elimination. Several of the structural changes made in the synthetic congeners have resulted in interference with this process. As a result, circulation of the active form is prolonged, and a larger percentage of the dose is eliminated in the urine unchanged. Only 3 percent of hydrocortisone, for example, is eliminated in the free unconjugated form, whereas 20–40 percent of prednisolone is eliminated as the free drug.[135]

Corticosteroids are the only currently available antiasthmatic agents that can reverse the bronchodilator unresponsive component of asthmatic airway obstruction. They increase the sensitivity of the airways to β-agonist bronchodilators,[136] beginning as soon as 1 hour after an intravenous dose in some patients,[137] and increase Po_2 in hypoxic patients as early as 3 hours after administration.[138] Clinically, production of the thick tenacious sputum peculiar to asthma is controlled, and mucosal edema appears to be decreased. They do not block the immediate skin test,[139] however, or initial bronchospasm resulting from antigen challenge.[105] Moreover, they do not inhibit exercise-induced bronchospasm,[140] nor do they appear to inhibit experimental bronchospasm provoked by inhalation of methacholine or histamine.

There is virtually no risk of serious toxicity with short-term (less than 2 weeks) use of daily oral or parenteral corticosteroids, even in high doses. Daily administration of even low doses for extended periods, however, is accompanied by a high risk of toxic effects, including suppression of endogenous adrenal function, cush-

ingoid changes in appearance, growth suppression, posterior subcapsular cataracts, aseptic necrosis of the femoral head, and osteoporosis.

The risks of long-term corticosteroid therapy can be minimized by the use of prednisone, prednisolone, or methylprednisolone (but not longer acting agents such as triamcinolone or dexamethasone) as a single dose every other morning.[141–144] The introduction of inhaled beclomethasone dipropionate was first enthusiastically endorsed as a corticosteroid regimen without systemic effect, but subsequent data have demonstrated that this inhaled agent differs little from alternate-day prednisone with regard to suppressive effects on the HPA axis.[27] Although occasional patients may experience some fullness of the face and excessive weight gain from appetite stimulation with alternate-day prednisone, most do not exhibit clinically important changes, and the serious metabolic effects, including growth suppression and bone demineralization associated with daily prednisone, have not been seen.[145] Inhaled beclomethasone dipropionate, on the other hand, has been associated with oral moniliasis manifested clinically as thrush and occasionally by hoarseness. This is readily responsive to treatment with a mycostatin mouthwash, however, and rarely requires stopping the medication. An additional nuisance is coughing stimulated by inhaling fluorocarbon propelled aerosolized powder; this generally can be prevented by preceding the beclomethasone with an inhaled bronchodilator. Both alternate-day prednisone and inhaled beclomethasone dipropionate are indicated solely for prophylaxis in patients who frequently respond inadequately to bronchodilators; neither is sufficient for treatment of acute exacerbations.

Guide to Treatment

Once a diagnosis of asthma is made, therapeutic decisions require classification of the asthma as intermittent or chronic. The therapeutic strategy for intermittent asthma is the education of the patient or family to intervene rapidly and effectively when acute symptoms develop, but the extended symptomatic periods that characterize the clinical course of intermittent asthma make maintenance prophylactic medication unnecessary. On the other hand, patients with chronic asthma, that is, those with frequently recurring or continuous symptoms, require mea-

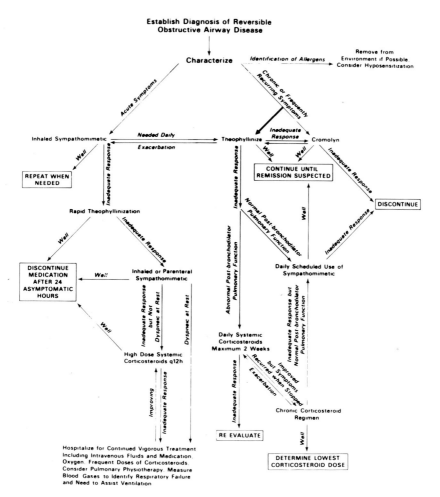

Figure 16-7. Criteria for selection and sequence of drug therapy used for the management of asthma. From Weinberger M, Hendeles L: Pharmacotherapy of asthma. *Am J Hosp Pharm* 33:1071, 1976. With permission.[183]

sures to prevent the return of symptoms, in addition to contingency measures to deal with occasional acute symptoms when they still occur (Fig. 16-7).

Acute Symptoms

Acute symptoms of asthma are most effectively relieved initially by prompt use of an inhaled sympathomimetic bronchodilator such as metaproterenol, albuterol, or terbutaline. The standard dose is two inhalations from the metered dose inhaler separated by 1 or 2 minutes. The same medications also can be delivered by a compressed air–driven nebulizer. Metaproterenol, 10 mg, or terbutaline, 1 mg, are commonly used doses when delivered by compressed air driven open nebulizer. A dose of 2 mg of terbutaline can be used for more severe symp-

toms, and doses can be repeated frequently if the patient is being carefully monitored in the hospital. Equipotent doses of albuterol (salbutamol) or fenotenol would be equally acceptable when available. Repeat doses at 4-hour intervals are acceptable for home use. Parenteral sympathomimetic bronchodilators such as injectable terbutaline in a dose of approximately 0.01 mg/kg can be used if there is an inadequate response to inhaled medication, which usually occurs when the patient has sufficient airway obstruction that inhaled medication cannot be adequately delivered.

The primary bronchodilator for acute symptoms of asthma is thus inhaled or parenteral sympathomimetics. Theophylline can play an important adjunctive role, however, when added to the inhaled or parenteral β2-agonist therapy.

205

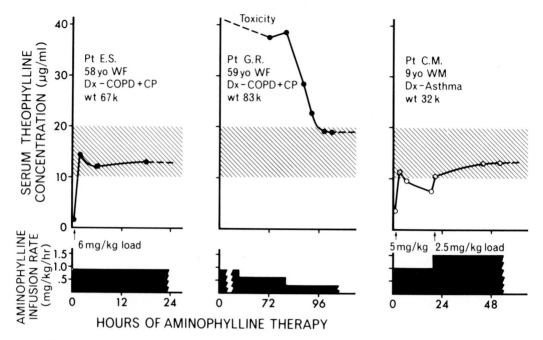

Figure 16-8. Intravenous theophylline (as aminophylline) dosage required to achieve and maintain serum theophylline concentrations in three patients. From Weinberger M, Matthay RA, Ginchansky EJ, et al: Intravenous aminophylline dosage: Use of serum theophylline measurement for guidance. *JAMA* 235:2110, 1976. With permission.[186]

To obtain efficacy from theophylline for acute bronchodilation, a loading dose should be used initially to rapidly attain serum concentrations between 10 and 20 μg/ml this should be followed by a sustaining infusion to maintain levels at this therapeutic range. Each milligram per kilogram of the loading dose will raise the serum theophylline concentration by about 2 μg/ml. This can be used for guidance in initial therapy. For example, if the patient has not received any prior theophylline, a 5 mg/kg loading dose will, on the average, attain a serum concentration of 10 μg/ml. Initial dose requirements can be calculated if prior theophylline was given. Ideally the serum theophylline concentration should then be measured before administration of theophylline, but this is not always practical when the patient is suffering from acute respiratory distress. While the appropriate continuous infusion is running, the change in serum concentration during the course of the infusion can then be used to guide adjustments of the infusion rate (Fig. 16-8). Use of inhaled or parenteral sympathomimetic bronchodilators should be repeated as needed for acute symptoms during the course of the theophylline

infusion. Most importantly, corticosteroid therapy should be begun as soon as it is apparent that a prompt and complete response to bronchodilators alone is not occuring. The empirically determined dosage extensively utilized at our institution is 10 mg of prednisone or the equivalent for children under 1 year of age, 20 mg for children 1–3 years old, 30 mg for children 3–12 years old, and 40 mg for adolescents and adults. Corticosteroids should be repeated as often as every 4–6 hours if the patient is in respiratory failure; 12-hour dosages generally sufficient under less critical conditions.

Chronic symptoms

For patients with frequently recurring or continuous symptoms of asthma, theophylline is the most effective single medication in preventing return of symptoms. The initial dosage of theophylline should be low, the lesser of 16 mg/kg/day or 400 mg/day, to ensure that the medication is well tolerated even though this dosage will be insufficient to attain therapeutic serum concentrations for all but a small percentage of patients. Subsequent incremental increases can then be

Initial Dose:

Weight: ___42___ kg

☒ Adults and children over 25 kg.........................200 mg at _7_ am and _7_ pm
☐ Children 20 to 25 kg.................................150 mg at ___ am and ___ pm
☐ Children 15 to 20 kg.................................100 mg at ___ am and ___ pm

Increase Dose After 3 Days If Tolerated To:

☒ Adults and children over 35 kg.........................300 mg at _7_ am and _7_ pm
☐ Children 25 to 35 kg.................................250 mg at ___ am and ___ pm
☐ Children 20 to 25 kg.................................200 mg at ___ am and ___ pm
☐ Children 15 to 20 kg.................................150 mg at ___ am and ___ pm

Attention: Decrease dose to **Initial Dose** if the increased dose is not tolerated because of headaches or stomach upset (nausea, vomiting, diarrhea)

Increase Dose After 3 More Days If Tolerated To:

☒ Adults and children over 40 kg.........................400 mg at _7_ am and _7_ pm
☐ Children 35 to 40 kg.................................350 mg at ___ am and ___ pm
☐ Children 30 to 35 kg.................................300 mg at ___ am and ___ pm
☐ Children 20 to 30 kg.................................250 mg at ___ am and ___ pm
☐ Children 15 to 20 kg.................................200 mg at ___ am and ___ pm

CHECK SERUM CONCENTRATION BETWEEN 3 AND 8 HOURS AFTER A DOSE WHEN NONE HAVE BEEN MISSED OR ADDED FOR AT LEAST 3 DAYS.

Serum Theophylline Concentration ___14___ mcg/ml

Patient: _James Jones_

If serum theophylline is: **Directions:**

OK—   10 to 20 mcg/ml ....Maintain dose if tolerated. **RECHECK SERUM THEOPHYLLINE CONCENTRATION AT 6 TO 12 MONTH INTERVALS.***

TOO HIGH—20 to 25 mcg/ml ....Decrease doses by 50 mg.
        25 to 30 mcg/ml ....Skip next dose and decrease subsequent doses by 25% to the nearest 50 mg.
        Over 30 mcg/ml ....Skip next 2 doses and decrease subsequent doses by 50%. **RECHECK SERUM THEOPHYLLINE.**

TOO LOW— 7.5 to 10 mcg/ml...............Increase dose by 25% to the nearest 50 mg.**
        5 to 7.5 mcg/ml...............Increase dose by 25% to the nearest 50 mg and **RECHECK SERUM THEOPHYLLINE FOR GUIDANCE IN FURTHER DOSAGE ADJUSTMENT.**

*Finer adjustments in dosage may be needed for some patients.
**Dividing the daily dosage into 3 doses administered at 8-hour intervals may be indicated if symptoms occur repeatedly at the end of a dosing interval.

Figure 16-9. Oral theophylline dosage guide with a slow-release formulation suitable for 12-hour dosages and available in 50-mg increments. This is a reproduction of part of a two-page form; the second page is a duplicate copy for the patient indicating the number of each size tablets to be taken. This dosage schedule has been incorporated into current FDA approved package inserts.

made at 3-day intervals, as long as the medication is tolerated, until age-specific mean doses are attained.[178] The dosage should be lowered in the presence of any adverse effects. Serum concentrations performed on blood drawn at the time of estimated peak serum concentration for the product used can provide guidance for the final dosage (Fig. 16-9). Whereas the initial dosage that rapidly attains serum concentration is associated with a high frequency of minor adverse complaints, this procedure of initial doses with subsequent titration is associated with an exceedingly low frequency of even transient complaints (Table 16-3).

Cromolyn provides an alternative medication for the control of chronic asthma. Although less effective on the average, many patients will dramatically respond to this medication; it has the least risk for serious toxicity of any medication used for asthma. Cromolyn may be a preferred first drug when the psychosocial situation creates a likelihood of potentially dangerous noncompliance with theophylline or the measurement of serum concentrations or when the patient is either intolerant or, because of other aspects of the clinical situation, is likely to be intolerant of theophylline. The addition of cromolyn to theophylline is only occasionally associated with additive effect.

Inhaled β_2-agonists should be used promptly for any breakthrough symptoms that occur, and regularly scheduled use of longer acting inhaled β_2-agonists is indicated for patients with bronchodilator-responsive symptoms recurring with sufficient frequency to warrant additional preventive measures. All patients, regardless of age,

Table 16-3 *Serum Theophylline Measurements and the Frequency of Adverse Effects Elicited by the History at the Time of Initial Blood Sampling in Sequentially Selected Ambulatory Patients Whose Dose was Titrated Over 9 Days as Previously Described (see Figure 9).*

Serum Concentration	Number of Children	Number of Adults	Percentage with Adverse Effects	
			Children	Adults
< 10	29	12	0	0
10–19.9	258	38	1.9	7.9
≥ 20	61	6	28	67

*From Hendeles L, Weinberger M, Wyatt R: *Am J Dis Child* 1978; 132:876.[178]

who have had emergency care requirements should have the means of delivering an inhaled β₂-agonist at home. Metered dose inhalers are generally sufficient for older children, as long as adequate instruction is given and reinforced each time the patient is seen. A compressed air–driven nebulizer is more appropriate for younger children. In unusual circumstances, if the patient has had life-threatening episodes of asthma characterized by sudden onset, it is appropriate to provide the parents with the means and instruction for delivery of a parenteral β₂-agonist such as terbutaline.

Finally, corticosteroids are often essential to prevent emergency medical care when the patient becomes unresponsive to bronchodilators. Because of the delay in onset of action, the use of corticosteroids should be begun promptly when incomplete responsiveness to the addition of the inhaled β₂-agonists is apparent. An incomplete response is defined as failure to return to normal even after a repeat dose or when the duration of effect is less than 4 hours. Oral doses of 10 mg of prednisone or prednisolone or equivalent doses of methylprednisone should then be initiated twice daily for children under 1 year old, 20 mg twice daily for children 1–3 years of age, 30 mg twice daily for children 3–12 years of age, and 40 mg twice a day for adolescents and adults. Corticosteroids should be continued until the patient has been totally well for 24 hours; Normal postbronchodilator pulmonary function can be used to document maximal effect and should be used for guidance when possible. Daily prednisone at these doses is rarely needed beyond 7–10 days, and often shorter periods than that are sufficient.

For patients who repeatedly become unresponsive to bronchodilator medication, mainte-nance corticosteroids are needed. Alternate-day prednisone or one of the new generation of inhaled corticosteroids such as beclomethasone dipropionate are both acceptably safe regimens for long-term usage. In general, initial mainte-nance steroid therapy should be at a dose somewhat higher than is likely to be needed to minimize the risk of breakthroughs. If the patient is well, reductions in dosage can then be made at about 2-week intervals to determine the lowest dose needed for a sufficient degree of control of the disease to allow normal sleep and daytime functioning. Choices between the two steroids are based on the ability to deliver the inhaled steroid with the metered dose inhaler along with considerations of convenience and cost. For the occasional patient who experiences repeated airway irritation from use of the metered dose inhaler, alternate-day prednisone becomes the medication of choice. For the minority of patients who experience appetite stimulation and consequent excessive weight gain with alternate-day prednisone, the inhaled steroid becomes preferable. Otherwise, the relative advantages of each should be explained to the patient or family and then an informed decision made. Even when maintenance corti-costeroids are needed, additional contingency measures for breakthrough symptoms may still require short bursts of oral corticosteroids in the doses described for exacerbations.

Injections of allergenic extracts have only a limited indication for the treatment of asthma. They generally are not indicated for symptoms that are only intermittent and easily controllable with acceptable medication but are worth considering in the presence of clear-cut exacerbations of asthma associated with specific inhalant allergy seasons. Seasonality, however also can be caused by viral respiratory tract infections that predominate in the spring and fall. Thus the history needs to closely correlate with skin tests, and the physician making decisions for allergy shots needs to be familiar with the aerobiology of the locale.

Using these various measures, most patients with asthma can be kept free of symptoms most of the time. Specifically, patients should seldom have the asthma interfere with sleep, and normal activities. Even athletics should rarely be interrupted by wheezing, coughing, or shortness of breath. Emergency care requirements and hospitalization should, with rare exceptions, be avoided. In fact, the current therapy of asthma has made this disease one of the most controllable of chronic illnesses.

CYSTIC FIBROSIS (AND OTHER DISEASES ASSOCIATED WITH CHRONIC PURULENT BRONCHITIS AND BRONCHIECTASIS)

Cystic fibrosis is the major disease causing chronic purulent bronchitis and bronchiectasis. Although the pulmonary disease of cystic fibrosis and chronic purulent bronchitis and bronchiectasis of other causes are associated with progressive destruction of airways and surrounding lung tissue, extraordinary progress has been made during recent years in increasing the quality of life and longevity of these patients. The pathophysiologic mechanism of this group of diseases involves defective mucociliary transport in association with chronic bronchiolar obstruction and chronic bacterial lower respiratory tract infection. Progressive damage to the bronchi results in bronchiectasis. This is a nearly universal component of cystic fibrosis.[146] Patients with immotile cilia syndrome and immunoglobulin deficiency disease also develop this type of chronic lung disease, although often at a slower rate than occurs with cystic fibrosis and as a result of different etiology. Additionally, there is a group of patients who can only be characterized as having idiopathic purulent bronchitis and bronchiectasis. This may be familial, sometimes associated with sweat chloride values that are intermediate between normal and those which are diagnostic for cystic fibrosis. These patients, however, have no extrapulmonary manifestations of cystic fibrosis.

Microbiology of the Lower Respiratory Tract

Predominant organisms reported in the sputum of patients with cystic fibrosis have been *Staphylococcus aureus* and *Pseudomonas aeruginosa*. The increasing frequency of *P. aeruginosa* has been apparent in association with the use of antibiotics and longer survival of the patients. In addition, normal oropharyngeal commensal flora have been identified in the lower respiratory tract of patients with cystic fibrosis through the bronchoscope and at postmortem examination.[147,148] The repetitive and frequent recovery of high concentrations of *Haemophilus* species, *Staphylococcus epidermidis,* α-hemolytic streptococci, nonhemolytic streptococci, Neisseria species, and diphtheroids[149-151] suggests that the ecology of lower respiratory tract flora of patients with cystic fibrosis is complex. It seems unlikely that these organisms always represent contamination with oropharyngeal secretions, since their concentration in saliva, after rinsing the mouth with water, is substantially less than that found in sputum.[151] Moreover, these organisms repeatedly may be recovered from some patients.

Characterization of the lower respiratory tract flora in patients with cystic fibrosis is essential if specific antibiotic therapy is to be used. Unfortunately, organisms recovered from sputum or even bronchial secretions obtained with bronchoscopy may include the many organisms that make up the normal oropharyngeal flora, as well as organisms that are truly from the lower respiratory tract which may therefore be potentially pathogenic.[152,151] Transtracheal aspiration has been a traditional reliable means of bypassing the microorganisms that inhabit the upper respiratory tract flora, but the risks for children exceed those for adults, making this means impractical for repeated culturing. Lung aspiration has been another means of sampling the normally sterile lung. Unfortunately, an attempt of this procedure in three patients was not associated with any microbial growth despite subsequent demonstrable improvement in pulmonary tests and respiratory symptoms while undergoing antimicrobial therapy (unpublished data).[153] In addition, bacteria may be irregularly distributed throughout pulmonary secretions, and streaking a thick, tenacious glob of sputum on agar may not give representative information.

To minimize the sampling problems associated with multiple microfoci of infection embedded within sputum, the potential contamination of sputum by clinically irrelevant oropharyngeal flora, and the problem of differing rates of bacterial growth, quantitative cultures of homogenized sputum samples have potential usefulness in identifying the lower respiratory tract flora of patients with cystic fibrosis. The technology of quantitative cultures of homogenized sputum has been available for almost 30 years,[154–157] and this procedure has been employed in a few reports with cystic fibrosis.[158–160] A variety of mucolytic agents have been employed for homogenization of sputum, including acetylcysteine, ethylenediaminetetraacetic acid, sonication, and others. The authors have employed 2-percent acetylcysteine because of its apparent lack of toxicity to the pathogens expected to be found in sputum from patients with cystic fibrosis.

Organisms commonly found in saliva from patients with cystic fibrosis included both oropharyngeal commensal organisms and those associated with lower respiratory tract illness. The authors limit the degree of oropharyngeal contamination by washing the mouth out with water before collecting sputum. This appears to reliably decrease colony counts to less than 10^4 colony-forming units/ml. An analogous procedure has been to wash the sputum samples themselves with a stream of water in a tea strainer.[161] It is also wise to examine the collected specimen closely to observe for sputum and microscopically to document the presence of neutrophils.

After rinsing the mouth with water and collecting the sputum, the problem associated with differential rates of growth for various organisms can be managed by transporting the collected sputum sample on ice to the laboratory for examination within 10–20 minutes. Prompt dilution in 2-percent acetylcysteine and phosphate-buffered saline, followed by vigorous mixing with glass beads, prepares the sputum for subsequent dilution and plating.[162] The dilution procedure can be simplified by using a calibrated 0.001-ml platinum loop. By employing a semisolid medium and the homogenized specimen, the problem of overgrowth by more rapidly growing organisms is obviated. Specimens present at $>10^6$ colony-forming units are enumerated and speciated by the usual microbiologic means[163] and then may be tested for antimicrobial susceptibility. Using this method, microbiologic flora present in saliva are less likely to be attributed to

Table 16-4 *Isolation of Bacteria from Homogenized Sputum**

Organism	Frequency of Recovery[†]		
	Patient 1	Patient 2	Patient 3
S. aureus	6/6	0/6	6/6
S. epidermidis	0/6	1/6	1/6
P. aeruginosa	0/6	6/6	0/6
H. influenzae	6/6	6/6	2/6
Streptococcus			
α-Hemolytic	2/6	6/6	4/6
Nonhemolytic	0/6	2/6	1/6
Neisseria sp.	0/6	5/6	0/6

*Modified from Myers MG, Koontz FP, Weinberger M: Lower respiratory infections in patients with cystic fibrosis. In Lloyd-Still J (ed): *A Textbook on Cystic Fibrosis.* Littleton, Mass., John Wright/PSG Inc. (In press.) With permission.[164]
[†]Number of sputa with less than or equal to 10^6 colony-forming units/ml and the number tested at monthly intervals.

sputum, and sputum flora can be demonstrated to be highly stable in the same patients (Table 16-4).

In a comparison of qualitative and quantitative sputum cultures, *H. influenzae* was commonly not identified in the qualitative culture even though it averaged 2×10^8 colony-forming units/ml and quantitative culture with individual cultures ranging up to 7×10^{10} culture-forming units/ml (Table 16-5). This study treated both sputum samples identically, that is, keeping the sputum on ice and placing it on culture plates within 20 minutes. With routine handling of sputum when hours at room temperature may elapse before plating, even *Staphylococcus* organisms may be overgrown by *Pseudomonas* organisms and not identified on the culture. In addition, species often considered normal oropharyngeal flora by qualitative culture such as α-hemolytic streptococci, *S. epidermidis*, *Neisseria* species, and diphtheroids were frequently present at colony counts exceeding 10^6 colony-forming units/ml and thus were likely to have come from the lower respiratory tract. Histologically, microfoci of organisms consistent with these "normal flora" also have been observed in sputum from patients culturing these organisms.[164]

Table 16-5 *Comparison of Culture of 97 Sputa from Patients with Cystic Fibrosis**

Organism	Organisms Recovered from Culture		
	Both	Qualititative Only[†]	Quantitative Only[‡]
S. aureus	37	2	3
H. influenzae	11	2	29
P. aeruginosa	65	3	4
Oral commensal flora	68	24	1

*Modified from Myers MG, Koontz FP, Weinberger M: Lower respiratory infections in patients with cystic fibrosis. In Lloyd-Still J (ed): *A Textbook on Cystic Fibrosis*. Littleton, Mass., John Wright/PSG Inc. (In press.) With permission.[164]
[†]Present or absent.
[‡]Present in greater than or equal to 10^6 colony-forming units/ml, absent in less than 10^6 colonly-forming units/ml.

Antimicrobial Therapy

With the advent of the "antibiotic era" it quickly became apparent to physicians caring for children with cystic fibrosis that antimicrobial agents could alter the outcome of acute lower respiratory tract exacerbations.[165,166] Improved survival, although partly attributable to the improved diagnosis of patients with less severe disease, is in large measure attributable to antibiotics.[167–171]

Although there is little debate over the potential value of antibiotics, there has often been inadequate justification for the selection, dosage, and end points for antibiotic therapy in the patient with cystic fibrosis. The primary indication for antibiotic therapy of lower respiratory tract disease in otherwise normal children is acute pyogenic pneumonia with *S. pneumoniae* and *H. influenzae*. These generally result in lobar or lobular alveolar infiltrates. Children with cystic fibrosis are not at particular risk for pneumococcal infection and the pathophysiologic process is not that of a pyogenic pneumonia. In fact, the infection is not predominately in the lung parenchyma per se but is in the airway, resulting in mucous production and airway obstruction. Because of the host-defense abnormality, antibiotic therapy, by selectively killing susceptible bacteria, has the potential to alter the flora that has colonized the lower respiratory tract and thereby select out resistant organisms. Eventually, most patients become colonized by mucoid strains of *P. aeruginosa* with all the potential for antibiotic resistance associated with that organism.

Thus antibiotics ameliorate, they do not cure.

Nonetheless, they decrease morbidity and improve survival. Once the limitations of antibiotic therapy are understood, the basic principles of antimicrobial therapy are the same for cystic fibrosis as for other diseases. When the potential bacterial pathogen has been identified, initial antibiotic selection can be made based on expected sensitivities. Drugs effective against *S. aureus* include penicillins such as dicloxacillin, all of the cephalosporins, and a few miscellaneous agents such as clindamycin and lincomycin. Resistance of *staphylococci* to these antibiotics has so far been rare. *Haemophilus* species have generally been sensitive to penicillin derivatives such as ampicillin, amoxicillin, carbenicillin, ticarcillin, and becampicillin. In recent years, β-lactamase–producing strains of *Haemophilus* species have been seen with increasing frequency; alternative choices have then been required. These have included the sulfa drugs, the trimethoprim-sulfamethoxazole combination, chloramphenicol, and possibly some of the progeny among the new generations of cephalosporins.

The choice of antibiotics remains limited for *P. aeruginosa*, and rapid development of resistance to multiple antimicrobials is common. Although in vitro sensitivities of naive patients often indicate sensitivity to various antibiotics, resistance generally develops rapidly to all oral antibiotics. Generally, treatment of the *Pseudomonas* infection, when judged necessary, requires parenteral therapy with a combination of a synthetic penicillin such as carbenicillin or ticarcillin and one of the aminoglycoside antibiotics. Because of the narrow therapeutic index for the aminoglycosides and the variable degree of sensitivity of the *Pseudomonas* organisms, expected patterns of sensitivity based on specific identification of the organism provide a degree of guidance to therapy, but determination of the minimal inhibitory concentration provides a useful guide for therapy by indicating both the optimal choice of the specific aminoglycoside and the desired minimal serum concentration.

Antibiotic Delivery

The oral route is convenient, may avoid hospitalization, and is therefore of potential value for *Staphylococcus* and *Haemophilus* species.[162] There is little reason, however, to expect oral antibiotics to be effective for *Pseudomonas* infections. Moreover, even for the penicillins and cephalosporins, oral doses may not attain blood levels as high as that which can effectively be attained with parenteral therapy. This problem especially may be compounded in patients with cystic fibrosis where malabsorption is part of the clinical problem, and therapeutic effect therefore may be decreased because of lower antibiotic blood levels.[172] Since the infection in cystic fibrosis is in relatively loculated areas, such as the mucous membranes and bronchiectatic lesions in the airways, doses of antibiotics need to be high enough not only to exceed the minimal inhibitory concentration of the organism in the circulation where antibiotic levels are determined, but also must be sufficient to attain adequate therapeutic levels in the airway secretions where the primary site for colonization provides the seed for the infection.

Because of this anatomic location of the organism and the consequent limitation of antibiotic delivery to the site of the infection, even temporary elimination of the target bacteria in the sputum is likely only with the most sensitive organisms. Since the sensitivity of *Pseudomonas* organisms is often relative, only occasional transient elimination of these bacteria from the sputum is seen.

The dosage of most antibiotics greatly exceeds the minimum that might be needed while still allowing a large margin of safety. The aminoglycosides and chloramphenicol, however, have in common a narrow therapeutic index whereby the toxic dose does not greatly exceed the generally required therapeutic dose. Therapeutic drug monitoring is therefore essential for optimal safe use of these antimicrobial agents. The aminoglycosides combined with a synthetic penicillin effective against *Pseudomonas* organisms, such as carbenicillin or ticarcillin, are most important for cystic fibrosis because of their major role in the treatment of *Pseudomonas* infections.

"Standard" dosage recommendations for the aminoglycoside antibiotics generally have been inadequate (Table 16-6). Studies that have used traditional dosages of gentamicin and tobramycin, such as 5–7.5 mg/kg/day, even in combination with carbenicillin, appear to be associated with less evidence of clinical benefit in patients than the generally higher dosages needed to attain optimal peak serum concentration, whereas objective benefit clinically, physiologically, and bacteriologically has been seen with individualized doses guided by serum concentration. When gentamicin or tobramycin is given to provide peak levels near 10 μg/ml with troughs below 2 μg/ml, dosages commonly average about 12 mg/kg/day in four to six divided doses.

Initial dosages of tobramycin or gentamicin should be 2.5–3 mg/kg every 6 hours. This is best administered intravenously over 20–30 minutes by a constant infusion pump. Once the rate of infusion is set, it is repeated for all subsequent doses so that similar blood levels will be attained. Care must be taken to ensure that the full dose is consistently delivered and that part is not left in the intravenous tubing. This will result in a peak serum concentration being attained essentially at the end of the infusion. This initial peak, however, may not yet be in equilibrium with tissue levels. A brief period of rapid decrease in serum concentrations may therefore follow; the subsequent disappearance of aminoglycoside from serum follows a log linear pattern, at least to low serum concentrations where slow elimination of tissue-bound drug from previous doses may result in prolonged elimination of this residual aminoglycoside (Fig. 16-10).

Measurement of serum concentrations at 1, 2, and 3 hours after completion of the intravenous infusion allows extrapolation of the measurement to time zero (time of completion of the infusion), assuring complete distribution of the drug, and extrapolation to the time when the serum concentration decreases to under 2 μg/ml, which appears important for safety (Fig. 16-10). The dosage can then be adjusted proportionately to assure extrapolated peak concentrations of 8–12 μg/ml, and the dosage interval can be adjusted to

Table 16-6 *Summary of Studies Evaluating the Efficacy of Aminoglycoside Therapy for Cystic Fibrosis*

Reference	Dosage	Conclusions
Marks et al.[179]	Gentamicin, 4.5–5 mg/kg/day Carbenicillin, 400–600 mg/kg/day	No significant improvement
Beaudry et al.[180]	Gentamicin, 5 mg/kg/day in three doses Carbenicillin, 600 mg/kg/day in six doses	No significant benefit
Weintzen et al.[159]	Tobramycin, 2/mg/kg, three times a day	Some improvement
McCrae et al.[181]	Tobramycin, 5–12 mg/kg/day	Patients receiving dosages of 10 and 12 mg/kg/day had mean serum levels of 6.8 and 8.7 μg/ml; in some of these patients the *pseudomonas* infection was eradicated
Rabin et al.[158]	Tobramycin, 12–16 mg/kg/day, individualized doses and dosing intervals Carbenicillin, 600 mg/kg/day (100 mg/kg/Q4H)	Effective; response proportional to in vitro sensitivity
Cipolle et al.[182]	Tobramycin, variable	Doses need to be individualized and are often higher than recommended

provide levels under 2 μg/ml but not for excessive durations.

Although the use of appropriately selected antibiotics during acute exacerbations of pulmonary symptoms appears to be well established, there are less data related to the maintenance use of antibiotics for long-term therapy in an attempt to prevent progression of the pulmonary disease. For organisms such as *S. aureus* and *H. influenzae,* however, oral antibiotics are available for which development of resistance is uncommon and the maintenance of antibiotics appears to have a relative degree of efficacy. In one of the few controlled evaluations of this subject, an oral cephalosporin was associated with fewer hospitalizations, improved pulmonary function, and better weight gain than the placebo when each was given for alternating 3-month periods over 2 years.[162] This therapy was specific, however, for those patients who had *Staphylococcus* organisms cultured in significant colony counts from their sputum. The same results could reasonably be expected for patients having recurrent symptoms from *H. influenzae.*

Oral antibiotics are not effective for *Pseudomonas* organisms, however, and the indiscrimi-

nate use of antibiotics not specific for organisms identifiable from appropriately collected sputum is probably of no value and only exposes the patient to the potential risks of the drugs. Moreover, it is clear that many patients can have a relatively benign course for extended periods without maintenance antibiotics; the routine use of oral antibiotics in all patients with cystic fibrosis therefore is not justifiable exclusively on the basis of susceptible organisms alone. Although not established, it is possible that oral antistaphylococcal therapy may be associated with the earlier colonization of *Pseudomonas* organisms, thereby potentially complicating, rather than benefiting, the clinical course of the patient. It thus appears appropriate to select those patients with recurrent symptoms or deteriorating pulmonary function *and* susceptible organisms for maintenance antibiotic therapy and then maintain the therapy only until a definable clinical end point, such as decrease in the frequency of symptoms and deteriorating pulmonary function, is observed.

Rational alternatives to recurrent hospitalization or intravenous therapy when symptoms are associated primarily with isolation of *Pseudomo-*

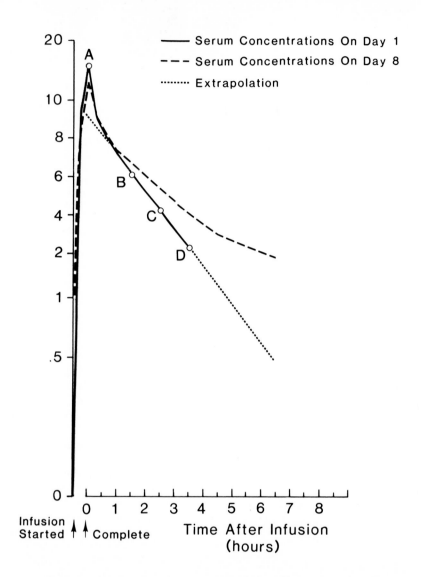

Figure 16-10. Serum concentration time curve after 2.5 mg of tobramycin on the first and eighth day of treatment in a young adult with cystic fibrosis. Because of the initial rapid distribution phase of elimination (*A* to *B*), measurement of serum concentration for determination of elimination half-life should be delayed until at least 60 or even 90 minutes after the dose has been administered (*B*) and repeated at hourly intervals (*C* and *D*). A least square linear regression can be performed (even small handheld calculators can do this), and the line can be extrapolated to below 2 μg/ml and back to time zero, that is, the time that dose administration was complete. This is illustrated on a semilog plot. The dosage can then be adjusted proportionately to attain projected serum concentrations at time zero to levels of 8–12 μg/ml; the dosage interval can be adjusted so that the next dose is administered shortly after the serum concentration falls below 2 μg/ml. Doses and dosing intervals to attain these serum concentrations vary and must be individualized for optimal and safe therapy. Care also must be taken to allow for the possibility of a prolonged terminal phase of degradation after multiple doses because of slowed elimination of residual tissue-bond drug (*dashed line*).

nas organisms from the sputum culture are limited. Recurrent illness in selected patients may be prevented by prophylactic treatment with intravenous antibiotics, for example, carbenicillin/ticarcillin and an aminoglycoside for 48–72 hours at monthly to weekly intervals, depending on the patient and the rapidity with which illness would otherwise occur. The administration of the antibiotics at home on an outpatient basis has also been used in some cases.

An alternative for maintenance suppressive therapy of *Pseudomonas* infection using aerosolized carbenicillin and gentamicin has recently been proposed.[173] In a double-blind randomized controlled study of 20 patients treated alternately for 6 months with the aerosolized antibioitic and placebo, subjective and objective benefit was associated with the aerosol therapy. Doses consisted of 1 g of carbenicillin and 80 mg of gentamicin administered by nebulizer morning and evening. Among the 20 patients included in the study, 7 courses of intravenous antibiotics were needed while patients were receiving the placebo and 3 were needed while receiving the antibiotic aerosol. Measurements of respiratory function were significantly improved in association with the maintenance antibiotic aerosol. The authors emphasized, however, that the bother, expense, and limited experience with this procedure justified it primarily for patients having the need for recurrent intravenous therapy or a deteriorating clinical condition in which *Pseudomonas* organisms are the primary infectious agent. Furthermore, they emphasized that *Pseudomonas* organisms continued to grow in the sputum of all patients, and prolonged usage might eventually select out resistant organisms.

Assessment of Antibiotic Therapy

The symptoms associated with exacerbation of lower respiratory tract infection for cystic fibrosis include increased coughing, sputum production, malaise, easy fatigability, and poor weight gain or weight loss, especially when not associated with the voracious appetite characteristic of the pancreatic insufficiency and consequent malabsorption. Increasing signs of airway obstruction, however, can appear even earlier, and measurement of pulmonary function provides a sensitive and objective means of identifying increasing airway disease. Low-grade fever is a variable and late sign, as are changes in the white blood cell count and chest roentgenogram.

The physiologic effects of airway disease that characterize cystic fibrosis are obstruction manifested by a decrease in the forced vital capacity, 1-second forced expiratory volume, and various flow-rate measurements. The easily measured peak expiratory flow rate is a relatively insensitive indicator of small airway disease in which much of the obstruction initially occurs. The optimal use of pulmonary function to assess the clinical course of cystic fibrosis includes the spirometric measurement of the vital capacity, 1-second forced expiratory volume, and flow rates and the plethysmographic measurement of the functional residual capacity, residual volume, and total lung capacity.

The progression of airway obstruction leads to ventilation/perfusion mismatching, which results in varying degrees of relative hypoxia, and progressive airway obstruction can lead to acute or chronic respiratory failure manifested by accumulating carbon dioxide. Thus the measurement of blood gases provides another important measurement of pulmonary function and is, in fact, the only pulmonary function that can be measured reliably on a routine clinical basis in children too young to perform spirometry and plethysmography. The serial comparison of flow-rate measurements, such as the $FEF_{25-75\%}$ or flow rates at 25, 50, and 75 percent of expiration, must be examined at isovolume conditions if values are to be used in assessment of the patient. Changes in vital capacity influence these traditional flow-rate measurements and can even, on occasion, give paradoxical results if these values are not calculated at isovolume conditions, that is, measurement of the flow rates at the same degree of expiration with regard to total lung capacity and not just vital capacity.

The use of pulmonary function measurements to assess the status of airway disease in cystic fibrosis is so superior to the use of subjective assessment alone or other indirect means of clinical assessment, including the use of a stethoscope and chest roentgenogram that the justification can be made for routine measurement of pulmonary function each time the patient is seen. Transcutaneous oxygen monitoring now can provide routine monitoring of Pao_2 as an additional measure of pulmonary function. The need for treatment can be identified because of an acute exacerbation of symptoms or progression of a consistent decrease in pulmonary function. Repeat measurements of pulmonary function during the course of treatment then can objectively examine efficacy and guide duration of treatment.

REFERENCES

1. Smith, JM: Epidemiology and natural history of asthma, allergic rhinitis and atopic dermatitis (eczema). In *Allergy: Principles and Practice* Middleton E, Reed CE, Ellis RF, (eds.), St. Louis: C. V. Mosby, 1978, pp. 633–658.

2. Connell JT, Bernoske D: *Evaluation of Rondec-T vs Its Components in Relieving the Symptoms of Allergic Rhinitis during the Ragweed Pollen Season.* (Report No. CP5362), Columbus, Ohio, Ross Laboratories, 1977.

3. Cook TJ, MacQueen DM, Wittig HJ, Thornby JI, Lantos RL and Virtue CM: Degree and duration of skin test suppression and side effects with antihistamines. *J Allergy Clin Immunol* 51:71–77, 1973.

4. Rhoades RB, Leifer KN, Cohan R. and Wittig HJ: Suppression of histamine induced pruritis by three antihistaminic drugs. *J Allergy Clin Immunol* 55:180–185, 1975.

5. Schaaf L., Hendeles L, Weinberger, M: Suppression of seasonal allergic rhinitis symptoms with daily hydroxyzine. *J Allergy Clin Immunol* 63:129–133, 1979.

6. Wong L, Hendeles L, Weinberger M: Placebo-controlled evaluation of hydroxyzine and chlorpheniramine for seasonal allergic rhinitis. *J Allergy Clin Immunol* 63:203, 1979.

7. Connell JT: A novel method to assess antihistamine and decongestant efficacy. *Ann Allergy* 42:278–285, 1979.

8. Empey DW, Bye C, Hodder M, Hughes DTD: A double-blind crossover trial of pseudoephedrine and triprolidine alone and in combination for the treatment of allergic rhinitis. *Ann Allergy* 34:41–46, 1975.

9. Anonymous: Cyproheptadine as an appetite stimulant. *Drug Ther Bull* 8:71–72, 1970.

10. King CTG, Weaver SA, Narrod SA: Antihistamines and teratogenicity in the rat. *J Pharmacol Exp Ther* 147:391–398, 1965.

11. Franks HM, Hensley VR, Hensley WF, Starmer GA, Teo RKC: The interaction between ethanol and antihistamines. 1:dexchlorpheniramine. *Med J Aust* 65(1):449–452, 1978.

12. Karlin J: The use of antihistamines in asthma. *Ann Allergy* 30:342–347, 1972.

13. Carruthers SG, Shoeman DW, Hignite CE, Azarnoff DL: Correlation between plasma diphenhydramine level and sedative and antihistamine effects. *Clin Pharmacol Ther* 23:375–382, 1978.

14. Albert KS, Hallmark MR, Sakmar E, Weidler DJ and Wagner J G: Pharmacokinetics of diphenhydramine in man. *J. Pharmacokinet Biopharm* 3:159–170, 1975.

15. Roth RP, Cantekin EI, Bluestone CD, Welch RM, and Cho Y W: Nasal decongestant activity of pseudoephedrine. *Ann Otol Rhinol Laryngol* 86:235–242, 1977.

16. Dressler WE, Meyers T, Rankell AS, London SJ, Poetsch C E: A system of rhinomanometry in the clinical evaluation of nasal decongestants. *Ann Otol Rhinol Laryngol* 86:310–317, 1977.

17. Lader MH, Sakalis G, Tansella M: Interactions between sympathomimetic amines and a new monoamine oxidase inhibitor. *Psychopharmacologia* 18:118–123, 1970.

18. Elis J, Laurence DR, Mattie H, Prichard BNC: Modification by monoamine oxidase inhibitors of the effect of some sympathomimetics on blood pressure. *Br Med J* 2:75–78, 1967.

19. Bickerman HA: Physiologic and pharmacologic studies on nasal airway resistance (R_N) (Dec. 8, 1971). *Proceedings of Conference on Current Research Methodology in the Evaluation of Proprietary Medicines* Washington, DC The Proprietary Association, 1971.

20. Weinberger M, Bronsky E: Interaction of ephedrine and theophylline. *Clin Pharmacol Ther* 17:585–592, 1975.

21. Weinberger MM, Bronsky EA: Evaluation of oral bronchodilator therapy in asthmatic children. *J Pediatr* 84:421–427, 1974.

22. Black MJ and Remsen KA: Rhinitis medicamentosa. *Can Med Assoc J* 122:881–884, 1980.

23. Norman PS, Winkenwerder WL, Agbayani BF, Migeon CJ: Adrenal function during the use of dexamethasone aerosols in the treatment of ragweed hay fever. *J Allergy* 40:57–61, 1967.

24. Michels MI, Smith RE, Heimlich EM: Adrenal suppression and intranasally applied steroids. *Ann ALlergy* 25:569–574, 1967.

25. Heroman WM, Bybee DE, Cardin MJ, Bass JW, Johnsonbaugh RE: Adrenal suppression and cushingoid changes secondary to dexamethasone nose drops. *J Pediatr* 96:500–501, 1980.

26. Handleman NI, Friday GA, Schwartz HJ, Kuhn FS, Lindsay DE, Koors PG, Moyer RP, Smith CS, Kemper CF, Nagel JR, Rosch J, Murphey S, Miller DL: Cromolyn sodium nasal solution in the prophylactic treatment of pollen-induced

seasonal allergic rhinitis. *J Allergy Clin Immunol* 59:237–242, 1977.

27. Wyatt R, Waschek J, Weinberger M, Sherman B: Effects of inhaled beclomethasone dipropionate and oral alternate-day prednisone on pituitary-adrenal function in children with chronic asthma. *N Engl J Med* 299:1387–1392, 1978.

28. Mygind N, Hansen I, Pedersen CB, Prytz S, Sorensen H: Intranasal beclomethasone dipropionate aerosol in allergic nasal diseases. *Postgrad Med J* 51(Suppl 4):107–110, 1975.

29. Vilsvik JS, Jenssen AO, and Walstad R: The effect of beclomethasone dipropionate aerosol on allergen induced nasal stenosis. *Clin Allergy* 5:291–294, 1975.

30. Chatterjee SS, Nassar WY, Wilson O, Butler AG: Intranasal beclomethasone dipropionate and intranasal sodium cromoglycate: a comparative trial. *Clin Allergy* 4:343–348, 1974.

31. Greenbaum J, Cockcroft D, Hargreave FE, Dolovich J: Sodium cromoglycate in ragweed-allergic conjunctivitis. *J Allergy Clin Immunol* 59:437–439, 1977.

32. Wald ER, Pang D, Milmoe GJ, Schramm VL Jr.: Sinusitis and its complications in the pediatric patient. *Pediatr Clin N America* 28:777–796, 1981a.

33. Shopfner CE, Rossi JO: Roentgen evaluation of the paranasal sinuses in children. *Am J Roentgenol Radium Ther Nucl Med* 118:176–186, 1973.

34. Swischuk LE, Hayden CK Jr., Dillard RA: Sinusitis in Children. *RadioGraphics* 2:241–252, 1982.

35. Towbin R, Dunbar JS: The paranasal sinuses in childhood. *RadioGraphics* 2:253–270, 1982.

36. Wald ER, Milmoe GJ, Bowen A, Ledesma-Medina J, Salamon N, Bluestone CD: Acute maxillary sinusitis in children. *New England J Med* 304:749–754, 1981b.

37. Rachelefsky GS, Goldberg M, Katz RM, Boris G, Gyepes MT, Shapiro MJ, Mickey MR, Finegold SM, Siegel SC: Sinus disease in children with respiratory allergy. *J Allergy Clin Immunol* 61:310–314, 1978.

38. Rachelefsky GS, Katz RM, Siegel SC: Chronic sinusitis in children with respiratory allergy: the role of antimicrobials. *J Allergy Clin Immunol* 69:382–387, 1982.

39. Maresh MM: Paranasal sinuses from birth to late adolescence; size of paranasal sinuses as observed in routine posteroanterior roentgenograms. *Am J Dis Child* 60:55–78, 1940.

40. Maresh MM, Washburn AH: Paranasal sinuses from birth to late adolescence; clinical roentgenographic evidence of infection. *Am J Dis Child* 60:841–861, 1940.

41. Revonta M: A-mode ultrasound of maxillary sinusitis in children (letter). *Lancet* 1:320, 1978.

42. Teele DW, Klein JO, Rosner BA: Epidemiology of otitis media in children. *Ann Otol Rhinol Laryngol* 89 (Suppl. 68):5–6, 1980.

43. Bluestone, CD: Recent advances in the pathogenesis, diagnosis, and management of otitis media. *Pediatr Clin N America* 28:727–755, 1981.

44. Bernstein JM, Ellis E and Li P: The role of IgE-mediated hypersensitivity in otitis media with effusion. *Otolaryngol & Head & Neck Surg* 89:874–878, 1981.

45. Liu YS, Lim DS, Lang RW: Chronic middle ear effusions. Immunochemical and bacteriological investigations. *Arch Otolaryngol* 101:278–286, 1975.

46. Chilton CA, Skipper BE: Antihistamines and alpha-adrenergic agents in treatment of otitis media. *Southern Medical Journal* 72:953–955, 1979.

47. Buchem FL, Dunk JHM, van't Hof MA: Therapy of acute otitis media: Myringotomy antibiotics or neither? and is your antibiotic really necessary? *Lancet* 2:883–887, 909–910, 1981.

48. Saah AJ, Blackwelder WC, Kaslow RA: Treatment of acute otitis media. *J Amer Med Assoc* 248: 1071–1072, 1982.

49. Perrin JM, Charney E, MacWhinney JB, McInerny TK, Miller RL, Nazarian LF: Sulfisoxasole as chemoprophylaxis for recurrent otitis media. A double-blind crossover study in pediatric practice. *N Engl J Med* 291:664–667, 1974.

50. Maynard JE, Fleshman JK, Tschopp CF: Otitis media in Alaskan Eskimo children. Prospective evaluation of chemoprophylaxis. *J Amer Med Assoc* 219:597–, 1972.

51. Shurin PA, Pelton SI, Donner A, Klein JO: Persistence of middle-ear effusion after acute otitis media in children. *N Engl J Med* 300:1121–1123, 1979.

52. Olson AL, Klein SW, Charney E, MacWhinney JB, McInerny TK, Miller RL, Nazarian LF, Cunningham D: Prevention and therapy of serous otitis media by oral decongestant: a double-blind study in pediatric practice. *Pediatrics* 61:679–684, 1978.

53. Persico M, Podoshin L, Fvadis M: Otitis media with effusion. A steroid and antibiotic therapeutic trial before surgery. *Ann Otol* 87:191–196, 1978.

54. Schwartz RH, Puglese J, Schwartz DM: Use of a short course of prednisone for treating middle ear effusions—a double-blind crossover study. *Ann Otol Rhinol Laryngol* 84 (Suppl 68):296–300, 1980.

55. Brown MJK, Richards SH, Ambegaoker AG: Grommets and glue ear: a five-year follow-up of a controlled trial. *Royal Society Med* 71:353–356, 1978.

56. Stolley PD: Asthma mortality: Why the United

States was spared an epidemic of deaths due to asthma. *AM Rev Resp Dis* 105:883–890, 1972.

56a. Inman, WHW, Adelstein AM: Rise and fall of asthma mortality in England and Wales in relation to use of pressurised aerosols. *Lancet* 2:279–284, 1969.

56b. Patrick PR, Tonge JI: Reply to letter to the editor. *Med J Aust* 2:668, 1966.

56c. Campbell AH: Mortality from asthma and bronchodilator aerosols. *Med J Australia* 1:386–391, 1976.

57. Collins JM, McDevitt DG, Shanks RG, Swanton JG: The cardio-toxicity of isoprenaline during hypoxia. *Br J Pharmacol* 36:35–45, 1969.

58. Dollery CT, Williams FM, Draffan GH: Arterial blood levels of fluorocarbons in asthmatic patients following use of pressurized aerosols. *Clin Pharmacol Ther* 15:59–66, 1974.

59. Conolly ME, Davies DS, Dollery CT: Resistance to beta-adrenoceptor stimulants (a possible explanation for the rise in asthma deaths). *Br J Pharmacol* 43:89 . . . 402, 1971.

60. Leferink JG, Wagemaker-Engles I, Maes RAA: Quantitative analysis of terbutaline in serum and urine at therapeutic levels using gas chromatography-mass spectrometry. *J Chromotog* 143:299–305, 1977.

61. Dulfano M, Glass P: Evaluation of a new beta₂ adrenergic receptor stimulant, terbutaline, in bronchial asthma. II. Oral comparison with ephedrine. *Curr Ther Res* 15:150–157, 1973.

62. Dusdieker L, Green M, Smith GD, Ekwo EE, Weinberger M: Comparison of orally administered metaproterenol and theophylline in the control of chronic asthma. *J Pediatr* 101:281–287, 1982.

63. Anderson S, Seale J, Rozea P, et al: Inhaled and oral salbutamol in exercise-induced asthma. *Am Rev Resp Dis* 114:493–500, 1976.

64. Nelson HS, Raine D, Doner C, Posey WC: Subsensitivity to the bronchodilator action of albuterol produced by chronic administration. *Am Rev Resp Dis* 116:871–878, 1977.

65. Plummer AL: The development of drug tolerance to beta₂ adrenergic agents. *Chest* 73: 949–957, 1978.

66. Chervinsky P, Belinkoff S: Comparison of metaproterenol and isoproterenol aerosols: Spirometric evaluation after two months' therapy. *Ann Allergy* 27:611–616, 1969.

67. Horrobin DF, Manku MS, Franks DJ, Hamet P: Methyl xanthine phosphodiesterase inhibitors behave as prostaglandin antagonists in a perfused rate mesenteric artery preparation. *Prostaglandins* 13: 33–40, 1977.

68. Brisson GR, Malaisse-Lagie F, Malaisse WJ: The stimulus-secretion coupling of glucose-induced insulin release. VII. A proposed site of action for

adenosine 3.5′-cyclic monophosphate. *J Clin Invest* 52: 232–241, 1972.

69. Weinberger M: Thephylline for treatment of asthma. *J Pediatr* 92:1–7, 1978.

70. Levy G, Koysooko R: Pharmacokinetic analysis of the effect of theophylline on pulmonary function in asthmatic children. *J Pediatr* 86:789–793, 1975.

71. Mitenko PA, Ogilvie RI: Rational intravenous doses of theophylline. *N Engl J Med* 289:600–603, 1973a.

72. Pollock J, Kiechel F, Cooper D, Weinberger M: Relationship of serum theophylline concentration to inhibition of exercise-induced bronchospasm and comparison with cromolyn. *Pediatrics* 60:840–844, 1977.

73. Bierman CW, Shapiro GG and Pierson WE: Acute and chronic theophylline therapy in exercise-induced bronchospasm. *Pediatrics* 60:845–849, 1977.

74. Ellis EF: Theophylline and derivatives. In *Allergy: Principles and Practice* Middleton E, Reed CE, Ellis EF (eds.): St. Louis, The C. V. Mosby Co., 1978, pp. 434–453.

75. Weinberger M, Hendeles L: Pharmacologic management of asthma, rhinitis, anaphylaxis, and urticaria. In Bierman CW, Pearlman DS (eds.), *Allergic Diseases in Infancy* Philadelphia: W. B. Saunders, 1980, pp. 328–329.

76. Weinberger M, Hendeles L, Bighley L: The relation of product formulation to absorption of oral theophylline. *N Engl J Med* 299:852–857, 1978.

77. Ridolfo AS, Kohlstaedt KG: A simplified method for the rectal installation of theophylline. *Am J Med Sci* 237:585–589, 1959.

78. Ellis EE, Koysooko R and Levy G: Pharmacokinetics of theophylline in children with asthma. *Pediatrics* 58:542–547, 1976.

79. Mitenko PA, Ogilvie RI: Pharmacokinetics of intravenous theophylline. *Clin Pharmacol Ther* 14: 509–513, 1973b.

80. Aranda JV, Sitar DS, Parsons WE, Loughnan PM, and Neims AH: Pharmacokinetic aspects of theophylline in premature newborns. *N Engl J Med* 295:413–416, 1976.

81. Arwood LL, Dasta JF, and Friedman C: Placental transfer of theophylline: Two case reports. *Pediatrics* 63:844–846, 1979.

82. Yurchak AM, Jusko WJ: Theophylline secretion into breast milk. *Pediatrics* 57:518–520, 1976.

83. Koysooko R, Ellis EF, Levy G: Relationship between theophylline concentration in plasma and saliva of man. *Clin Pharmacol Ther* 15:454–460, 1974.

84. Weinberger M, Ginchansky E: Dose-dependent kinetics of theophylline elimination in asthmatic children. *J Pediatr* 91:820–824, 1977.

85. Jenne J, Nagasawa HT, Thompson RD: Relationship of urinary metabolites of theophylline to serum theophylline levels. *Clin Pharmacol Ther* 19:375–381, 1976.

86. Mangione A, Imhoff TE, Lee RV, Shum LY, Jusko WJ: Pharmacokinetics of theophylline in hepatic disease. *Chest* 73:616–622, 1978.

87. Piafsky KM, Sitar DS, Rangno RE, Ogilvie RI: Theophylline kinetics in acute pulmonary edema. *Clin Pharmacol Ther* 21:310–316, 1977.

88. Vicuna N, McNay JL, Ludden TM, et al: Impaired theophylline clearance in patients with cor pulmonale. *Br J Clin Pharmacol* 7:33–37, 1979.

89. Weinberger M, Hudgel D, Spector S, Chidsey C: Inhibition of theophylline clearance by troleandomycin. *J Allergy Clin Immunol* 59:228–231, 1977.

90. Kozak PP, Cummins LH, Gillman SA: Administration of erythromycin to patients on theophylline. *J Allergy Clin Immunol* 16:149–151, 1977.

91. Prince RA, Wing DS, Weinberger M, Hendeles L, Riegelman S: Effect of erythromycin on theophylline kinetics. *J Allergy Clin Immunol* 68:427–431, 1981.

92. Klotz V, Reimann I: Delayed clearance of diazepam due to cimetidine. *N Engl J Med* 302:1012–1014, 1980.

93. Jackson JE, Powell JR, Wandell M, Bently J, Dorr R: Cimetidine decreases theophylline clearance. *Am Rev Respir Dis* 123:615–617, 1981.

94. Reitberg DP, Bernhard H, Schentag JJ. Alteration of theophylline clearance and half-life by cimetidine in normal volunteers. *Ann Int Med* 95:582–585, 1982.

95. Roberts RK, Grice J, Wood L, Petroff V, McGuffie C: Cimetidine impairs the elimination of theophylline and antipyrine. *Gastroenterology* 81:19–21, 1981.

96. Weinberger M, Smith G, Milavetz G, Hendeles L: Decreased theophylline clearance due to cimetidine. *N Engl J Med* 304:672, 1981c.

97. Koysooko R, Ellis EF, Levy G: Effect of ethanol on theophylline absorption in humans. *J Pharm Sci* 64:299–301, 1975.

98. Waxler SH, Schack JA: Administration of aminophylline (theophylline ethylenediamine). *J Am Med Assoc* 143:735–739, 1950.

99. Weinberger M, Hendeles L, Wong L: Relationship of formulation and dosing interval to fluctuation of serum theophylline concentration in children with chronic asthma. *J Pediatr* 99:145–152, 1981a.

99a. Weinberger M, Hendeles L: Current concepts: Slow-release theophylline—rationale and basis for product selection. *N Eng J Med.* 308:760–764, 1983.

100. Marshall R: Protective effect of disodium cromoglycate on rat peritoneal mast cells. *Thorax* 27:38–43, 1972.

101. Foreman JC and Mongar JL: Effect of calcium on dextran-induced histamine release from isolated mast cells. *Br J Pharmacol* 46:767–669, 1972.

102. Gold WM: Cholinergic pharmacology in asthma. In Austen KF, Lichtenstein LM (eds): *Asthma: Physiology, Immunopharmacology and Treatment.* New York, Academic Press, 1973, pp 169–184.

103. Jackson DM, Richards IM The further action of sodium cromoglycate. *Br J Pharmacol* 58:301–302, 1976.

104. Walker SR, Evans ME, Richards AJ, Paferson JW: The fate of (^{14}C) disodium cromoglycate in man. *J Pharm Pharmacol* 24:525–531, 1972.

105. Booij-Noord H, Orie NGM, DeVries K: Immediate and late bronchial obstructive reactions to inhalation of house dust and protective effects of disodium cromoglycate and prednisone. *J Allergy Clin Immunol* 48:344–354, 1971.

106. Altounyan REC: Inhibition of experimental asthma by a new compound—disodium cromoglycate "Intal." *Acta Allergol* 22:487–489, 1967.

107. Kolotkin BM, Lee CK, Townley TG: Duration and specificity of sodium cromolyn on allergen inhalation challenges in asthmatics. *J Allergy Clin Immunol* 53:228–297, 1973.

108. Basomba A, Romar A, Pelaez A, Villamanzo IG and Campos A: The effect of sodium cromoglycate in preventing aspirin-induced bronchospasm. *Clin. Allergy* 6:269–275, 1976.

109. Breslin ABX, Hendrick DJ, Pepys J: Effect of disodium cromoglycate on asthmatic reactions to alcoholic beverages. *Clin Allergy* 3:81–92, 1971.

110. Clark TS: Effect of disodium cromoglycate on exacerbations of asthma produced by hyperventilation. *Br Med J* 1:317–319, 1971.

111. Inoue S, Nishima S: Effects of disodium cromoglycate on airway histamine hypersensitivity and daily pulmonary function in asthmatic children, *In* Disodium cromoglycate: Papers presented at the Seventh International Congress of Allergology Special Sectional Meetings, Excerpta Medica, Int Congr Ser No. 211, Florence.

112. Rosenthal RR, Laube BL, Hood DB, Bleeker S, Permutt S, Norman PS: Inhibition of methacholine challenge by disodium cromoglycate. *Am Rev Resp Dis* 121 (Suppl.):90, 1980. Abstract.

113. Townley RG, Kang B, Lee CK, Kolotkin B: Effects of disodium cromoglycate on the intravenous infusion of histamine in asthmatics. *J Allergy Clin Immunol* 51:121–122, 1973.

114. Ryo, UY, Kang B, Townley RG: Cromolyn therapy in patients with bronchial asthma. *J Am Med Assoc.* 236:927–931, 1976.

115. Godfrey S: The physiological assessment of the

effect of DSCG in the asthmatic child. *Respiration (Suppl)* 27:353–356, 1970.

116. Blumenthal MN, Schoenwetter WF, MacDonald FM and McHugh RB: Cromolyn in extrinsic and intrinsic asthma. *J Allergy Clin Immunol* 52:105–114, 1973.

117. Brompton Hospital/Medical Research Council Collaborative Trial: Long-term study of disodium cromoglycate in treatment of severe extrinsic or intrinsic bronchial asthma in adults. *Br Med J* 4:383–388, 1972.

118. Anonymous: Acute safety studies—Clinical. *In Intal (Cromolyn Sodium—Fisons): A Monograph.* Fisons Corp., Bedford, Mass. 1973, pp. 81–83.

119. Toogood JH: Multi-centre surveillance of long-term safety of sodium cromoglycate. *Acta Allergol* 32(Suppl. 13):44–52, 1977.

120. Settipane GA, Klein DE, Boyd GK, Sturam JH, Freye HB, Weltman JK: Adverse reactions to cromolyn. *J Am Med Assoc* 241:811–813, 1979.

121. Scheffer AL, Ross EP, Goetzl EJ: Immunologic components of hypersensitivity reactions to cromolyn sodium. *N Engl J Med* 293:1220–1224, 1975.

122. Rinehart JJ, Sagone AL, Balcerzak SP, Ackerman GA, LoBuglio AF: Effects of corticosteroid therapy on human monocyte function. *N Engl J Med* 292:236–241, 1975.

123. Cline MJ, Melman KL: Plasma kinins and cortisol: A possible explanation of the anti-inflammatory action of cortisol. *Science* 153:1135–1138, 1966.

124. Hong SL, Levine L: Inhibition of arachidonic acid release from cells as the biochemical action of anti-inflammatory corticosteroids. *Proc Natl Acad Sci* 73:1730–1734, 1976.

125. Logsdon PJ, Middleton E, Jr, Coffey RG: Stimulation of leukocyte adenyl cyclase by hydrocortisone and isoproterenol in asthmatic and nonasthmatic subjects. *J Allergy Clin Immunol* 50:45–56, 1972.

126. Morris HG: Pharmacology of corticosteroids in asthma. In *Allergy: Principles and Practice.* Middleton E, Reed CE, Ellis EF, (eds), St. Louis: C. V. Mosby Company, 1978, pp. 464–480.

127. Sullivan TJ, Hallmark MR, Sakmar E, Weidler DJ, Earhart RH, Wagner JG: Comparative bioavailability: Eight commercial prednisone tablets. *J Pharmacokinet Biopharm* 4:157–172, 1976.

128. Novey HS, Beall G: Aerosolized steroids and induced Cushing's syndrome. *Arch Intern Med* 115: 602–605, 1965.

129. Siegel SC, Heimlich EM, Richards W, Kelley VC: Adrenal function in allergy. IV. Effect of dexamethasone aerosols in asthmatic children. *Pediatrics* 33:345–250, 1964.

130. Harris DMJ: Properties and therapeutic uses of some corticosteroids with inhanced topical potency. *Steroid Biochem* 6:711–716, 1975.

131. Meilke AW, Weed JA, Tyler FJ: Kinetics and interconversion of prednisolone and prednisone studied with new radioimmunoassays. *J Clin Endocrinol Metab* 41:717–721, 1975.

132. Brooks SM, Werk EE, Ackerman SJ, Sullivan I, Thrasher K: Adverse effects of phenobarbital on corticosteroid metabolism in patients with bronchial asthma. *N Engl J Med* 286:1125–1128, 1972.

133. Buffington GA, Dominguez JH, Piering WF, Hebert LA, Kauffman HM, Lemann J: Interaction of rifampin and glucocorticoids. *J Am Med Assoc* 236:1958–1960, 1976.

134. Petereit LB, Meikle AW: Effectiveness of prednisolone during phenytoin therapy. *Clin Pharmacol Ther* 22:912–966, 1977.

135. Sandberg AA, Slaunwhite WR, Jr: Difference in metabolism of prednisolone-C^{14} and cortisol C^{14}. *J Clin Endocrinol Metab* 17:1040–1050, 1957.

136. Arnaud A, Vervloet D, Dugue P, Orechek J and Charpin J: Treatment of acute asthma: Effect of intravenous corticosteroids and beta$_2$ adrenergic agonists. *Lung* 156:43–48, 1979.

137. Ellul-Micallef R and Fench FF: Effect of intravenous prenisolone in asthmatic with diminished adrenergic responsiveness. *Lancet* 2:1269–1270, 1975.

138. Piersen WE, Bierman CW, Kelley VC: A double-blind trial of corticosteroid therapy in status asthmaticus. *Pediatrics* 54:782–788, 1974.

139. Galant SP, Bullock J, Wong D, Maibach HI: The inhibitory effect of antiallergy drugs on allergen and histamine-induced wheal and flare response. *J Allergy Clin Immunol* 51:11–21, 1973.

140. Konig P, Jaffe P, Godfrey S: Effect of corticosteroids on exercise-induced asthma. *J Allergy Immunol* 54:14–19, 1974.

141. Ackerman GL, Nolan CM: Adrenocortical responsiveness after alternate-day corticosteroid therapy. *N Engl J Med* 278:405–409, 1968.

142. Easton JG, Busser RJ, Neimlich EM: Effect of alternate-day steroid administration on adrenal function allergic children. *J Allergy Clin Immunol* 48:355–360, 1971.

143. Falliers CJ, Chai H, Molk L, Bane H, Cardoso RR: Pulmonary and adrenal effects of alternate-day corticosteroid therapy. *J Allergy Clin Immunol* 49:156–166, 1972.

144. Harter JG, Novitch AM: Evaluation of steroid analogues in terms of suitability for alternate day steroid therapy. *J Allergy* 37:108–109, 1966.

145. Sadeghi-Nejad A, Senior B: Adrenal function function, growth, and insulin in patients treated with corticoids on alternate days. *Pediatrics* 43:277–283, 1969.

146. Esterley JR, Oppenheimer EH: Observations in cystic fibrosis of the pancreas. III. Pulmonary lesions. *J H Med J* 122:94–101, 1968.

147. Iacocca VF, Sivinga MS, Barbera GJ: Respiratory tract bacteriology in cystic fibrosis. *M J Dis Child* 106:115–124, 1963.

148. Huang NN, Loon ELV, Sheng KT: The flora of the respiratory tract of patients with cystic fibrosis of the pancreas. *J Pediatr* 59:512–521, 1961.

149. Kilbourn JP, Campbell RA, Grach JL, Willis MD: Quantitative bacteriology of sputum. *Am Rev Resp Dis* 98:810–818, 1968.

150. Pirtle JK, Monroe PW, Smalley TK, Mohr JA, Rhoades ER: Diagnostic and therapeutic advantages of serial quantitative cultures of fresh sputum in acute bacterial pneumonia. *Am Rev Resp Dis* 100: 831–838, 1969.

151. Monroe PW, Muchmore HG, Felton FG, Pirtle JK: Quantitation of micro-organisms in sputum. *App Microbiol* 18:214–220, 1969.

152. Dixon JMS, Miller DC: Value of dilute inocula in cultural examination of sputum *Lancet* 2: 1046–1048, 1965.

153. Myers M, Weinberger M: Unpublished data.

154. May JR: Bacteriology of chronic bronchitis. *Lancet* 2:534–537, 1953.

155. Lorian V, Khavari P, Gray N: Quantitative bacteriological analysis of sputum as a test of antibioitic efficacy. *App Microbiol* 15:564–565, 1967.

156. Loria DB: Uses of quantitative analyses of bacterial populations in sputum. *J Am Med Assoc* 182:1082–1086, 1962.

157. Thorsteinsson SV, Musher DM, Fagan T: The diagnostic value of sputum culture in acute pneumonia. *J Am Med Assoc* 182:1082–1086, 1975.

158. Rabin HR, Harley FL, Bryan LE, Elfring GL: Evaluation of a high dose tobramycin and ticarcillin treatment protocol in cystic fibrosis based on improved susceptibility criteria and antibiotic pharmacokinetics. *Proc 8th International Congress on Cystic Fibrosis,* 370–375, 1980.

159. Weintzen R, Prestidge CB, Kramer RI, McCracken GH, Nelson JD: Acute pulmonary exacerbations in cystic fibrosis. A double-blind trial of tobramycin and placebo therapy. *Am J Dis Child* 134:1134–1138, 1980.

160. Marino JT, Beaudry PH: Antibiotic treatment of cystic fibrosis (letter). *J Pediatr.* 98: 511, 1981.

161. Bartlett JG and Finegold SM: Bacteriology of expectorated sputum with quantitative culture and wash technique compared to transtracheal aspirates. *Am Rev Resp Dis* 117, 1019–1027, 1978.

162. Loening-Baucke VA, Mischler E, Myers MG: A placebo-controlled trial of cephalexin therapy in the ambulatory management of patients with cystic fibrosis. *J. Pediatr* 95:630–637, 1979.

163. Lennette EH, Spaulding EH, Truant JP: *Manual of Clinical Microbiology,* Ed. 2. American Society for Microbiology, Washington, D.C.

164. Myers MG, Koontz FP, Weinberger M: Lower respiratory infections in patients with cystic fibrosis. In J. Lloyd-Still (ed.). *A Textbook on Cystic Fibrosis.* John Wright, PSG, Inc. (in press).

165. Di Sant'Agnese PA, Andersen DH: Celiac syndrome. IV. Chemotherapy of infections of the respiratory tract associated with cystic fibrosis of the pancreas; observations with penicillin and drugs of the sulfanomide group, with special reference to penicillin aerosol. *Am J Dis Child* 72:17–61, 1946.

166. Shwachman H, Crocker AC, Foley G, Patterson PR: Aureomycin therapy in the pulmonary involvement of pancreatic fibrosis (mucoviscidosis). *N Engl J Med* 41:185–192, 1949.

167. Shwachman H, Redmond A, Khaw KT: Studies in cystic fibrosis. Report of 130 patients diagnosed under 3 months of age over a 20-year period. *Pediatr* 46:335–343, 1970.

168. Warwick WJ, Munson S: Life table studies of mortality. In *Cystic Fibrosis, Part I, Physiology and Pathophysiology of Serous Secretion, Clinical Investigations and Therapy.* Proc. of 4th International Conference on Cystic Fibrosis; pp. 353–367, 1966.

169. Shwachman H, Kulczycki LL: Long-term study of 105 patients with cystic fibrosis. *Am J Dis Child* 96:6–15, 1958.

170. Phelan PD, Allan JL, Landau LI, Barnes GL: Improved survival of patients with cystic fibrosis. *Med J Aust* 1:261–263, 1979.

171. Huang NN, Macri CN, Girone J, Sproul A: Survival of patients with cystic fibrosis. *Amer J Dis Child* 120:289–295, 1970.

172. Guggenbichler JP, Kienel G: Bioavailability of oral antibiotics in cystic fibrosis. *Monogr Paediat* 10:34–40, 1979.

173. Hodson ME, Penketh ARL, Batten JO: Aerosol carbenicillin and gentamicin treatment of *Pseudomonas aeruginosa* infection in patients with cystic fibrosis. *Lancet* 2:1137–1139, 1981.

174. Chiou WL, Athanikar NK, Huang S: Long half-life of chlorpheniramine. *N Engl J Med* 300: 501, 1979.

175. Fouda HG, Hobbs DC, Stambaugh JE: Sensitive assay for determination of hydroxyzine in plasma and its human pharmacokinetics. *J Pharm Sci* 68:1456–1458, 1979.

176. Mullarkey MF, Hill JS, Webb DR: Allergic and nonallergic rhinitis: their characterization with attention to the meaning of nasal eosinophilia. *J Allergy Clin Immunol* 65:122–126, 1980.

177. Weinberger M, Hendeles L, Ahrens R: Pharmacologic management of reversible obstructive airways disease. *Ped Clin NA* 28:47–75, 1981b.

178. Hendeles L, Weinberger M, Wyatt R: Guide to oral theophylline therapy for the treatment of chronic asthma. *Am J Dis Child* 132:876–880, 1978.

179. Marks MI, Prentice R, Swarson R, et al: Carbenicillin and gentamicin: Pharmacologic studies in patients with cystic fibrosis and *Pseudomonas* pulmonary infections. *J Pediatr* 71:822–828, 1971.

180. Beaudry PH, Marks MI, McDougall D, et al: Is anti-*Pseudomonas* therapy warranted in acute respiratory exacerbations in children with cystic fibrosis? *J Pediatr* 97:144–147, 1980.

181. McCrae WM, Raeburn JA, Hanson EJ: Tobramycin therapy of infections due to *Pseudomonas aeruginosa* in patients with cystic fibrosis: Effect of dosage and concentrations of antibiotic in sputum. *J Infect Dis* 134:S191–193, 1976.

182. Cipolle RJ, Seifert RD, Zaske DE, Strate RG: Systematically individualizing tobramycin dosage regimens. *J Clin Pharmacol* 20:570–580, 1980.

183. Weinberger M, Hendeles L: Pharmacotherapy of asthma. *Am J Hosp Pharm* 33:1071–1080, 1976.

184. Hendeles L, Bighley L, Richardson RH, Helper CD, Carmichael J: Frequent toxicity from IV aminophylline infusions in critically ill patients. *Drug Intell Clin Pharm* 11:12–18, 1977.

185. Hambleton G, Weinberger M, Taylor J, Cavanaugh M, Ginchansky E, Godfrey S, Tooley M, Bell T and Greenberg S: Comparison of cromoglycate (cromolyn) and theophylline in controlling symptoms of chronic asthma. (1977). *Lancet* 1:381–385.

186. Weinberger M, Matthay RA, Ginchansky EJ, Chidsey CA, Petty T: Intravenous aminophylline dosage: Use of serum theophylline measurement for guidance. *J Am Med Assoc* 235:2110–2113, 1976.

187. Weinberger, M, Hendeles, L: Commentary: Role of dialysis in the management and prevention of theophylline toxicity. *Dev Pharmacol Ther* 1:26–30, 1980.

17

Oxygen Transport Prenatally and Postnatally

Barry Fisher

A primary function of the cardiopulmonary system is the transport and exchange of oxygen and carbon dioxide. Complex mechanisms exist for oxygen transport from the external environment to the cellular level to meet body metabolic requirements, as well as for the removal of carbon dioxide from the body. This chapter will review these various processes for both the fetus and newborn.

The transport of oxygen in humans depends on the presence of hemoglobin. The amount of oxygen dissolved in plasma is small, being 0.003 ml/mm Hg of partial pressure of oxygen (Po_2). If the Po_2 is 100 torr, the amount of dissolved oxygen in plasma is 0.3 ml. On the other hand, hemoglobin carries 1.36 ml of oxygen for each gram of hemoglobin. If the hemoglobin concentration is 15 g/dL, the oxygen-carrying capacity is 20.4 ml/dL. The total oxygen carried for each 100 ml of blood with a hemoglobin concentration of 15 g/dL is that bound to hemoglobin (20.4 ml) plus that dissolved in plasma (0.3 ml) or 20.7 ml/dL. In this example, 98.5 percent of transported oxygen is bound to hemoglobin. If no changes are made other than increasing the Po_2 from 100 to 400 torr, the amount of oxygen bound to hemoglobin would remain unchanged, but the amount of oxygen that would be dissolved in plasma increases to 1.2 ml/dL (400×0.003). The amount of additional oxygen transported for each 100 ml is therefore only 0.9 ml, despite the fact that the Po_2 has been quadrupled (Table 17-1).

This concept assumes added significance when oxygen transport in patients is considered. Similar calculations performed on a patient with a hemoglobin concentration of 7.5 g/dL reveals that 10.2 ml of oxygen are bound to hemoglobin

for each 100 ml of blood. The total amount of oxygen transported for each 100 ml of blood is therefore 10.2 + 0.3 or 10.5 ml of oxygen for each 100 ml of blood with a hemoglobin concentration of 7.5 g/dL.

Under normal circumstances, the arteriovenous difference for oxygen (A-V O_2 difference) averages 5 ml of oxygen for each 100 ml of blood. For a 70-kg man with a cardiac output of 5 L/min, this translates to an oxygen consumption ($\dot{V}o_2$) of 250 ml/min. If a 70-kg anemic patient with a hemoglobin concentration of 7.5 g/dL were to maintain an A-V O_2 difference of 5 ml/dL, a $\dot{V}o_2$ of 250 ml/min could only be sustained if the cardiac output is doubled to 10 L/min. The only other mechanism available for maintaining a $\dot{V}o_2$ of 250 ml/min would be increased extraction of oxygen from hemoglobin (increased A-V O_2 difference) with subsequent lowering of the mixed venous oxygen tension ($P\bar{v}o_2$). Because of the sigmoidal shape of the oxyhemoglobin dissociation curve, it is progressively more difficult to extract oxygen from hemoglobin below a P_ao_2 of 40 torr (see later discussion). Consequently, the most physiologically cost-effective mechanism available for increasing the amount of transported oxygen in the presence of an inadequate hemoglobin concentration is increasing the hemoglobin concentration and not increasing the (1) cardiac output, (2) A-V O_2 difference, or (3) concentration of inspired oxygen.

THE HEMOGLOBIN MOLECULE

The complex biology of hemoglobin has been extensively studied, both structurally and functionally. The elegant studies of Perutz and

Table 17-1 *Oxygen-Carrying Capacity*

Hemoglobin (g/dL)	ml O_2 bound to hemoglobin	ml O_2 in plasma	Total ml O_2 in blood
7.5 (Po_2 = 100 torr)	10.2	0.3	10.5
7.5 (Po_2 = 400 torr)	10.2	1.2	11.4
15 (Po_2 = 100 torr)	20.4	0.3	20.7
15 (Po_2 = 400 torr)	20.4	1.2	21.6

co-workers[1-3] helped elucidate the molecular structure of hemoglobin using x-ray diffraction. Detailed reviews[4-9] describe the physiologic and pathophysiologic mechanisms of hemoglobin. The hemoglobin molecule consists of four polypeptide chains, each surrounding a heme molecule (a porphyrin ring with an iron atom at its center). Normal adult hemoglobin (Hb A) consists of two α-chains of 141 amino acids each and two β-chains of 146 amino acids each (Fig. 17-1) Twenty different amino acids are present in these polypeptide chains, with their amino acid sequence being genetically determined. In fetal hemoglobin (Hb F) a γ-chain is substituted for each β-chain. γ-Chains also contain 146 amino acid residues, but differ sequentially from β-chains at 39 loci. Hb F is designated α_2, γ_2, rather than α_2, β_2 for Hb A.

In addition to amino acid sequencing, the three-dimensional geometric structure of these polypeptide chains is determined by helical segments and bends. α-Chains have seven helical segments and six structural bends, whereas β-chains have eight helical segments and seven structural bends. γ-Chains likewise, have seven bends and are geometically similar to β-chains except for differing nitrogen terminal groups. The porphyrin heme molecule consists of four pyrrole rings with a central iron atom. Iron can accept electrons from up to six ligands (oppositely charged ions or neutral substances). In the hemoglobin molecule, there are four bonds with the porphyrin ring (one bond for each pyrrole ring), one bond with a single particular polypeptide chain, and one bond with oxygen. Hemoglobin thus consists of four heme molecules each bound to a single polypeptide chain, which are then geometrically arranged in a three-dimensional configuration.

If there were two available binding sites on each iron atom for oxygen, the resultant combination would be irreversible oxygen binding, and hemoglobin would be ineffective as a transport vehicle for oxygen. Since oxygen binds to one iron site on each of two heme molecules, the iron-oxygen bond is now reversible and hemoglobin is able to serve as an effective oxygen transporter.

The four polypeptide-heme subunits are arranged tetrahedrally with the vertical and horizontal axes intersecting at a central water-filled cavity. Oxygenated hemoglobin exists in the tense state, or T state, where salt bridges hold the four units tightly together and interfere with oxygen's ability to bind to the available iron-binding sites within the porphyrin ring (Fig. 17-2). When oxyhemoglobin is present, however, the four subunits (polypeptide chain plus heme molecule) are loosely bound (fewer salt bridges), and oxygen readily binds to the hemoglobin molecule. This is referred to as 'he R state, or relaxed state. The more relaxed the hemoglobin molecule, the greater the affinity of hemoglobin for oxygen. The reaction of one subunit of hemoglobin with oxygen alters both the position of the iron atom within the porphyrin ring and the geometric configuration of the hemoglobin molecule. This configurational change within the hemoglobin molecule increases its oxygen affinity and changes the molecule from the T to the R state. This concept is referred to as heme—heme interaction and suggests that the initial oxygen molecule is the most difficult to bind to hemoglobin. Binding of subsequent oxygen molecules is then progressively easier. Similarly, as oxygen is extracted from hemoglobin, it becomes progressively more difficult for this extraction to take place. It is these physiochemical properties which

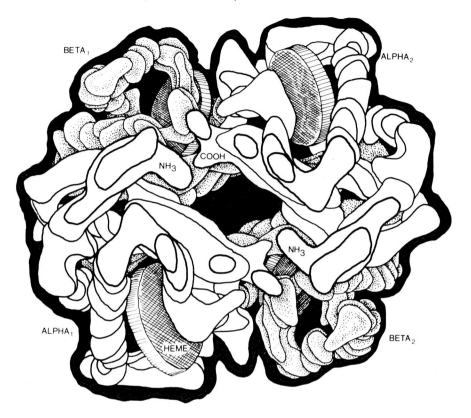

Figure 17-1. Complete molecule of hemoglobin is made up of four subunits, each of which consists of one polypeptide chain and one heme. There are two kinds of subunit, designated α (*white*) and β (*gray*), which have different sequences of amino acid residues but similar three-dimensional strucures. The β-chain also has one short extra helix. The four subunits, seen here in two views, are arranged at the vertexes of a tetrahedron around an axis of twofold symmetry. Each heme lies in a separate pocket at the surface of the molecule

give hemoglobin its unique sigmoidal oxygen dissociation curve.

A third physical state of hemoglobin is referred to as the S state. This is a state where the T state is stabilized by the binding of 2,3 diphospho-glycerate (2,3-DPG) to hemoglobin. As will be discussed subsequently, 2,3-DPG favors the unloading of oxygen to the tissues by decreasing hemoglobin's affinity for oxygen. The 2,3-DPG molecule fits into the top of the three-dimensional hemoglobin tetrahedron in a fashion comparable to the way a cork fits into the top of a bottle. The addition of 2,3-DPG to the hemoglobin tetrahedron interferes with oxygen's ability to combine with deoxyhemoglobin.

PHYSIOLOGY OF HEMOGLOBIN

An effective way to evaluate the oxygen-binding characteristics of hemoglobin is to consider the P_{50}. P_{50} is defined as the partial pressure of oxygen at which hemoglobin is 50 percent saturated with oxygen (Fig. 17-3). At a pH 7.40, a Pco_2 of 40 torr, and a temperature of 37°C, the P_{50} of Hb A is 26.6 torr. With increasing oxygen affinity, the oxyhemoglobin dissociation curve shifts to the left and the P_{50} falls. Conversely, with decreasing oxygen affinity, the oxyhemoglobin dissociation equilibrium is shifted to the right and the P_{50} increases. Several factors affect the shift of the oxyhemoglobin dissociation equilib-

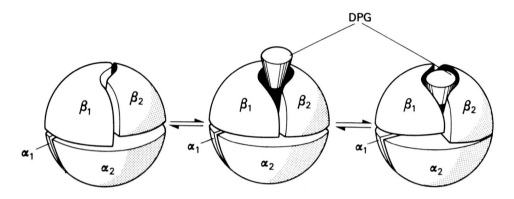

Figure 17-2. R, T, and S states of the Hb A molecule. Diagram showing the four subunits of Hb A ($\alpha_2\beta_2$). In the R state the subunits are more free to react with oxygen than in the T state. The T state is stabilized by the addition of 2,3-DPG, yielding the S state. From Strang LB: *Neonatal Respiration— Physiological and Clinical Studies,* Oxford, England, Blackwell Scientific Publications, 1977, p 141.

rium to the right: (1) increased P_{CO_2}, (2) increased acidosis (a decreased pH-level), (3) increased temperature, and (4) increased 2,3-DPG. The shift of the oxyhemoglobin dissociation curve to the right caused by an increased P_{CO_2} or a decreased pH is known as the *Bohr effect.* The Bohr effect increases the oxygen gradient between hemoglobin and the tissues and favors the unloading of oxygen to the cellular level. As hydrogen ions and carbon dioxide are picked up from the tissues, the pH of hemoglobin decreases slightly, favoring further oxygen unloading. Similarly, increased concentrations of 2,3-DPG also shift the oxyhemoglobin dissociation equilibrium to the right, resulting in increased oxygen unloading to the tissues. For example, if the P_{CO_2} is raised to 80 torr, as might occur in acute respiratory failure, the P_{50} increases to 39 torr. The P_{50} decreases toward 22 torr when hyperventilation is employed to reduce cerebral blood flow in disease states associated with increased intracranial pressure, such as bacterial meningitis or near drowning. The P_{50} can be calculated from the P_{O_2} and the saturation of a venous blood sample using the Severinghouse formula:

$$\text{Estimated } P_{50} = 26.6 \frac{P_{O_2}}{P_{O_2} \text{ sat}}$$

and P_{O_2} sat is obtained by reading the saturation of P_{O_2} from the standard oxyhemoglobin dissociation curve. In addition, one can use the Severinghouse slide rule[10] (which uses the above equation) or the Canizaro nomogram[11] (Fig. 17-4). The P_{50} thus effectively describes the position of the oxyhemoglobin dissociation equilibrium.

If one examines a model of the circulation, deoxyhemoglobin arrives at the pulmonary capillary bed with a physical gradient favoring the unloading of carbon dioxide from hemoglobin to the alveoli and the loading of oxygen from the alveoli to hemoglobin. In the case of oxygen, there is a large pressure gradient favoring the diffusion of oxygen from the alveoli to hemoglobin. As oxygen binds to hemoglobin, hemoglobin's oxygen affinity increases, and the oxyhemoglobin dissociation curve shifts to the left. The unloading of carbon dioxide to the alveoli and the simultaneous loading of oxygen from the alveoli is referred to as the *Haldane effect.*

When oxygenated hemoglobin arrives at the systemic capillary bed, oxygen is released to the tissues because of the wide oxygen gradient, where hydrogen ions, carbon dioxide, and heat are picked up. This further shifts the oxyhemoglobin dissociation equilibrium to the right, favoring additional oxygen unloading to the tissues (Bohr effect). As hemoglobin becomes more acidic, the oxygen dissociation equilibrium is shifted farther to the right, favoring even greater oxygen unloading to the tissues.

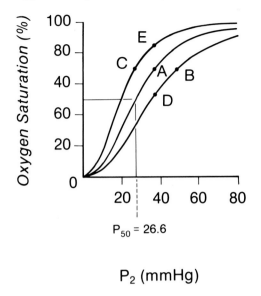

Figure 17-3. Oxyhemoglobin dissociation curve. The middle curve is the standard curve at 37°C and a pH of 7.4. It has a P_{50} of 26.6 mm Hg. *Point A* represents $P\bar{v}o_2$ in a subject with a normal P_{50}. *Points B* and *C* show the changes in Po_2 caused by altering mixed venous saturation, whereas *points D* and *E* show the changes in saturation that occur if $P\bar{v}o_2$ remains constant as oxygen affinity changes. From Thomas HM, Lefrak SS, Irwin RS, et al: The oxyhemoglobin dissociation curve in health and disease. *Am J Med* 57:331, 1974. With permission.

2,3–DPG

The observation that the oxygen affinity of Hb A in solution is greater than the oxygen affinity of the intact fresh erythrocyte has long suggested that the intact red cell contains a substance or substances capable of interracting with hemoglobin to decrease its oxygen affinity.[12] Valtis and Kennedy[13] in 1954 demonstrated that blood stored in a blood bank had increasing oxygen affinity with aging. This increase in oxygen affinity is now known to be due to a progressive decrease in intraerythrocyte 2,3–DPG concentrations to values as low as 10 percent of initial levels when blood is stored for 21 days. The classic simultaneous studies in 1967 by Benesch and Benesch[14] and Chanutin and Curnish[15] demonstrated that several inorganic phosphates were each capable of altering the oxygen affinity of Hb

A. The greatest effect on lowering oxygen affinity was found when the inorganic phosphate 2,3–DPG became bound to deoxyhemoglobin. The 2,3–DPG anion does not bind well to oxyhemoglobin and therefore does not interfere with oxygen uptake in the lung. When oxygen diffuses from oxyhemoglobin toward the tissues, producing a narrower A-V O_2 gradient, deoxyhemoglobin is formed, 2,3–DPG binds to it, and the oxyhemoglobin dissociation equilibrium shifts to the right. This shift to the right permits additional oxygen to be released from hemoglobin to the tissues (wider A-V O_2 content) with no change in the Po_2 (Fig. 17-5).

The concentration of 2,3–DPG in the normal human red cell averages 4.5 + 0.7 mol/ml of red blood cells. Certain conditions, such as high altitude,[16,17] cyanotic congenital heart disease,[18–20] chronic liver disease,[21] anemia,[22,23] and hyperthyroidism[24] are associated with increased levels of 2,3–DPG. In each of these situations

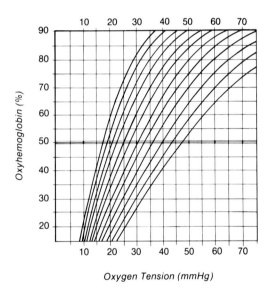

Figure 17-4. The Canizaro nomogram for the calculation of P_{50}. The point on the nomogram corresponding to the measured Po_2 and saturation of a sample of venous blood is faced to the line representing 50-percent saturation. The intersect represents the estimated P_{50}, for example, $P\bar{v}o_2 = 39$ mm Hg, oxygen saturation = 65 percent, $P_{50} = 31$ mm Hg. From Canizaro PC, et al: A technique for estimating the position of the oxyhemoglobin dissociation curve. *Ann Surg* 180, 364, 1974. With permission.

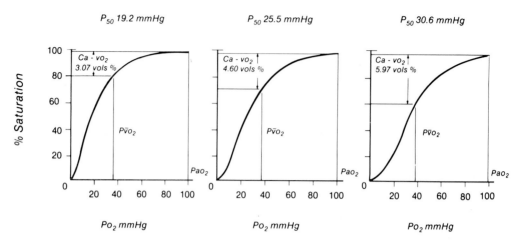

Figure 17-5. The effect of different positions of the oxyhemoglobin dissociation curve (curves associated with different P$_{50}$ values) on saturation and arteriovenous oxygen content. Note that the arteriovenous oxygen content (Ca–v̄o$_2$) increases with progressive rightward displacement of the P$_{50}$ despite the fact that Pv̄o$_2$ is kept constant. From McConn R: The oxyhemoglobin dissociation curve in acute disease. *Surg Clin North Am* 55: 627, 1979. With permission.

elevated 2,3–DPG concentrations facilitate increased oxygen delivery to the tissues, producing a rightward shift of the oxyhemoglobin dissociation equilibrium. The situation with respect to lung disease is even more complicated. In 1969 Oski et al.[18] reported elevated levels of 2,3–DPG, as well as an increased P$_{50}$, in patients with chronic pulmonary disease associated with hypoxemia. Weiss and Desforges[25] demonstrated that acute asthmatic patients with hypoventilation (Pco$_2$ of 37 torr or greater) had low levels of 2,3–DPG and a variably left-shifted oxygen dissociation curve. The effect of a lowered pH on the position of the oxyhemoglobin dissociation curve (Bohr effect) as a result of acute respiratory acidosis and hypoxemia tended to temper these leftward shifts, however. The anticipated increase in 2,3–DPG and P$_{50}$ in patients with pulmonary disease associated with hypoxemia was found to be unpredictable. The proposed mechanism for this variable 2,3–DPG response appears to be related to the observation that glycolysis (necessary for the synthesis of 2,3–DPG) is decreased or stopped in the presence of acidosis.[9] Conversely, Chapman et al.[26] and Minakami and Yoshikawa[27] have demonstrated that alkalosis stimulates erythrocyte glycolysis and increases 2,3–DPG synthesis. Since the intraerythrocyte pH rises slightly relative to the

plasma pH when hemoglobin becomes deoxygenated, it has been postulated that this resultant mild intraerythrocyte alkalosis may be sufficient to stimulate 2,3–DPG synthesis.

When blood poor in 2,3–DPG is transfused into healthy persons, there is a rapid rise in recipient 2,3–DPG concentrations with levels reaching 50–60 percent of normal within 24 hours. Full restoration of 2,3–DPG levels usually takes 6–10 days.[28,29] The physiologic impact of transfusing multiple units of acid citrate dextrose (ACD) blood that have been stored for varying lengths of time resulted in a P$_{50}$ averaging 19 torr and 2,3–DPG levels that were one third of predicted normal. This lowering of P$_{50}$ with its resultant increase in oxygen affinity can be avoided by transfusing with fresh frozen blood.

Hechtman et al.[30] have reported that the use of ACD anticoagulant in blood is associated with a more rapid decrease in 2,3–DPG levels than is citrate phosphate dextrose (CPD) anticoagulated blood. A preliminary study by these investigators on the use of ACD blood during cardiopulmonary bypass resulted in a decrease in P$_{50}$ from 25.1 to 19.4 torr. This was associated with a decrease in the mean Pv̄o$_2$ from 43 to 27 torr, implying a decrease in oxygen reserves. The gradient between mean oxygen tension in the capillaries and tissues serves as the driving force for oxygen delivery. As this gradient narrows, so does the rate of oxygen diffusion to the tissues.

Widening of the A-V O_2 difference or lowering of the $P\bar{v}o_2$ has great clinical significance. For the heart, coronary sinus blood is $P\bar{v}o_2$. There is normally a wide A-V O_2 difference in the heart with coronary sinus $P\bar{v}o_2$ averaging between 23 and 29 torr. When a normal A-V O_2 difference cannot be achieved in the heart (most often as the result of hypoxia), the heart changes from a user to a producer of lactate. Myocardial performance decreases, and net cardiac output falls. By raising the fraction of inspired oxygen, hemoglobin becomes fully saturated and dissolved oxygen increases. Oxygen availability to the myocardium increases, and myocardial performance improves. Dennis et al.[31] demonstrated that myocardial performance curves were reduced after cardiopulmonary bypass with ACD anticoagulated blood and that these performance curves returned to normal within 24–48 hours postoperatively, apparently because of the restoration of 2,3–DPG levels to normal.

When red blood cells were anticoagulated with CPD, 2,3–DPG averaged 70 percent of baseline levels compared to 10 percent of baseline levels for red cells suspended in ACD anticoagulant. The use of CPD anticoagulated blood for cardiopulmonary bypass resulted in no decrease in myocardial performance or $P\bar{v}o_2$.[32] Because of near-normal 2,3–DPG levels found in CPD anticoagulated blood, oxygen availability was nearly normal and capable of meeting body oxygen demands in this latter group of patients.

Biochemical manipulation of the position of the oxyhemoglobin dissociation curve to increase the availability of oxygen to the tissues is an intriguing therapeutic advance. Miller et al.[33] have reported that treatment of blood with inosine pyruvate and phosphate after allopurinol to control hyperuricemia in humans was associated with rapid and significant increases in 2,3–DPG concentrations and the P_{50}. Clinical use of concepts discussed in this section could soon be part of our usual therapeutic armamentarium.

In 1930 Anselmino and Hoffman[34] observed that the oxygen affinity of freshly drawn fetal blood (P_{50} = 19–21 torr) was greater than freshly drawn maternal blood (P_{50} = 26.6 torr). Allen, Wyman, and Smith[35] reported in 1953 that oxygen affinities were comparable when fetal and adult hemoglobin was dialysed against the same surrounding medium. Subsequent reports[36–38] have demonstrated that fetal deoxyhemoglobin has a lower affinity for 2,3–DPG than does adult deoxyhemoglobin, presumably due to the fact that 2,3–DPG binds to histidine on the β-chain of Hb A, which is absent in Hb F. Delivoria-Papadopoulos, Roncevic, and Oski[39] reported that the P_{50} was increased from 18 to 28 torr after exchange transfusion with fresh blood in a premature infant with idiopathic respiratory distress syndrome. They suggested that this rightward shift of the oxyhemoglobin dissociation curve produced by the increase in P_{50} contributed to the infant's clinical improvement and subsequent survival. The beneficial effect of transfusion with fresh adult blood in a sick premature infant appears to be due to the replacement of Hb F with Hb A. Decreased 2,3–DPG has also been reported in infants with meconium aspiration.[40]

In almost all species of mammals studied to date, the oxyhemoglobin dissociation curve for fetal blood is shifted to the left of maternal blood, indicating that Hb F has a lower P_{50} and a higher oxygen affinity than Hb A. This increased oxygen affinity of Hb F has been considered a biologic advantage for the fetus, since it permits fetal blood to take up oxygen across the placenta and saturate Hb F at a lower oxygen tension.[41,42] For example, at a pH of 7.40 and Pco_2 of 40 torr, a Po_2 of 60 torr corresponds to a saturation of 90 percent with Hb A, whereas a Po_2 of 48 torr results in a saturation of 90 percent with Hb F at the same pH and Pco_2. At first glance, this increased oxygen affinity of Hb F appears to be a disadvantage for oxygen unloading toward the fetal tissues. The oxyhemoglobin dissociation curve for Hb F is very steep, however, and a small decrease in Po_2 results in a large decrease in saturation, partially offsetting the disadvantage of increased oxygen affinity.

Various other physiologic adaptations also aid in promoting oxygen transport from the maternal circulation to the fetal circulation and from there to the fetal tissues. During pregnancy, both the maternal circulating blood volume and red blood cell mass increase, but the red blood cell mass increases less rapidly than the blood volume. These physiologic adaptations result in an apparent "maternal anemia" where the total oxygen carrying capacity is increased, but the oxygen capacity for each deciliter is decreased. This relative "maternal anemia" has the biologic advantage of shifting the maternal oxyhemoglobin dissociation curve to the right, favoring oxygen unloading toward the fetal tissues. Increased maternal 2,3–DPG levels, which rise an average of 30 percent during pregnancy,[43] are probably the cause of this rightward shift of the maternal oxyhemoglobin dissociation curve.

In addition, maternal cardiac output increases during the first trimester as much as 30–60 percent above prepregnancy levels and serves as a major compensatory mechanism to provide more oxygen for each unit of time for transfer to the fetus across the placenta.[44-46] Maternal uterine blood flow also increases dramatically during pregnancy to provide additional maternal oxygen for placental transfer to the fetus. Towell and Liggins[47] reported that uterine blood flow averaged 13 percent of cardiac output in pregnant ewes within 4 weeks of term and that placental blood flow accounted for 85 percent of uterine blood flow. In the human, uterine blood flow increases from approximately 50 ml/min in the nonpregnant state to approximately 600 ml/min at term. Uterine blood flow seems to be constant on a flow per kilogram basis throughout pregnancy, with blood flow increasing as uterine size increases.[48-50]

The A-V O_2 difference of placental blood is approximately 5 ml/dL of maternal placental blood flow.[51] This observation has suggested that human placental blood flow at term is between 400 and 600 ml/min. If the maternal oxygen-carrying capacity decreases to less than 6 ml/dL of maternal blood (hemoglobin less than 4 g/dL), fetal hypoxemia will invariably result unless compensatory mechanisms are invoked. These mechanisms include increased maternal 2,3–DPG levels as a result of "maternal anemia" and/or increased maternal placental blood flow or increased placental surface area with resultant increased diffusing capacity.[52]

Conditions that decrease maternal blood flow to the placenta (maternal hypertension, placental abruption, maternal supine hypoventilation syndrome, and spinal anesthesia) interfere with oxygen delivery to the fetus, as do conditions that adversely affect the placental tissue or decrease the surface area of the placental tissue (multiple placental infarcts and postdatism). There does not appear to be a placental oxygen gradient when the high intrinsic oxygen consumption of the placenta is considered.[53]

Maternal hyperventilation during pregnancy, probably due to the effect of progesterone on the respiratory system,[54,55] produces a mild respiratory alkalosis that is partially compensated by a metabolic acidosis (the result of increased metabolism during pregnancy). The resultant lowered maternal P_{CO_2} maintains a wide CO_2 gradient between the maternal and fetal circulations, thereby keeping the fetal P_{CO_2} in an optimal range.[56] During labor, maternal hyperventilation increases dramatically (either spontaneously or induced), and a maternal pH above 7.6 is not uncommon. This would result in a significant leftward shift of the maternal oxyhemoglobin dissociation curve unless compensatory mechanisms such as increased maternal metabolic activity occur. Fetal asphyxia as the result of maternal hyperventilation has been reported,[54] since maternal respiratory alkalosis is associated with decreases in uterine blood flow of up to 25 percent, and fetal oxygenation has been shown to decrease an equivalent amount.[57]

Total hemoglobin concentration increases throughout gestation[58] in the fetus, favoring oxygen diffusion across the placenta. The fraction of Hb A in fetal blood increases as gestation proceeds (particularly in the third trimester), so that the P_{50} of the newly born infant is approximately 19 torr. The increasing concentrations of Hb A in fetal blood favors oxygen unloading to the fetal tissues, especially during the last trimester when metabolic activity is greatest. The increasing proportion of Hb A as gestation increases and the great increase in Hb A postnatally (P_{50} = 27.4 torr by 6 months of age) also increases the effectiveness of 2,3–DPG, which preferentialy binds to Hb A compared to Hb F.

The pH of fetal blood is approximately 0.1 pH unit lower than that of adult blood.[59] This lower pH aids in shifting the fetal oxyhemoglobin dissociation curve to the right, as well as facilitating oxygen release to the fetal tissues. The lower pH of fetal blood may also facilitate oxygen transport across the placenta by lowering the pH of maternal blood passing through the intervillous space (Bohr effect). This would produce a rightward shift of the maternal oxyhemoglobin dissociation curve, favoring oxygen unloading from the maternal circulation to the fetal circulation. As Hb F accepts oxygen, it becomes more alkalotic, thereby increasing its oxygen affinity. When oxygenated Hb F passes through the fetal circulation, however, it becomes relatively acidotic and a Bohr relationship with the fetal tissues develops and oxygen diffuses to them. Fetal temperature is greater than maternal temperature by 0.5–1.0°.[60] This small increase in

fetal temperature also minimally favors oxygen transport first from the maternal circulation to the fetal circulation and from there to the fetal tissues.

REFERENCES

1. Muirhead H, Cox JM, Mazzarella L et al: Structure and function of hemoglobin III: three-dimensional Fourier synthesis of human deoxyhaemoglobin at 5.5A resolution. *M Mol Biol* 28:117, 1967.
2. Perutz MF: The structure and function of haemoglobin. Harvey Lectures, Series 63, 1967–68, p 213.
3. Perutz MF: Hemoglobin structure and respiratory transport. *Sci Am* 239:92, 1978.
4. Roughton FJW: Transport of oxygen and carbon dioxide, in Fenn WO, Rahn H (eds): *Handbook of Physiology,* Washington, DC, American Physiological Society, Vol 1: *Section 3, Respiration,* p 767, 1964.
5. Michel CC: The transport of oxygen and carbon dioxide by the blood, in Widdicombe JD (ed): *MTP International Review of Science:* Respiratory Physiology, London, Butterworth & Co, Ltd, 1974, p. 67.
6. Shapiro BA: *Clinical Application of Blood Gases.* Chicago, Year book Medical Publishers, Inc, 1973.
7. Winters RW, Engel K, Dell RB: *Acid-Base Physiology in Medicine,* Cleveland, London Co, 1967.
8. Winters RW: Studies of acid-base disturbances. *Pediatrics* 39:700, 1967.
9. Thomas HM, Lefrak SS, Irwin RS, et al: The oxyhemoglobin dissociation curve in health and disease. *Am J Med* 57:331, 1974.
10. Severinghouse JW: Blood gas calculator. *J Appl Physiol* 21:1108, 1966.
11. Canizaro PC, Nelson JL, Hennessy JL, et al: A technique for estimating the oxyhemoglobin dissociation curve. *Ann Surg* 180:364, 1974.
12. Oski FA, Delivoria-Papadopoulos M: The red cell, 2,3–Diphosphoglycerate, and tissue oxygen release. *J Pediatr* 77:941, 1970.
13. Valtis DJ, Kennedy AC: Defective gas-transport function of stored red-blood cells. *Lancet* 1:119, 1954.
14. Benesch R, Benesch RE: The effect of organic phosphates from the human erythrocyte on the allosteric properties of hemoglobin. *Biochem Biophys Res Commun* 26:162, 1967.
15. Chanutin A, Curnish RR: Effect of organic and inorganic phosphates on the oxygen equilbrium of human erythrocytes. *Arch Biochem Biophys* 121:96, 1967.
16. Lenfant C, Torrence J, English E, et al: Effect of altitude on oxygen binding by hemoglobin and on organic phosphate levels. *J Clin Invest* 47: 2652, 1968.
17. Eaton JW, Brewer GJ, Grover RF: Role of red cell

2,3–diphosphoglycerate in the adaptation of man to altitude *J Lab Clin Med* 73: 603, 1969.
18. Oski FA, Gottlieb AJ, Delivoria-Papadopoulos M, et al: Red cell 2,3–diphosphoglycerate levels in subjects with chronic hypoxemia. *N Engl J Med* 280: 1165, 1969
19. Morge M, Cassels DE, Holder M: The position of the oxygen dissociation curve of the blood in cyanotic congenital heart disease. *J Clin Invest* 29:1098, 1950.
20. Lenfant C, Ways P, Aucutt C, et al: Effect of chronic hypoxia on the O_2-Hb dissociation curve and respiratory gas transport in man. *Respir Physiol* 7:7, 1969.
21. Mulhausen R, Astrup P, Kjeldsen K: Oxygen affinity of hemoglobin in patients with cardiovascular disease, anemia and cirrhosis of the liver. *Scand J Clin Lab Invest* 19:291, 1967.
22. Torrence J, Jacobs P, Restrepo A, et al: Intraerythrocyte adaptation to anemia. *N Eng J Med* 283: 165, 1970.
23. Richards DW, and Strauss ML: Oxyhemoglobin dissociation curves of whole blood in anemia. *J Clin Invest* 4: 105, 1927.
24. Miller WW, Delivoria-Papadopoulos M, Miller LD, et al: Increased release of oxygen from hemoglobin in hyperthyroidism: control by red cell 2,3—diphosphoglycerate. *JAMA* 211:1824, 1970.
25. Weiss EB, Desforges JF: Oxyhemoglobin affinity in bronchial asthma: chronic stable state, acute, and status asthmaticus. *Chest* 62: 709, 1972.
26. Chapman RG, Hennessey MA, Waltersdorph AM, et al: Erythrocyte metabolism: V. Levels of glycolytic enzymes and regulation of glycolysis. *J Clin Invest* 41: 1249, 1962.
27. Minakami S, Yoshikawa H: Studies on erythrocyte glycolysis: III. The effects of active cation transport, pH, and inorganic phosphate concentration on erythrocyte glycolysis. *J Biochem* 59: 145, 1966.
28. Valeri CR, Hirsch N: Restoration in vivo of erythrocyte adenosine triphosphate, 2,3–diphosphoglycerate, potassium ion, and sodium ion concentrations following the transfusion of acid-citrate-dextrose-stored human red cells. *J Lab Clin Med* 73:822, 1969.
29. Beutler E, Wood L: The in vivo regeneration of red cell 2,3–diphosphoglyceric acid (DPG) after transfusion of stored blood. *J Lab Clin Med* 74: 300, 1979.

30. Hechtman HB, Grindlinger GA, Vegas AM, et al: Importance of oxygen transport in clinical medicine. *Crit Care Med* 7:419, 1979.

31. Dennis RC, Hechtman HB, Berger RL, et al: Transfusion of 2,3–DPG enriched red blood cells to improve cardiac function. *Ann Thorac Surg* 25:17, 1978.

32. Miller H, Ayres SM, Gregory JJ, et al: Hemodynamics, coronary blood flow and myocardial metabolism in coronary shock: response to l-norepinepherine and isoproterenol. *J Clin Invest* 49:1885, 1970.

33. Miller LD, Sugarman HJ, Cromie WJ et al: *Administration of Inosine in Man, in Preservation of Red Blood Cells.* Washington, DC, National Academy of Sciences, 1973, p 253–262.

34. Anselmino KT, Hoffman F: Die Ursachen des Icterus Neonatorum. *Arch Gynak* 143:477, 1930.

35. Allen DW, Wyman T, Smith CA: The oxygen equilibrium of fetal and adult human hemoglobin. *J Biol Chem* 203:84, 1953.

36. Bauer C, Ludwig I, Ludwig M: Different effects of 2,3–diphosphoglycerate and adenosine triphosphate on oxygen affinity of adult and fetal human hemoglobin. *Life Sci* 7:1339, 1968.

37. Bunn HF, Briehl RW: The interaction of 2,3–diphosphoglycerate with various human hemoglobins. *J Clin Invest* 49: 1088, 1970.

38. Oski FA, Miller W, Delivoria-Papadopoulos M, et al: The effects of deoxygenation of adult and fetal hemoglobin on the synthesis of red cell 2,3–diphosphoglycerate and its in vivo consequences. *J Clin Invest* 49: 400, 1970.

39. Delivoria-Papadopoulos M, Roncevic NP, Oski FA: Postnatal changes in oxygen transport of term, premature, and sick infants: the role of red cell 2,3–diphosphoglycerate and adult hemoglobin. *Pediatr Res* 5:235, 1971.

40. Morris FH, Brumley GW: Erythrocyte 2,3–diphosphoglycerate concentrations in umbilical venous blood from normal and meconium stained infants. *Am J Obstet Gynecol* 119:998, 1974.

41. Towell ME: Fetal respiratory physiology in perinatal medicine, in Goodwin JW, Godden JO, Chance GW (eds): *The Basic Science Underlying Clinical Practice,* Baltimore, The Williams & Wilkins Co, 1976, p 171–176.

42. Strang LBL: Oxygen transport in blood, in *Neonatal Respiration: Physiological and Clinical Studies* Oxford, England, Blackwell Scientific Publications, 1977, p. 138.

43. Rorth M, Bille-Brate NE: 2,3-Diphosphoglycerate and creatine in the red cell during pregnancy. *Scand J Clin Lab Invest* 28: 271, 1971.

44. Ueland K, Novy MJ, Metcalfe J: Cardio-respiratory responses in pregnancy and exercise in normal women and patients with heart disease. *Am J Obstet Gynecol* 115: 4, 1973.

45. Kerr MG: Cardiovascular dynamics in pregnancy and labor. *Br Med Bull* 24: 19, 1968.

46. Lees MM, Taylor SHJ, Scott DB, et al: A study of cardiac output at rest throughout pregnancy. *J Obstet Gynaecol Br Commonw* 74: 319, 1967.

47. Towell ME, Liggins GC: The effect of labour on uterine blood flow in the pregnant ewe. *QJ Exp Physiol* 61 (1): 23, 1976.

48. Assali NS, Rauramo L, Peltonen T: Measurement of uterine blood flow and uterine metabolism: VIII. Uterine and fetal blood flow and oxygen consumption in early human pregnancy. *Am J Obstet Gynecol* 103:19, 1969

49. Metcalfe J, Romney SL, Ramsey LH, et al: Estimation of uterine blood flow in normal human pregnancy at term. *J. Clin Invest* 34: 1632, 1955.

50. Jansson, I: ^{133}Xenon clearance in the myometrium of pregnant and non-pregnant women. *Acta Obstet Gynecol Scand* 48: 302, 1969.

51. Metcalfe J, Baitels H, Moll W: Gas exchange in the pregnant uterus. *Physiol Rev* 47: 782, 1967.

52. Beischer NA, Sivasamboo R, Vohra S, et al: Placental hypertrophy in severe pregnancy anemia. *J Obstet Gynaecol Br Commonw* 77: 398, 1970.

53. Campbell AGM, Dawes GS, Fishman AP, et al: The oxygen consumption of the placenta and fetal membranes in the sheep. *J Physiol (Lond)* 182:439, 1966.

54. Pronse CM, Goensley EA: Respiratory and acid-base changes during pregnancy. *Anesthesiology* 26: 381, 1964.

55. Pernoll ML, Metcalfe J, Kovach PA, et al: Ventilation during rest and exercise in pregnancy and postpartum. *Respir Physiol* 25:295, 1975.

56. Matalon SV, Manning PJ, Bernie BJ, et al: The effects of change of maternal Pao_2 and $Paco_2$ on the fetal Pao_2 and $Paco_2$—in vivo study. *Respir Physiol* 32:51, 1978.

57. Moya F, Morishima HO, Shnider SM, et al: Influence of maternal hyperventilation on the newborn infant. *Am J Obstet Gynecol* 91: 76, 1965.

58. Barcroft J: *Researches on Prenatal Life, vol 1,* Oxford, England, Blackwell Scientific Publication, 1946.

59. Jacobson L, Rooth G: Interpretative aspects on the acid-base composition and its variation in fetal scalp blood and maternal blood during labour. *J Obstet Gynaecol Br Commonw* 78: 971, 1971.

60. Walker D, Walker A, Wood C: Temperature of the human fetus. *J Obstet Gynaecol Br Commonw* 76:503, 1969.

18

Pulmonary Function Testing in Infants and Small Children

Barry Fisher

INTRODUCTION

Pulmonary function testing provides a quantitative method for assessing normal and pathologic pulmonary physiology while permitting the natural history or the response to therapy of a disease process to be observed. The majority of pulmonary function tests currently available can generally be performed on children above 6 years of age without modification. Great strides have been made during the past 20 years to adapt existing techniques or design new methods for studying both normal and abnormal pulmonary physiology in children from the newborn period through early childhood. The differences between obstructive and restrictive pulmonary diseases encountered in a pediatric population both clinically and physiologically will be reviewed in this chapter. Also discussed in this chapter are the methods used to make these observations in the laboratory.

Knowledge of prenatal and postnatal development of the lungs aids in understanding the pathophysiologic processes of restrictive and obstructive lung diseases. The increasing severity of obstructive pulmonary disease during the first eight extrauterine years of life suggests that postnatal development of the lungs may play a contributory role. The development of interstitial fibrosis (as occurs with viral interstitial pneumonitis and the fibrotic component of cystic fibrosis) results in poorer compliance and decreased expansion of the lungs (restrictive disease). This results in a decreased lung volume with decreased pulmonary reserve and poorer net gas exchange.

GROWTH AND DEVELOPMENT OF LUNGS

Intrauterine embryology of the human lung has been well described.[1-6] The progressive branching of cartilage-containing airways appears to be complete by 25 weeks of gestation,[3] with the same number of cartilage-containing bronchi (conducting airways) present at 25 weeks of gestation as during adult life. Bucher and Reid[7] have reported extensive branching of epithelial-lined respiratory bronchioles and alveoli after 25 weeks of gestation that is virtually complete by 8 years of age. Growth of the lung after 25 weeks of gestation thus occurs primarily in the respiratory or gas exchange portions. Growth of the conducting airways[8,9] involves increases in diameter and length without the formation of new conducting tissue elements. Branching of the conducting airways is asymmetrical, resulting in airways with varying numbers of generations and length. Peripheral branching of the gas-exchange portions of the lung becomes progressively more symmetrical as the result of the massive proliferation of respiratory bronchioles and alveoli postnatally.[10-14] Dunnill[11] has reported that respiratory bronchioles and alveoli undergo massive proliferation postnatally, with their numbers increasing approximately tenfold by adulthood. Concomitant with this proliferation is a 27 times increase of the air-tissue interface that provides the milieu for the rapid exchange of oxygen and carbon dioxide between the air-containing spaces of the lung and the pulmonary capillary bed. This increase in air-tissue interface also accounts for the extensive physiologic reserve capacity of the lungs.

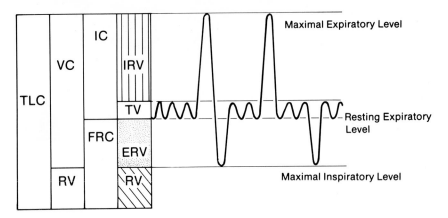

Figure 18-1. Subdivisions of the lung.

DIVISIONS OF THE LUNG

To understand obstructive and restrictive changes, it is necessary to be familiar with the various subdivisions of the lungs (Fig. 18-1). The total lung capacity (TLC) is the amount of air present in the lung at the end of a maximal inspiratory effort. It is the sum of the maximal amount of air that can be voluntarily moved (vital capacity, or VC) and the amount of air remaining in the lungs after a maximal expiratory effort (residual volume, or RV). Under normal circumstances the VC is approximately 75 percent, and the RV is approximately 25 percent of the TLC. Tidal volume (TV) is the usual amount of air moved with each breath and averages 7 cc/kg/ breath. In normal individuals, the TV is found near the midpoint of the VC. From end expiratory TV to the expiratory end of the VC is the expiratory reserve volume (ERV). This volume represents the maximal volume of air that can be exhaled after a normal tidal expiration.

Functional residual capacity (FRC) is the volume of air remaining in the lungs at the end of a tidal expiration. FRC is the sum of ERV and RV. Inspiratory reserve volume (IRV) is the maximal volume of air that can be inspired after end tidal inspiration. Inspiratory capacity (IC) is the maximal amount of air that can be inspired after end tidal expiration and is the sum of TV and IRV. RV can be obtained by measuring FRC and subtracting ERV. TLC can be calculated by adding either IC and FRC or VC and RV.

In summary, then, there are four primary volumes (TV, RV, IRV, and ERV) that do not overlap and four standard capacities (TLC, VC,

IC, and FRC), each of which includes two or more of the primary volumes. By convention, various points on the lung subdivision graph are defined with volume or capacity names. For example, the end tidal expiration point is often referred to as the *FRC point.* This means that the gas-containing compartment below this point is the FRC. Similarly the maximal expiratory point of the VC may be referred to as the *RV point.*

OBSTRUCTIVE AND RESTRICTIVE LUNG DISEASE

This next section concerns itself with a clinicophysiologic description of obstructive and restrictive lung disease. Obstructive lung disease is a classification of diseases associated with a normal to moderately increased TLC, obstruction of airflow during expiration, and an increased RV after maximal expiration. In its most severe forms, inspiratory airway obstruction also may be present.

Since TLC remains normal to moderately increased in obstructive lung disease, the physiologic changes result primarily from a redistribution of the compartments of the lung (Fig 18-2). With increasing airway obstruction RV increases and VC decreases. The conducting airway cross-sectional diameter is normally smaller during expiration than during inspiration. Disease states associated with a decreased conductive airway cross-sectional diameter (asthma, cystic fibrosis, bronchiolitis) therefore have a potential increase in RV with each successive inspiration. As a result VC decreases as RV increases. Associated with

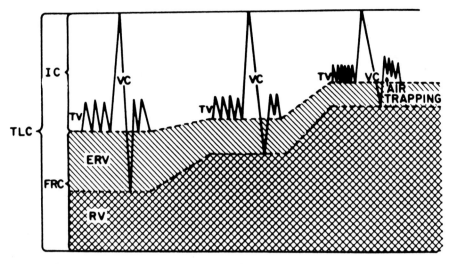

Figure 18-2. Progression of pulmonary function changes in patients with obstructive lung disease of increasing severity. The increase in FRC and decrease in ERV are due to the obstructive disease process that results in an even greater use in RV. The VC and FEV_1/FVC may be reduced to as little as 25–30 percent or less, whereas the RV/TLC ratio may increase to 0.70–0.75 percent or greater with the most severe disease. From Matthews LW, Doershuk CF: *Mod Probl Pediatr* 10:237, 1967. With permission.

this decrease in VC there is a nonlinear increase in respiratory rate. A reduction in the alveolar component of the TV without change in the conductive component of the TV accounts for the decrease in TV seen in progressive obstruction. In severe airway obstructive disease, minute alveolar ventilation generally is decreased while total minute ventilation may be normal or increased.

As the TV is displaced upward toward the inspiratory end of the VC, the lung becomes less compliant, and respiratory effort increases to move the same volume of air. The dyspnea associated with obstructive airway disease thus becomes understandable. The severity of inspiratory intercostal and subxiphoid retractions parallel the decrease in lung compliance. As the diaphragms are displaced downward by the increasing RV, the diaphragmatic contribution to the normal inspiratory increase in lung volume is diminished. In an attempt to compensate for this decreased inspiratory contribution of the diaphragms, intercostal muscles vigorously contract, and suprasternal muscles elevate the entire thorax. However, these latter maneuvers are not as effective as the normal diaphragmatic contribution to inspiration. As the effectiveness of respiration is decreasing, the work of breathing is increasing.

As the severity of airway obstructive disease increases, VC decreases even further, with ERV decreasing proportionately more than IC. The adequacy of gas exchange continues to decrease as the alveolar or gas exchange component of TV is further reduced. This results in a progressive mismatch of alveolar ventilation and capillary perfusion. As the TV progressively nears the maximal inspiratory point of TLC, respiratory effort increases, and the patient's ability to effectively exhale is reduced. A simple clinical experiment demonstrates the difficulties these patients encounter as they struggle to breathe. If we were to perform a maximal inspiratory effort and then not exhale, we begin to experience how these patients feel all the time. If we then try to do tidal breathing at maximal inspiration, the difficulty and inadequacy of ventilation at this position of the lung volume curve is appreciated.

Clinically these patients develop progressive tachypnea and dyspnea at rest. Intercostal, subxiphoid, and suprasternal retractions appear with increasing disease severity. On auscultation, prolongation of expiration with or without wheezing is usually heard. Airflow during expiration is generally decreased, but airflow throughout ventilation also can be reduced. Rales and rhonchi are often heard. Occasionally, one hears moist, popping sounds suggestive of opening and closing of small airways during the various phases of respiration. Hypoxemia generally develops early with subsequent carbon dioxide retention. Clinical signs of pulmonary overinflation include an increase in the anteroposterior diameter of the chest, hyperresonance to percussion, and depression of the diaphragms. Roentgenologically the lungs appear overinflated, there is widening of the intercostal spaces, and the ribs assume a progressively more horizontal position. The diaphragms become depressed and flattened. Retrosternal air (another sign of pulmonary overinflation) also can be seen on lateral chest roentgenograms. The cardiac silhouette generally appears normal to small in size compared to the increased size of the lungs. Even when cardiac enlargement is present, it generally appears mild. In disorders such as allergic bronchopulmonary aspergillosis or cystic fibrosis, peribronchial cuffing is usually present, probably the result of chronic inflammation and scarring.

Restrictive pulmonary disease is present when there is decreased compliance of the lungs, chest wall, or both. Examples of retrictive lung diseases include the fibrotic component of cystic fibrosis, interstitial fibrosis, and viral interstitial pneumonias. Chest wall diseases that may result in restrictive pulmonary disease include kyphoscoliosis, pectus deformities, and thoracic surgery with subsequent pleural scarring.

The pathophysiologic mechanism of restrictive lung disease is a decreased TLC as the result of intrinsic lung disease or external compression of the lung prohibiting full expansion. Lung volumes tend to be reduced symmetrically, but the RV may be increased in some cases because of the inability to produce a maximal expiratory effort. Flow rates may be either normal or reduced, but when corrected for the ratio of the forced expiratory volume in 1 second (FEV_1) to the forced vital capacity with maximally forced expiratory effort (FVC), flow rates may be either normal or increased. The distinction between obstructive and restrictive lung disease is characterized by a reduced FEV_1/FVC in the former and a normal or increased FEV_1/FVC in the latter. In restrictive lung disease, the RV/TLC ratio may be either normal or increased. If RV is increased and TLC is decreased, the resultant RV/TLC ratio would be increased. By contrast, in obstructive lung disease, TLC is normal to

increased, with RV being disproportionately increased. This, too, results in an increased RV/TLC ratio. The in-laboratory distinction between obstructive and restrictive disease when an increased RV/TLC ratio is present is that the TLC is normal to increased in obstructive disease, but it is reduced in restrictive disease.

The compliance of the lung (C_L) is decreased in both obstructive and restrictive lung disease. In normal lungs, TV is near the midpoint of the TLC where C_L is greatest. When TV is moved either up or down the TLC, the C_L decreases and the work of ventilation increases.

In summary, then, obstructive lung disease is present when TLC is normal to increased, VC and C_L are decreased, and RV/TLC is increased. Restrictive lung disease is associated with a decreased TLC, VC, C_L, and a normal or increased RV/TLC ration (Fig. 18-3).

PULMONARY FUNCTION TESTS

Spirometry

Flow rates and volume can be measured using a spirometer. Time is generally divided into 1-second intervals on the x axis, whereas volume is measured on the y axis. Since flow ($\dot{V}$) is volume per unit of time, timed volume measurements represent flow rates and relate to the tone and cross-sectional diameter of the airways. FEV_1 is the forced expiratory volume in 1 second measured from the peak of inspiration, and FEV_3 represents the forced expiratory volume in 3 seconds. Some laboratories also measure $FEV_{0.5}$ and $FEV_{0.75}$. Normal standards are available for these measurements in adults.[15-17] Standards for children from various studies have been collated by Polgar and Promadhat.[18]

Spirometry requires patient cooperation and results are effort dependent. Results generally improve somewhat with experience in performing this test. It has become the standard pulmonary function study to measure the health of the airways and parenchyma, however.

Flow-Volume Loops

By performing several mathematical manipulations and replotting the results, spirometry can be converted to a measure of flow ($\dot{V}$) versus volume (V) with expiratory flow rates that are independent of patient cooperation. The expira-

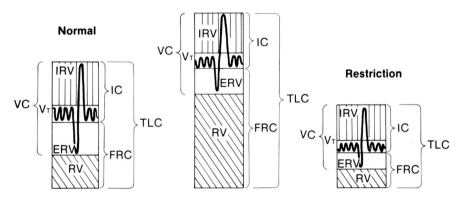

Figure 18-3. Graphic representation of the subdivisions of the lung in the normal state and in obstructive and restrictive disease. From Netter F: *Clinical Symposia* © CIBA Pharmaceutical Co., Division of CBA-Geigy Corp. 31:37, 1979. With permission.

tory slope of a flow-volume loop provides a reproducible signature of pulmonary dynamics in any individual at any particular time. Flow is a measurement of the volume for a unit time. By plotting $\dot{V}$ on the y axis and V on the x axis, a flow-volume loop is described. By convention inspiratory flow is downward, and expiratory flow is upward. Similarly the TLC point is to the left, and the RV point is to the right.

Figure 18-4 is the schematic representation of a normal flow-volume loop. Tidal ventilation is seen in the center (*point A*) followed by a maximal inspiratory effort (*point B*). The patient is then asked to exhale as hard, fast, and completely as possible. *Point C* is referred to as the peak expiratory flow rate (PEFR) and is an effort-dependent variable. The expiratory slope from PEFR to the RV point is effort independent. This slope defines the tone of the airways and is reproducible regardless of the patient's expiratory effort. If the expiratory effort is submaximal, the PEFR will be less, but the expiratory slope will be the same (*point C* to *point D*). Time can also be measured during this study with point B representing time 0. *Point E* is the FEV_1, and *point F* represents FEV_3. Classic spirometry also can be obtained from a flow-volume loop.

The maximal midexpiratory flow rate (MMEFR) is the flow at 50 percent of exhaled VC. This is also referred to as $\dot{V}_{max50\%VC}$. $\dot{V}_{max25\%VC}$ represents the maximum expiratory

flow rate at 25% of VC. Flow rate standards are available.[18–21] It is generally believed that flow beyond $\dot{V}_{max25\%VC}$ represents small airway flow in the normal state. In obstructive lung disease, the contributions of small airway tone are believed to represent a greater percentage of the expiratory slope with the effects seen earlier. Figure 18-5 is a reproduction of the flow-volume loop from a patient with severe obstructive airway disease. The VC is reduced, as is the PEFR (*point A*). Since small airway tone is the major contributor to airway obstruction, the maximal flow that can be generated in a patient with severe obstructive airway disease is reduced. The initial spike primarily represents the contribution of the large airways, and the very prolonged expiration from *point B* to *point C* at low flows is believed to represent the severity of the small airway obstruction. *Points D* and *E* represent FEV_1 and FEV_3, respectively. MMEFR or $\dot{V}_{max50\%VC}$ is represented by *point F* and is substantially reduced from the expected $\dot{V}_{max50\%VC}$ (*point G*).

Milder forms of airway obstruction are seen in Figure 18-6. *Panel A* represents mild airway obstructive disease, whereas *panel B* represents a moderate form of airway obstructive disease.

In summary, then, spirometry and flow-volume loops quantitate volume and flow characteristics of lung disease by measuring the magnitude and dynamic characteristics of the VC, the height of the PEFR, and the expiratory slope. $\dot{V}_{max50\%VC}$ or MMEFR is progressively reduced as airway

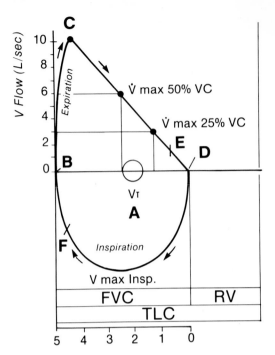

Figure 18-4. The normal flow-volume loop. From Andrews JL: *Med Clin North Am* 63:35, 1979. With permission.

obstruction increases. The contribution of small airway tone to the expiratory slope of the flow-volume loop increases as the degree of obstruction increases. In maximal obstructive airway disease there is a long, slow expiratory phase at very low flow rates representing small airway obstruction preceded by a reduced PEFR.

Flow-volume loops also are helpful in evaluating restrictive and extrathoracic airway obstructive changes. Figure 18-7 is a representation of a flow-volume loop seen in severe restrictive lung disease. The overall shape of the loop is normal, but it is miniaturized. The dotted lines represent the predicted normal flow-volume loop. The VC, PEFR, and flow rates at varying percentages of the exhaled, measured VC are all dramatically reduced on an absolute basis, but are normal to increased when the FEV_1/FVC is considered.

Figure 18-8, *Panel A,* is a schematic representation of a flow-volume loop characteristic of fixed extrathoracic inspiratory and expiratory airway obstructive diseases. Fixed extrathoracic airway obstruction includes any fixed obstruction above the carina. Representative diseases include epiglottitis, enlarged tonsils, and tracheal

stenosis. Variable extrathoracic obstruction (Fig. 18-8, *Panel B*) can be seen with polyps of the vocal cords or trachea.

Volume of Isoflow

Flow-volume loops provide estimates of the small airway contribution to expiratory airflow. In a normal individual, flow from $\dot{V}_{max25\%VC}$ to RV is believed to represent the small airway contribution to the maximum expiratory flow rate (MEFR) curve (Fig. 18-4). In severe obstructive lung disease (asthma, cystic fibrosis), it is believed that increased small airway tone is the dominant factor contributing to the greatly reduced expiratory slope of the MEFR curve after a reduced PEFR spike (Fig. 18-7).

If flow-volume loops are obtained after the patient breathes 80 percent helium and 20 percent oxygen and then are superimposed on a standard flow-volume loop (obtained while breathing room air), the expiratory slopes merge (Fig. 18-9) at a point referred to as the point of identical flow (PIF) or the isoflow point (VisoV̇). It has been shown that small airway flow is virtually independent of the density of the gas mixture being breathed, whereas large airway flow is gas-density dependent. Consequently, maximum expiratory flow rates obtained while the patient breathes a mixture of 80 percent helium and 20 percent oxygen are consistently higher than the flow rates obtained at any given

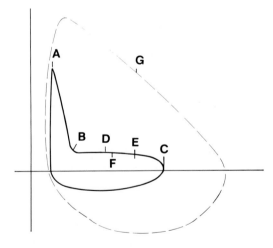

Figure 18-5. A flow-volume loop from a patient with severe airway obstructive disease (*solid line*) compared with predicted normal curve (*dashed line*).

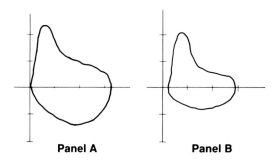

Panel A   **Panel B**

Figure 18-6. *Panel A,* Patient with mild airway obstructive disease. *Panel B,* Patient with moderate airway obstructive disease. Note that the VC, PEFR, and MMEFR in *panel B* is smaller than *panel A.*

volume when room air is breathed. Flow rates become identical when the small airway contribution to the MEFR curve begins.

Figure 18-10 demonstrates the increased percentage contribution of the small airways to the MEFR curve in a patient with severe asthma, a condition associated with an increased small airway contribution to forced expiration. Fox et al.[22] showed that the PIF was increased in 15 patients with cystic fibrosis compared to 24 control subjects, a finding compatible with mild small airway obstruction in this group of patients who had normal MMEFR values on standard flow-volume loops.

Crying Vital Capacity

Still another adaptation of the flow-volume or MEFR curve permitting flow studies in infants and small children is the crying vital capacity (CVC). McCarthy and Spock[23] have shown a maximal variation of 17.65 percent between obtained values over a 5-day period with repeated measurements in normal babies. When children with bronchiolitis or failure to thrive were studied over a 4-day period, however, the maximal variation for CVC determinations increased to 35.3 percent. The maximal percent variation in this population was significantly larger for PEFR as well (68.3 percent).

In another study evaluating CVC, Krauss et al.[24] showed that CVC was reproducible (r = 0.78) and that it was decreased in premature infants with hyaline membrane disease. This decrease in CVC correlated well with a decrease in helium dilution–measured FRC. Both values

returned toward normal as the infants recovered from the disease (Fig. 18-11).

Lung Volumes

The previous section has described spirometry and the flow characteristics of the FEV. The various measurements of flow and volume with their relationship to obstructive and restrictive disease have already been described. This section describes static lung volume measurements and their application to infants and small children.

The classic method for measuring FRC or the amount of air left in the lungs at the end of a tidal expiration uses the closed-circuit helium dilution method. Any inert gas that is neither consumed nor produced can be used as the reference gas, but helium has become the most commonly used. This method only measures lung volume in free

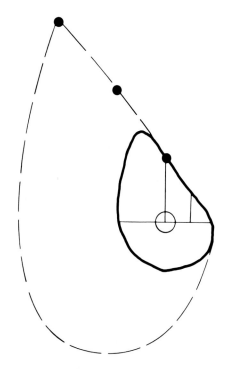

Restriction

Figure 18-7. Flow-volume loop from a patient with severe restrictive lung disease (*solid line*) compared with predicted normal loop (*dashed line*). From Andrews JL: *Med Clin North Am* 63:35, 1979. With permission.

Extrathoracic Obstruction

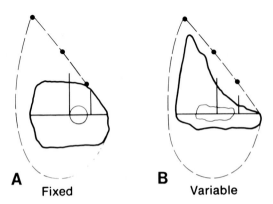

A Fixed   **B** Variable

Figure 18-8. *Panel A,* Flow-volume loop from a patient with fixed extrathoracic obstruction (*solid line*) compared with predicted normal loop (dotted line). *Panel B,* Flow-volume loop from a patient with variable extrathoracic obstruction. From Andrews JL: *Med Clin North Am* 63:35, 1979. With permission.

communication with the mouth. It is therefore ineffective in assessing airway obstruction or gas trapping. To measure both obstructed and unobstructed gas, it is necessary to measure the total thoracic gas volume (TGV) using plethysmography. Obstructed or trapped gas can be calculated by subtracting helium-measured FRC from plethysmographically measured TGV. Trapped gas is defined as that lung volume not in free communication with the mouth and generally increases as the severity of airway obstructive disease increases.

Helium Dilution Technique

The conventional technique for measuring FRC uses a spirometer filled with 10 percent helium in either air or oxygen. The patient is connected to the spirometer via a unidirectional rebreathing circuit. Carbon dioxide is absorbed using soda ash, and the initial spirometer volume is kept constant (steady baseline) by adding air or oxygen at the same rate that carbon dioxide is absorbed. A helium meter is also attached in line, and rebreathing is continued until a new helium steady state is achieved. A lower helium concentration indicates that helium equilibrium between the unknown volume of the patient's lung and the known volume of the spirometer has occurred. Then by calculating the volume of air needed to lower the helium concentration to the

new lower measured level, FRC is obtained. The equation for calculating FRC follows:

$$He_{inital} \times V_{spirometer} = He_{final} \times (V_{spirometer} + FRC)$$

Solving for FRC, the equation becomes:

$$FRC = \frac{V_{spirometer} \times (He_{final} - He_{initial})}{He_{final}}$$

Steady-State Nitrogen Washout Technique

The open-circuit nitrogen washout technique is another dilution technique that employs the complete displacement of nitrogen by breathing 100 percent oxygen. All exhaled air is collected with the volume and nitrogen concentration of the sample measured. The total expired amount of nitrogen collected is equal to the volume of nitrogen in the lung before the test. The following equation describes the calculation of FRC using this technique:

$$V_{expired\ air} \times [N_2]_{expired\ air} = FRC \times [N_2]\ \text{initially in lung}$$

Rearrangement gives:

$$FRC = \frac{V_{expired\ air} \times [N_2]_{expired\ air}}{[N_2]\ \text{initially in lung}}$$

Plethysmography

TGV is the total volume of air left in the lungs at the end of a tidal expiration, both obstructed and unobstructed. TGV is measured in a total body plethysmograph according to the technique described by Dubois et al. in 1956.[25] This technique is based on Boyle's law where $P_1V_1 = P_2V_2$ at constant temperature.

The technique for measuring TGV is to occlude the airway using a shutter at end tidal expiration with the patient enclosed in a constant-volume pressure plethysmograph. At a state of no flow, it is assumed that mouth pressure (P_m) is the same as alveolar pressure (P_A). This assumption has recently been questioned by Helms[26] who demonstrated that mouth pressure does not estimate P_A at low lung volumes because of small airway closure. In situations where low lung volumes are encountered, measurements of esophageal pressure result in a more representative assessment of TGV.

When the test subject inspires against the airway-occluding shutter, the airway and alveolar pressure fall below atmospheric and TGV in-

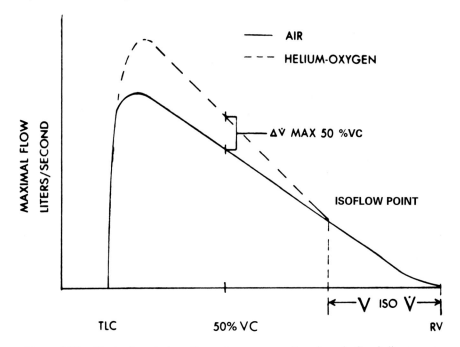

Figure 18-9. Maximal expiratory flow-volume curves after air and after helium-oxygen breathing. The percentage change in the flow at 50 percent VC after breathing helium and oxygen is expressed as $\dot{V}_{max50\%VC}$. The volume of isoflow (Viso$\dot{V}$) is determined where the helium and oxygen and air curves intersect and frequently is expressed as a percentage of the VC. From Lough MD, Doershuk CF, Stern RC: *Pediatric Respiratory Therapy,* ed 2. Chicago, Year Book Medical Publishers Inc, 1979.

creases. This increase in TGV is reflected by an increase in box pressure (P_b), since the plethysmograph is sealed and the volume of gas represented by that increase in box pressure cannot be dissipated.

During an expiratory effort against the shutter-occluded airway, alveolar and airway pressure rise above atmospheric pressure, resulting in a decrease in TGV. Associated with this decrease in TGV, the box pressure decreases and the air outside the thorax, but within the plethysmograph, decompresses to occupy a larger cubic area.

When the airway is occluded by the shutter, P_m is recorded on the y axis of a cathode ray oscilloscope with expiration being upward ($+$ changes) and inspiration downward ($-$ changes). Simultaneously, P_b is measured on the x axis with expiration to the left and inspiration to the right.

A decrease in TGV (expiratory effort against a closed shutter) is associated with a negative change in box pressure, whereas an inspiratory effort against the closed shutter is associated with

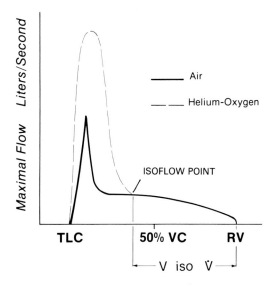

Figure 18-10. Representative Viso$\dot{V}$ curve from a patient with severe asthma. Note that isoflow point occurs during the first half of the maximally expired VC.

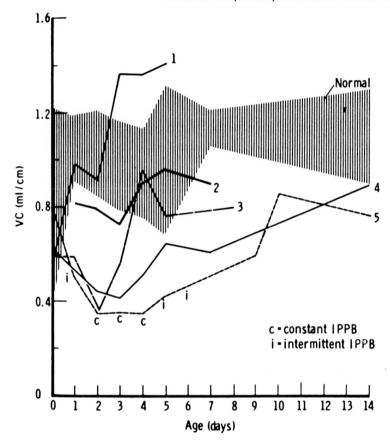

Figure 18-11. Crying vital capacity (CVC) versus age in infants 33–34 weeks old. *Hatched area,* Normal range; *lines,* 5 infants with hyaline membrane disease; *IPPB,* intermittent positive pressure breathing. From Krauss AN, Klain DB, Dahms BB, et al: Vital capacity in premature infants. *Am Rev Respir Dis* 108:1361, 1973. With permission.

a subatmospheric increase in TGV and an increase in P_b (associated with a decreased box volume).

Rather than measuring the actual linear deflection of mouth and box pressures, the angle theta (θ) formed by them is measured (Fig. 18-12). The slope of this relationship is tangential with $\tan \theta = Y/X$ or $\Delta P/\Delta V$.

Boyle's law can be rewritten as:

$$PV = (P + \Delta P)(V + \Delta V)$$

where P = Atmospheric pressure in cm H_2O (atmospheric pressure in mm Hg $\times$ 1.36) $-$ 47 cm H_2O vapor pressure.

V = The initial gas volume in the thorax, that is, TGV

ΔP = The change in alveolar pressure (ΔP_m) during panting efforts against the closed shutter

ΔV = The change in TGV (ΔP_b) resulting from gas compression or expansion by panting against a closed shutter

Since TGV measurements are made during expiration, ΔP_b is a negative deflection, and ΔP_m is a positive deflection. The above equation can now be rewritten as:

$$PV = (P + \Delta P)(V - \Delta V)$$

or

$$PV = PV - P\Delta V + \Delta PV - \Delta P\Delta V$$

or

$$0 = -P\Delta V + \Delta PV - \Delta P\Delta V$$

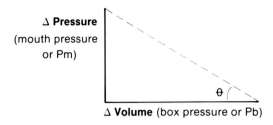

Figure 18-12. Angle θ represents the relationship between mouth pressure (Pm) and box pressure (Pb) for determination of plethysmographic TGV.

Since $\Delta P \Delta V$ is a very small number relative to the volume of the plethysmograph, it can be removed without influencing the result.

Rearrangement yields: $\Delta PV = P\Delta V$

solving for V:

$$V = \frac{P\Delta V}{\Delta P}$$

which converts to:

$$V = \frac{P \times \Delta \text{ Box pressure (Pb)}}{\Delta \text{ Mouth pressure (Pm)}}$$

or even better

$$V = \frac{P \times \Delta Pb}{\Delta Pm}$$

The tangent of the angle θ on the cathode ray oscilloscope = tan = $\Delta P/\Delta V$ therefore:

$$V = P \times \frac{1}{\tan \theta} \times \frac{\text{Box pressure calibration}}{\text{Mouth pressure calibration}}$$

The theory and technique for measuring plethysmographic lung volumes has just been reviewed. This method is easy to perform and is reproducible for patients above 5 or 6 years in age.

Various adaptations of this method to smaller children have been made. The modification employed by the author was initially described by Doershuk and Matthews.[27] Using this technique, the infant is studied in the supine position, either asleep in the postprandial state or using sedation with chloral hydrate, 60 mg/kg given orally or methohexital (Brevital) 5–8 mg/kg intramuscularly. Previous work has demonstrated no change in results when sedation is used.[27,28] A form-fitting mask of the face is used with a face seal made with aquaphor. The mouth is kept closed and measurements are made through the nares. Care must be taken not to occlude the nares with aquaphor or to compress them with the mask.

Increasing nasal airway resistance with increasing age does not interfere with TGV measurements, since TGV values do not differ significantly when measured either nasally or through the mouth.[29] A solenoid-triggered shutter occludes the airway at end tidal expiration, and the tangential angle describing $\Delta Ph/\Delta Pm$ is measured from a cathode ray oscilloscope.

This technique can also be adapted to infants with tracheostomies. Rather than using a face mask, an elbow, 15-mm universal adaptor is fitted to the tracheostomy and measurements are made as described above. At this point, an overestimating error is being made for length-related normal values because the volume of the nasoorolaryngeal airway is not being subtracted. Since infants and small children with tracheostomies generally do not have normal lung volumes, no normal standards are available. Standard predicted normal values therefore are used. The author calculates predicted normal values using the regression equation

$$TGV = 2.04 \times Ht^{2.7361} \times 10^{-6}$$

reported by Matthews and Doershuk,[30] where Ht = height in centimeters. Reproducible results are easily obtained, and the greatest value of these studies are comparisons over time in the same patient. Several other investigative groups have also reported normal TGV values for both premature and full-term neonates. Results range between 23 ml/kg within 20 minutes of birth and 40.6 cc/kg at 120 days of age with a mean of 32.34 ml/kg.[28,31–35]

Beyond the newborn period, however, the highest correlation has been found between body length and the TGV.[28] Even in the newborn period, the correlation between lung volume and length has proven valuable. Plethysmographically measured TGV values between 1.7–2.0 cc/cm of body length have been reported for infants with a birth weight above 1.75 kg.[35,36]

Airway resistance. The total body plethysmograph provides a method for measuring airway resistance (Raw) that is believed to be the most direct and accurate estimate of airway obstruction. Spirometry affords an indirect measure of Raw by evaluating flow rates. The implication is that Raw is increased when flow rates are decreased or when flow rates at a percent of VC are reduced on a flow-volume loop.

In the plethysmograph, Raw is the ratio of P_A over airflow when airflow is measured during successive respirations using the pneumotachometer and P_A is the same as Pm at a state of no flow (shutter-occluded airway).

Lung volume has a significant effect on Raw measurements. Consequently, it is helpful to measure Raw at a standard lung volume, so that reasonable comparisons over time can be made both on the same patient and on different patients. In general, Raw is measured at end tidal expiration, which is the FRC point (the point when the airway is occluded to measure alveolar pressure). Normally Raw is increased at smaller lung volumes and is normal or decreased at larger lung volumes. In obstructive lung disease with pulmonary overinflation, however, Raw increases because the airways are stretched and the mean airway cross-sectional diameter decreases. Measurements of Raw during a quiescent phase of chronic asthma are frequently elevated, but results are almost always elevated during acute exacerbations.

During the first 6 years of life, Raw decreases, presumably because of the extrauterine development of the gas-exchange portions of the lung. Developed gas-exchange units (alveoli) have a higher compliance than immature pulmonary tissue. Nasal Raw increases during the first 5 or 6 years of life, and measurements obtained nasally in a plethysmograph are somewhat higher than simultaneous measurements obtained orally.[29,37] In the adult, Raw averages 0.5–1.0 cm $H_2O/L/sec$ at an FRC of approximately 2.5 L, whereas the average Raw is 5 cm $H_2O/L/sec$ at a lung volume approximating 0.67 L by 6 years of age.

Total respiratory resistance. In 1970 Goldman et al.[38] reported a simplified method for measuring total respiratory resistance using the technique of forced oscillations. Total respiratory resistance includes not only the flow resistance of the lung tissues and airways (total pulmonary resistance), but also the flow resistance of the chest wall. The forced oscillations technique was originally described by Dubois et al.[39] and is useful because it eliminates the need for an esophageal balloon, as well as the body plethysmograph. It also requires little cooperation from the subject.

Wohl, Stigol, and Mead[40] used a modification of the forced oscillatory technique to measure total respiratory resistance in infants and children up to 15 months of age. The method included use of a sine wave of pressure produced by loudspeakers and applied to the

respiratory system at the latter resonant frequency. The pressures were those required to overcome the elastic and inertial impedance of the respiratory system and are dissipated in overcoming flow resistance. Flow was measured via a face mask. These subjects were studied unsedated during nasal breathing. Twenty-eight healthy newborns (mean age = 3.6 days) had a mean total pulmonary resistance during inspiration of 69 ± 25 cm $H_2O/L/sec$ and a mean total pulmonary resistance during expiration of 97 ± 52 cm $H_2O/L/sec$. This compares to 29 studies carried out on normal infants 1–15 months of age (mean age = 29.4 weeks) where the values for mean inspiratory and expiratory respiratory resistances were both 46 ± 17 cm $H_2O/L/sec$.

In 20 hospitalized patients with bronchiolitis ages 1–17 months, (mean age = 5.9 months), these investigators found that the respiratory frequency was increased and the TV was decreased, resulting in a minute volume comparable to that seen in healthy infants. Total respiratory resistance was increased during both inspiration and expiration in bronchiolitis with the ratio of inspiratory/expiratory time decreased to 0.68 from a normal of 0.75. In Krieger's patients[41] the ratio of inspiratory/expiratory time was increased to 0.93, whereas Phelan, Williams, and Freeman[42] found the mean ratio to be 0.72 during the acute stages of bronchiolitis and 0.71 after recovery. The mean inspiratory resistance during the acute states of bronchiolitis in this latter study was 93 ± 75 cm $H_2O/L/sec$ with a mean expiratory resistance of 152 ± 57 cm $H_2O/L/sec$. Two of seven patients studied 2 or more months later still had elevated resistances for both inspiration and expiration, whereas another patient who had become too large to study had continuing clinical evidence of obstruction.

Total pulmonary resistance. Total pulmonary resistance (Rp) is the sum of Raw and lung tissue resistance (Rlt). Krieger[43] determined Rp using a plethysmograph where airflow rather than airway pressure was measured so that the Rlt also could be considered. The calculated mean value for Rp measured nasally on 24 sedated, hospitalized children 1–24 months of age was 29 ± 20 cm $H_2O/L/sec$. Phelan, Williams, and Freeman[42] used a comparable method except that a pneumotachometer was used for airflow measurements and showed that Rp decreased with increasing body

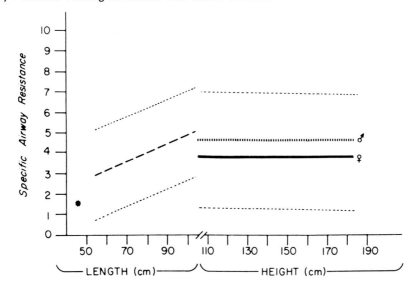

Figure 18-13. SRaw versus length SRaw for newborns (*star*), young children (*dashed line*), older females (*solid line*), and males (*dotted line*) are related to length. The 95-percent confidence limits are shown by the lighter dotted lines. Beyond age 6 years the SRaw remained stable through the period of body growth, unlike lung value and CL. The females consistently had a lower SRaw. From Charnock EL, Fisher BJ, Doershuk CF: Development of the Respiratory System, in Lough D, Doershuk CF, Stern RC (eds): *Pediatric Respiratory Therapy,* ed 2. Chicago, Year Book Medical Publishers Inc, © 1979. With permission.

length and lung volume in 38 healthy infants between 4 and 46 weeks of age.

Frank, Mead, and Wittenberger[44] reported that Rlt accounted for 15 percent of Rp in adults while Bachofen and Duc[45] reported that Rlt accounted for 29 percent of Rp in 10 healthy children between 7 and 11 years of age. In healthy newborns, Rlt was increased to 40 percent of Rp.[46] These results are expected when one considers that the majority of the massive proliferation of alveolar or gas-exchange portions of the lung occur during infancy and childhood.

Specific airway resistance. Specific airway resistance (SRaw) is the product of lung volume at which Raw is measured times Raw. As can be seen from Figure 18-13, this value is essentially a constant after 6 years of age. Females consistently have a lower SRaw than males after age 6, but the difference widens to 1 cm $H_2O/L/sec$ with puberty. This calculated value therefore may be helpful in dating puberty in the female. The presumed hormonal changes responsible for this sexual difference are not known.

SRaw has proven valuable in assessing the severity of pulmonary disease in cystic fibrosis patients. Figure 18-14 demonstrates the results in three groups of patients with varying clinical scores.[29] Those patients with the lowest clinical scores (most severe clinical pulmonary disease) had the most significant, consistent elevation of SRaw.

When lung volume is plotted against Raw, a nonlinear relationship is found. To overcome this nonlinearity, conductance (Gaw) is plotted against lung volume. Gaw is the reciprocal of Raw and specific conductance (SGaw) is the ratio of Gaw divided by the lung volume (TGV) at which Gaw is measured (SGaw = Gaw/TGV). With progressive obstructive abnormalities SGaw decreases and SRaw increases. Numerically and conceptually, it is easier to compare serial measurements of SRaw than SGaw. In the author's laboratory SRaw is generally used.

SRaw also permits easy comparison when the results of cystic fibrosis therapy are assessed.[47] Figure 18-15 shows the results of TGV, Raw, and SRaw studies on 27 children studied at the time of diagnosis and again at the end of 2 weeks of therapy. Statistically significant improvement in

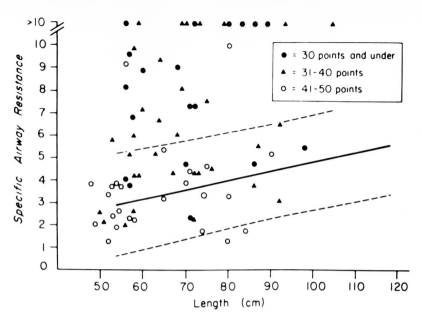

Figure 18-14. SRaw versus length for 77 patients with cystic fibrosis between 1 month and 5 years of age at the time of diagnosis. Patients are grouped by clinical scores. Scores under 30 are associated with the most severe pulmonary disease clinically and roentgenologically and scores above 40 points are associated with the mildest pulmonary disease. The solid line represents the mean SRaw value at any length, and the dotted lines represent the ninety-fifth percentile confidence limits. From Doershuk CF, Fisher BJ, Matthews LW: Specific airway resistance from the perinatal period into adulthood. *Am Rev Respir Dis* 109:452, 1974. With permission.

$\overline{m}$ age at diagnosis = 10.89 months

	TGV	Raw	SRaw
number	27	27	27
diagnosis	141.2 ± 46.3 (76-249)	35.0 ± 16.8 (9-59.1)	8.91 ± 5.7 (2.4-26.5)
follow up	117.8 ± 54.1 (78-241)	25.9 ± 13.4 (9.6 - 49.3)	6.2 ± 4.4 (2.2-19.1)
p value	<0.05	<0.015	<0.05

a) TGV is in % of predicted normal
b) Raw and SRaw are absolute values
c) Values in parentheses are ranges

Figure 18-15. TGV, Raw, and SRaw studies on 27 children at the time of diagnosis of cystic fibrosis and again after 2 weeks of hospital treatment.

246

m̄ age at diagnosis = 8.68 months

	TGV	Raw	SRaw
number	22	22	22
diagnosis	128.3 ± 29.4 (81-230)	39.4 ± 11.6 (12.9-58.0)	7.2 ± 4.9 (2.4-23.9)
follow up	99.6 ± 25.4 (59-181)	11.6 -5.7 (4.9 - 23.8)	4.3 ± 2.4 (1.1-9.4)
p value	0.005	0.005	0.015

a) TGV is in % of predicted normal
b) Raw and SRaw are absolute values
c) Values in parentheses are ranges

Figure 18-16. TGV, RAW, and SRaw studies on 22 children at the time of diagnosis of cystic fibrosis and again after 1 year of therapy.

all values are apparent. Figure 18-16 demonstrates the long-term improvement in TGV, Raw, and SRaw values for 22 children with cystic fibrosis studied initially at the time of diagnosis and again after 1 year of treatment. Not all the abnormal results reverse to normal with growth or treatment, since some abnormalities appear to be fixed or to progress, even at this early age.

Compliance. C_L is defined as a change in volume for each unit change in pressure ($C_L = \Delta V/\Delta P$). This relationship relies upon the pressure needed to overcome the elasticity of the lung and thereby change the lung volume. Over the normal range of TV this relationship is nearly linear. As TLC is approached, however, a progressively greater pressure is needed to effect a given volume change. The C_L therefore decreases as lung volume increases. The technique for determining C_L includes measurement of transpulmonary or esophageal pressure using an esophageal balloon or fluid-filled catheter with simultaneous determinations of airflow and lung volume.

Krieger and Whitten[48] measured C_L using a total body plethysmograph in 24 hospitalized normal children 1–24 months of age. FRC was not measured; however, an estimated FRC was used to determine the mean specific compliance (compliance/unit of FRC) of 0.0384 ± 0.0097 ml/cm H_2O/ml of lung volume. This value was less than that observed in newborns by Chu et al.[49] In their study, Krieger and Whitten observed a

significant decrease in C_L in infants with bronchiolitis followed by a rapid return to normal values after recovery. Phelan, Williams, and Freeman[42] used a method similar to that of Krieger and also observed a decrease in C_L in infants with bronchiolitis. Phelan and Williams[50] measured specific compliance (compliance/unit of FRC) in 38 healthy infants between 4 and 46 weeks of age and found a mean value of 0.056 ± 0.01 ml/cm H_2O/ml of lung volume, a value similar to the specific compliance values found in both newborns and adults.[17,48]

Griffin et al.[51] used a total body plethysmograph to measure C_L in children with congenital heart disease. In patients with ventricular septal defects or patent ductus arteriosus who had pulmonary artery pressures that were one half of systemic pressure or greater, a decreased C_L was generally seen. If the pulmonary artery pressure was less than one half of systemic pressure, C_L was usually not decreased. No simultaneous measurements of lung volume were made in this study.

There appears to be a relationship between increased SRaw values in patients with congenital heart lesions[52] associated with increased pulmonary artery pressure, high pulmonary blood flow, and decreased C_L. Our preliminary evaluation of plethysmographic lung volume (TGV) and Raw measurements with calculation of (SRaw) on over 50 infants with left-to-right shunt congenital heart lesions[52] showed that SRaw was generally increased with high-pressure, high-flow lesions, whereas the SRaw was consistently normal when pulmonary artery pressures were less than one half of systemic pressure, regardless of pulmonary flow. Since TGV was generally increased proportionately more than Raw to yield an increased SRaw, it appears that increased lung tissue resistance might be an abnormal parameter in these patients. Increased lung tissue resistance would also help explain the decreased CL frequently seen in these patients.

REFERENCES

1. Kikkawa Y: Morphology and morphologic development of the lung, in Scarpelli EM (ed): *Pulmonary Physiology of the Fetus, Infant and Child,* Philadelphia, Lea & Febiger, 1975. pp. 37–60.
2. Hodson WA: Development of the Lung, in Leafant C (ed): *Lung Biology in Health and Disease,* New York, Marcel Dekker Inc, 1975, pp. 3–261.
3. Weibel ER: *Morphometry of the Human Lung,* New York, Academic Press Inc, 1963.
4. Horsfield K, Cumming G: Morphology of the bronchial tree in man. *J Appl Physiol* 24:373, 1968.
5. Charnock EL, Fisher BJ, Doershuk CF: Development of the respiratory system, in Lough D, Doershuk CF, Stern RC (eds): *Pediatric Respiratory Therapy,* ed 2. Chicago, Year Book Medical Publishers Inc, 1979.
6. Charnock EL, Doershuk CF: Developmental aspects of the human lung. *Pediatr Clin North Am* 20:275, 1973.
7. Bucher U, Reid L: Development of the intrasegmental bronchial tree. *Thorax* 16:207, 1961.
8. Engel S: *Lung Structure,* Springfield, Ill, Charles C Thomas Publisher, 1962.
9. Fearon B, Whalen JS: Tracheal dimensions in the living infant. *Ann Otol Rhinol Laryngol* 76:964, 1967.
10. Emery JL, Mithal A: The number of alveoli in the terminal respiratory unit of man during late intrauterine life and childhood. *Arch Dis Child* 35:544, 1960.
11. Dunnill MS: Postnatal growth of the lung. *Thorax* 17:329, 1962.
12. Emery JL, Wilcock PF: The postnatal development of the lung. *Acta Anat* 65:10, 1966.
13. Reid L: The embryology of the lung, in deRench AVS, Porter R (eds): *CIBA Foundation Symposium on Development of the Lung,* London, JA Churchill, 1967, pp 109–124.
14. Davies G, Reid L: Growth of the alveoli and pulmonary arteries in childhood. *Thorax* 25:669, 1970.
15. Kory RC, Callahan R, Boren HG, et al: The Veterans Administration—Army Cooperative Study of Pulmonary Function: I. Clinical spirometry in normal men. *Am J Med* 30: 243, 1961.
16. Miller WF, Johnson RL, Wu N: Relationship between maximal breathing capacity and timed expiratory capacities. *J Appl Physiol* 14:510, 1959.
17. Comroe JH, Forster RE, Dubois AB, et al: *The Lung: Clinical Physiology and Pulmonary Function Tests,* Chicago, Year Book Medical Publishers Inc, 1962.
18. Polgar G, Promadhat V: *Pulmonary Function Testing in Children: Techniques and Standards,* Philadelphia, WB Saunders Co, 1971.
19. Bass H: The flow-volume loop: normal standards and abnormalities in chronic obstructive lung disease, *Chest* 63:171, 1973.
20. Kundson RJ, Slatin RC, Lebowitz MD, et al: The maximum expiratory flow-volume curve, *Am Rev Respir Dis* 113:587, 1976.
21. Zapletal A, Motoyama EF, Van de Woestijne KP, et al: Maximum expiratory flow-volume curves and airway conductance in children and adolescents. *J Appl Physiol* 267:308, 1969.
22. Fox WW, Bureau MA, Taussig LA, et al: Helium flow-volume curves in the detection of early small airway disease. *Pediatrics* 54:293, 1974.
23. McCarthy MM, Spock A: Crying pulmonary functin tests in infants and young children. (In press.)
24. Krauss AN, Klain DB, Dahms BB, et al: Vital capacity in premature infants. *Am Rev Respir Dis* 108:1361, 1973.
25. Dubois AB, Botelho SY, Bedell GN, et al: A rapid plethysmographic method for measuring thoracic gas volume. *J Clin Invest* 35:322, 1956.
26. Helms P: Problems with plethysmographic estimation of lung volume in infants and young children. *J Appl Physiol* 53:698, 1982.
27. Doershuk CF, Matthews LW: Airway resistance and lung volume in the newborn infant. *Pediatr Res* 3:128, 1969.
28. Doershuk CF, Downs TD, Matthews LW, et al: A method for ventilatory measurements in subjects 1 month—5 years of age: normal results and observations in disease. *Pediatr Res* 4:165, 1970.
29. Doershuk CF, Fisher BJ, Matthews LW: Specific airway resistance from the perinatal period into adulthood. *Am Rev Respir Dis* 109:452, 1974.
30. Matthews LW, Doershuk CF: Measurement of pulmonary function in cystic fibrosis. *Mod Probl Paediatr* 10:237, 1967.
31. Klaus M, Tooley WH, Weaver KH, et al: Lung volume in the newborn infant. *Pediatrics* 30:111, 1962.
32. Nelson NM, Prod'hom SL, Cherry RB, et al:

Pulmonary function in the newborn infant: V. Trapped gas in the normal infant's lung. *J Clin Invest* 42:1850, 1963.

33. Auld PAM, Nelson NM, Cherry RB, et al: Measurement of thoracic gas volume in the newborn infant. *J Clin Invest* 42:476, 1973.

34. Lacourt G, Polgar G: Development of pulmonary function in late gestation: I. The functional residual capacity of the lung in premature children. *Acta Paediatr Scand* 63:81, 1974.

35. Ronchetti R, Stocks J, Keith I, et al: An analysis of a rebreathing method for measuring lung volume in the premature infant. *Pediatr Res* 9:797, 1975.

36. Krauss AN, Auld PAM: Pulmonary gas trapping in premature infants. *Pediatr Res* 5:10, 1971.

37. Polgar G, Kong G: The nasal resistance of newborn infants. *J Pediatr* 67:557, 1965.

38. Goldman M, Knudson RJ, Mead J, et al: A simplified measurement of respiratory resistance by forced oscillation. *J Appl Physiol* 28:113, 1970.

39. Dubois AB, Brody AW, Lewis DH, et al: Oscillation mechanics of lungs and chest in man. *J Appl Physiol* 8:587, 1955.

40. Wohl MEB, Stigol LC, Mead J: Resistance of the respiratory system in healthy infants and infants with bronchiolitis. *Pediatrics* 43:495, 1969.

41. Krieger I: Mechanics of respiration in bronchiolitis. *Pediatrics* 33:45, 1964.

42. Phelan PD, Williams HE, Freeman M: The disturbances of ventilation in acute viral bronchiolitis. *Aust Paediatr J* 4:96, 1968.

43. Krieger I: Study on mechanics of respiration in infancy. *Am J Dis Child* 105:439, 1963.

44. Frank NR, Mead J, Whittenberger JL: Comparative sensitivity of four methods for measuring changes in respiratory flow resistance in man. *J Appl Physiol* 31:934, 1971.

45. Bachofen H, Duc G: Lung tissue resistance in healthy children. *Pediatr Res* 2:119, 1968.

46. Polgar G, String ST: The viscous resistance of the lung tissues in newborn infants. *J Pediatr* 69:787, 1966.

47. Fisher BJ, Doershuk C, Matthews L: Serial pulmonary function studies in infants and young children with cystic fibrosis. *Am Rev Respir Dis* 117:292, 1978.

48. Krieger I, Whitten CF: Work of respiration in bronchiolitis. *Am J Dis Child* 107:386, 1964.

49. Chu JS, Dawson P, Klaus M, et al: Lung compliance and lung volume measured concurrently in normal full-term and premature infants. *Pediatrics* 35:525, 1964.

50. Phelan PD, Williams HE: Ventilatory studies in healthy infants. *Pediatr Res* 3:425, 1969.

51. Griffin AJ, Ferrara JD, Lax JO, et al: Pulmonary compliance: an index of cardiovascular status in infancy. *Am J Dis Child* 123:89, 1972.

52. Fisher BJ, Doershuk CF: Unpublished observations, 1972.

19

Diagnostic Pulmonary Radiology in Children

Michael T. Gyepes

According to legend, Dr. Merryl Sossman, Harvard's great professor of radiology, had a stethoscope framed and kept it in the reading room of the Peter Bent Brigham Hospital. "Obsolete instrument," it said underneath, "used before the advent of x rays."

It is readily apparent that the art of physical diagnosis has not disappeared. Fingers, ears, and, yes, stethoscopes are still very much with us. This is particularly impressive considering the spectacular developments in radiology in the past decade. The specialty that was once called roentgenology is about to be renamed again, this time to diagnostic imaging.

In the course of these changes certain techniques fell by the wayside. For example, few use *stereo chest radiography* nowadays, because computed tomography (CT) provides a much better spatial picture of the lungs, a third dimension. *Fluoroscopy of the chest* is still useful in certain situations: evaluating diaphragmatic motion, getting a dynamic picture of a swinging mediastinum, or simply confirming whether a suspicious nodule is real or not, before committing the patient to a more extensive workup. In some situations, before undertaking traditional tomogrphy fluoroscopy might be helpful in estimating the location, that is, the depth, of the lesion in question.

Diagnostic pulmonary radiology in children can be divided into the following in seven sections:

I would like to thank my colleague Dr. A.S. Rappoport for reviewing this chapter and for his excellent suggestions.

1. The airways
2. The barium swallow and esophagram
3. The chest roentgenogram and conventional tomography
4. CT
5. Lung scanning
6. Bronchography
7. Angiography

Ultrasound will not be treated in detail; the lungs do not yield themselves to ultrasound imaging because of their air content. This is not to say, however, that ultrasound plays no role in diagnosis of thoracic disease.[1,2] Structures contiguous with the diaphragm or a fluid-filled pleural space can be imaged by ultrasound and valuable information obtained (Fig. 19-1) Echocardiography plays an increasingly important part in evaluating the heart and great vessels. This, however, is done through the "acoustic window" of the chest wall, not the lungs.

THE AIRWAYS

Two common problems in the evaluation of the upper airways[3–11] are the availability of proper films and familiarity with the normal anatomy. It is unwise to try to assess the upper airways on chest films, even if they include the area. The single lateral view of the neck provides only part of the information needed. Both views should always be obtained. In infants or small children proper immobilization is absolutely necessary to get films without rotation. In addition we use a special filter for the anteroposterior (AP) view and a high kilovoltage (KV) technique, which enhance the soft tissues and dimin-

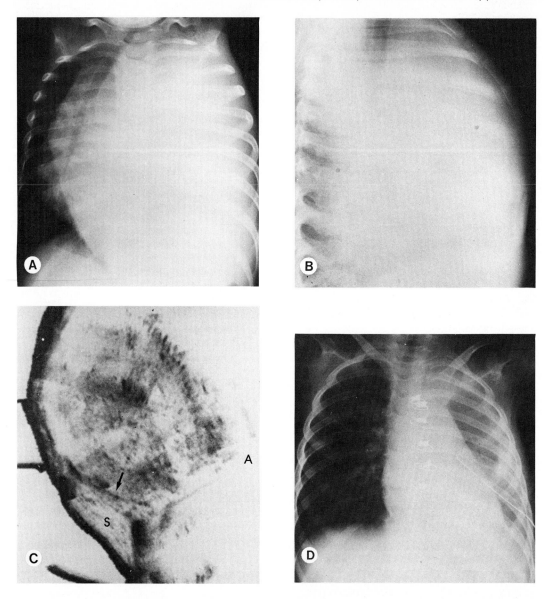

Figure 19-1. Pleural effusion versus thoracic mass. **(A),** AP view of the chest shows significant displacement of the heart, trachea, and mediastinum to the right. **(B),** The lateral view is of no help in resolving the diagnostic dilemma. **(C),** Lateral gray-scale ultrasound clearly shows that the lesion is a solid mass (by the character of the internal echos) and also its relation to the diaphragm (*arrow*). S, Spleen; *A,* anterior. **(D),** Postoperative chest film after virtually all the tumor (small cell sarcoma) was removed. (Courtesy Dr. J. Patel.)

ish interference from the bony structures. The normal anatomy of the upper airways is illustrated in Figures 19-2 and 19-3. In a patient with croup the normal smooth arch of the subglottic region becomes effaced by edema. Croup is due to subglottic edema and the diagnosis is primarily made on the AP film. The lateral film shows the usually normal epiglottis and varying degree of haziness in the trachea (Figs. 19-4 and 19-5).

In contradistinction to croup, in epiglottitis the subglottic region is usually normal. The epiglottis, however, is swollen and the vallecula is often

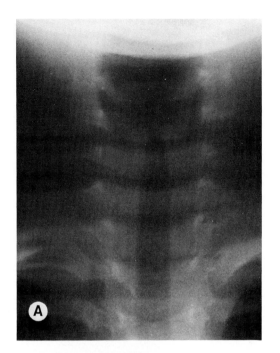

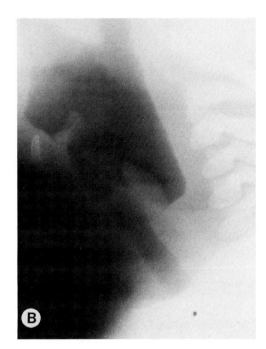

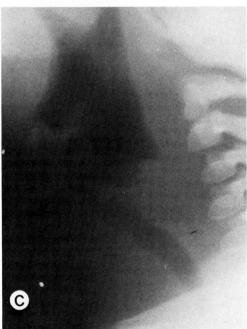

Figure 19-2. Normal upper airway. **(A),** Normal AP view with cords in abduction. **(B),** Normal lateral view in inspiration. **(C),** Normal lateral view in *expiration*. The anterior buckling of the trachea is normal in expiration.

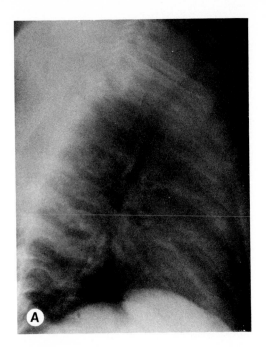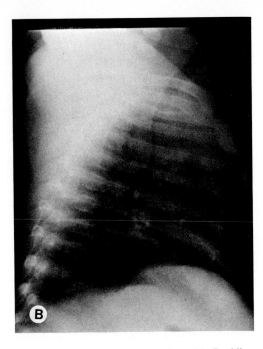

Figure 19-3. Normal buckling versus vascular ring. **(A)**, Normal anterior buckling of the trachea. **(B)**, Buckling and narrowing due to the presence of a vascular ring.

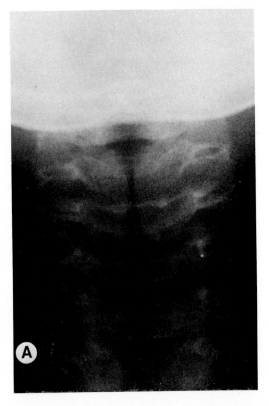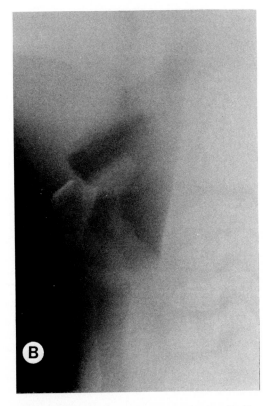

Figure 19-4. Croup. **(A)**, AP view shows elongation of the subglottic region and loss of the normal arch. **(B)**, The lateral view shows that the epiglottis is normal. The subglottic edema is rarely seen well on this view! This is the classic appearance of croup on the AP view.

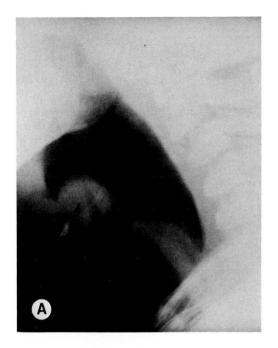
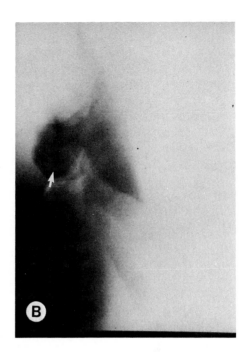

Figure 19-5. Epiglottitis versus croup (comparison of the lateral views). **(A)**, swollen, enlarged epiglottis (*arrow*) in epiglottitis. **(B)**, Normal epiglottis in a child with croup. Notice the small filled-in vallecula (white arrow) in front of the epiglottis on the left and the wide open, spacious vallecula on the right. The diagnosis of croup was confirmed on the AP view.

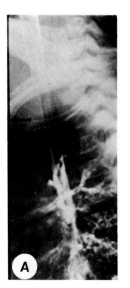
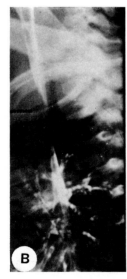

Figure 19-6. Tracheomalacia. Contrast tracheogram. The film on the left was taken in inspiration and shows a wide open, patent trachea. The film on the right was taken in expiration and shows complete collapse of the intrathoracic portion of the trachea. This infant had expiratory stridor and wheezing without bronchiolitis.

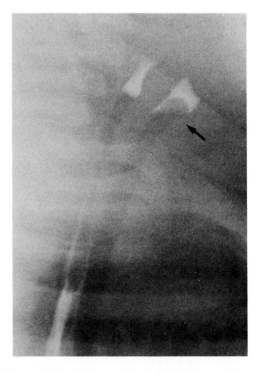

Figure 19-7. Trachea aspiration. Barium swallow shows contrast material aspirated into the trachea *(arrow).* child had chronic aspiration of unknown cause and repeated pulmonary infections.

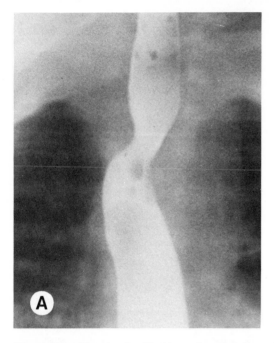 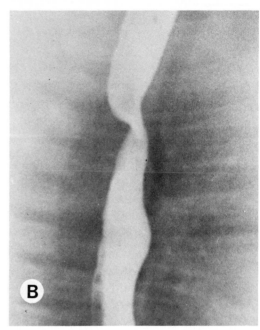

Figure 19-8.   Vascular ring (double aortic arch angiographically and surgically confirmed). **(A),** On the PA view the esophagus is indented both on the right and the left. **(B),** On the lateral view the esophagus is indented posteriorly, and the trachea is narrowed anteriorly. This appearance is usually caused by a double aortic arch (as was the case here) or a right aortic arch and a ductus diverticulum. Both are true rings and require surgical interruption.

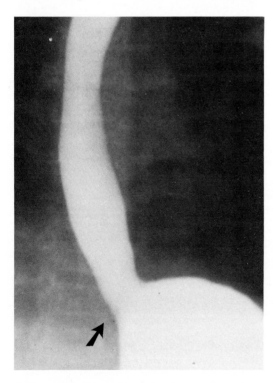

filled by the big epiglottis and surrounding edema. This is best seen on the lateral view (Fig. 19-5). The aryepiglottic folds are frequently also swollen. Sometimes croup and epiglottitis occur together, and this will be duly reflected on the films. Croup and epiglottitis are most commonly found in small children but they have been reported not only in older children but adults as well. The size of the adenoid gland is quite well outlined on the lateral view of the neck. Truly large adenoids occlude the nasopharyngeal airway. If they are associated with huge tonsils, chronic hypoxemia and even congestive heart failure may be the consequence.

Although epiglottis and croup are the most important causes of stridor in small children, there are other often baffling reasons for it. The radiologist can be of considerable help in evaluating the infant or child with stridor. The diagnosis of laryngomalacia can be made on fluoroscopy by demonstrating abnormal motion of the epiglottis and the aryepiglottic folds. This has to be recorded in motion (cinefluoroscopy), and recognizing it requires some experience. Also movement of the cords can be easily seen on fluoroscopy, either in the straight AP or the basal projection. The radiologic evaluation of a stridorous child should always include a barium

Figure 19-9.   Gastroesophageal reflux. Barium refluxed through the open gastroesophageal junction *(arrow)* all the way up to the pharynx.

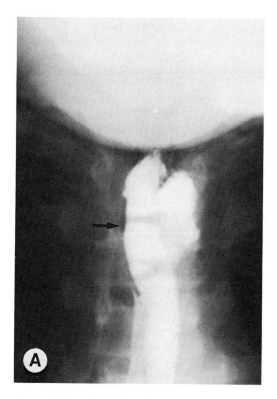 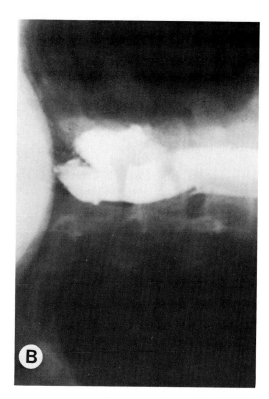

Figure 19-10. Foreign body in the esophagus. **(A),** Radiolucent foreign body *(arrow)* in the barium-filled esophagus. **(B),** The enlarged side view clearly shows that the foreign body is a tiny rocking horse. The foreign body was removed by esophagoscopy. The patient actually presented with hoarseness.

swallow. It only takes a few minutes to study the airways before introducing the barium, and it often pays handsome dividends in terms of diagnosis.

Unlike the upper airways, the lower airways (i.e., the trachea and main bronchi) require no special imaging technique. They are visible on every chest roentgenogram. In fact the smaller the child, the easier it is to see trachea and the carina on the AP film because the thymus provides an excellent background for contrast. Although intraluminal lesions are occasionally well seen in both the upper and lower airways, the most useful information that can be gleaned from the chest films regarding the trachea is its position, contour, and width. Perhaps the commonest source of error is to mistake the normal anterior or lateral buckling of the small child's pliable and overly long trachea for a pathologic condition. Infants "grow into their trachea." The trachea, like the other tubular organs (esophagus and colon), is ahead of the other organs in terms of longitudinal growth.

Congenital tracheal stenosis is extremely un-

common, and acquired stenosis is usually associated with prolonged intubation. Functional narrowing of the trachea, that is collapse of part or the entire intrathoracic trachea on expiration is due either to tracheomalacia or peripheral air trapping (Fig. 19-6). In the former the compliance of the trachea is high and the normal intrathoracic pressure variations are sufficient to cause significant narrowing of the trachea. In bronchiolitis, cystic fibrosis, or congestive heart failure the tracheal collapse is due to the high intrathoracic pressure, and there is nothing intrinsically wrong with the trachea itself. A narrow slitlike trachea on the lateral chest film is not normal and should be investigated, best by fluoroscopy, to evaluate tracheal dynamics.

THE BARIUM SWALLOW AND ESOPHAGRAM

A child of any age who has unexplained respiratory disease should have an esophagram.[12-20] The esophagram should always include a barium swallow, that is, a study of the oral and pharyngeal phase of deglutition. With rare exceptions the author uses barium as a contrast agent, unless there is danger of contrast extravasation into the mediastinum or pleural space. Feeding through a bottle (nipple) is well accepted by infants; occasionally one must resort to spoon feeding. Thicker, prepackaged contrast agents, such as Esophotrast, are excellent for coating the esophageal mucosa and assure prolonged opacification of the entire esophagus.

The barium swallow is the best, if not the only, way to demonstrate abnormalities of the swallowing mechanism. Of these *aspiration* into the airways is the most serious (Fig. 19-7). It is almost always caused by some form of neuromuscular dysfunction; children with cerebral palsy represent the largest group with this problem. There are silent aspirators with minor swallowing difficulties and recurrent pulmonary infections, however. Children with Riley-Day syndrome habitually aspirate.

X-ray film requisitions often give tracheoesophageal fistulas (TEFs) as the indication for an esophagram. TEFs without esophageal atresia are quite rare. Demonstrating them often takes patience and persistence, because they tend to be high and thin structures. The whole length of the esophagus must be well distended to be sure that a TEF does not escape detection.

The esophagram also plays an important part in the diagnosis of vascular rings. To be a real ring, a combination of vascular anomalies must have both an anterior and posterior component, as well as a structure on the right and left sides. It is much easier to visualize the lateral component of a ring on the well-opacified esophagus than the somewhat shadowy tracheal air column. The posterior component of the ring is only seen on the esophagram (Fig. 19-8).

During the past few years, gastroesophageal reflux (GER) became recognized as an important cause of respiratory disease in children (Fig 19-9). The literature on the subject is vast. It must be emphasized that the esophagram is only a survey tool in the diagnosis of GER. The very shortness of the fluoroscopic procedure (approximately 5–10 minutes) renders it a hit-and-miss proposition. Major reflux can be diagnosed on a properly performed study. Episodic, occasional reflux will naturally escape detection. The importance of the esophagram lies in demonstrating the presence of anatomic and functional abnormalities such as hiatus hernia, strictures, and abnormal motility.

It is the practice of pediatric radiologists to observe the barium through the stomach into the duodenum and to the ligament of Treitz even if only an esophagram is requested. Atypical pyloric stenosis, pylorospasm, and partial malrotation are occasionally responsible for what clinically might be present as a swallowing or respiratory problem. In the same vein, the foreign body in the esophagus, rather than in the airway could be the hidden cause of stridor in a minority of cases (Fig. 19-10).

THE CHEST ROENTGENOGRAM AND CONVENTIONAL TOMOGRAPHY

Universally referred to as the "chest x-ray" or the "chest film" the chest roentgenogram (to use its formal name at least once) is *the* most common radiologic examination, both in adult and pediatric radiology.[21–28] It is precisely for this reason that it should not be approached casually. Poor chest films have led to erroneous diagnoses far too often. With proper immobilization and modern equipment it is quite easy to get good films. Getting a film in proper inspiration is a question of training technicians. Expiratory films have been the source of as many errors as poorly positioned or "motion" films. There are at least two good uses of deliberately obtained expiratory films, however: (1) the detection of foreign bodies (Fig. 19-11) and (2) visualizing small pneumothoraces. Most prefer posteroanterior (PA) or AP and lateral films as a routine. The two films together give a quasi three-dimensional view of the chest. The old dictum about first localizing a pulmonary process before making a diagnosis still holds (Fig. 19-12).

AP views are preferred for infants and small children who cannot or will not sit or stand for a PA view. Unless one wishes to evaluate the heart size, there is no significant difference between the AP and PA views. Left lateral views are preferred to right views because of the heart's position.

Most AP films, particularly in infants, will be more apical lordotic than true AP in position. This is one good reason not to count ribs to decide whether a film was taken in proper inspiration or not. Knowing that the trachea buckles in expiration or looking for the position of the diaphragm in relation to the cardiac apex are more reliable indicators (Fig. 19-13).

Oblique views are never routine; there is relatively little use for them. Few places do

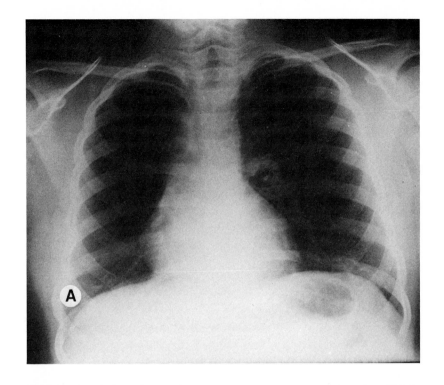

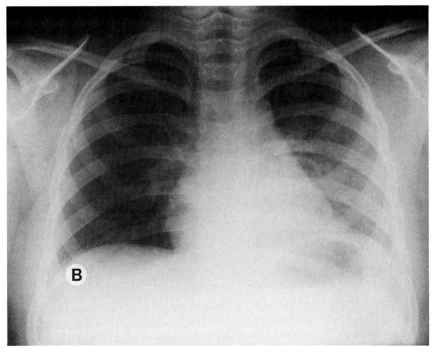

Figure 19-11. Foreign body in the right main bronchus. **(A),** The inspiratory film is essentially normal. **(B),** The expiratory film shows normal deaereation of the left lung and abnormal air trapping of the right lung. The expiratory film is deceptive; without the inspiratory film one would think that the pathologic condition was on the wrong side!

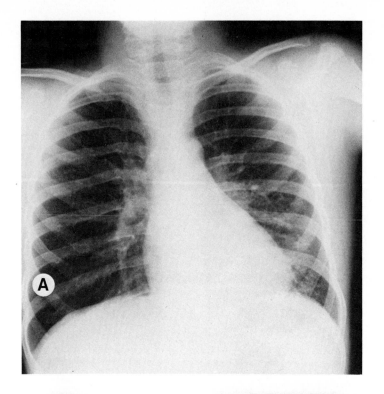

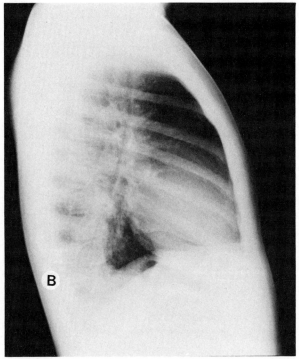

Figure 19-12. Hidden pneumonia. **(A),** On the AP view it is difficult to see the left lower lobe pneumonia. **(B),** The lateral view clearly shows the posterior, retrocardiac infiltrate, abutting on the diaphragm.

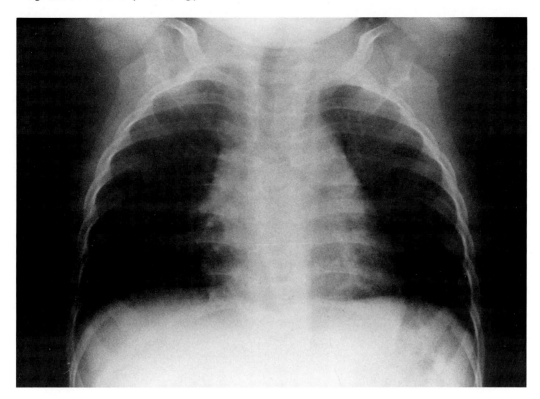

Figure 19-13. Expiratory film. The left hemidiaphragm is well above the apex of the heart. The trachea is buckled to the right. Both of these signs indicate that this is an expiratory film. The rib count is often unreliable on the chest films of small children.

four-view cardiac series nowadays. Oblique views can be useful in bringing out an elusive shadow and localizing it. Of course properly exposed oblique views are routinely used to fully visualize the ribs (Fig. 19-14).

There is little call for cross-table chest films but lateral decubitus views have several important applications. Both decubitus views are part of the so-called "obstructive series" that consist of inspiratory, expiratory, and lateral views. Between those five films one can usually lateralize a foreign body in the main bronchi. Another important use of decubituss film is in the detection and volume estimation of pleural effusion (Fig. 19-15). The lateral decubitus view also permits differentiation between a pneumothorax and pneumomediastinum. In the latter the air remains confined to the mediastinum, regardless of the patient's position.

Portable films are often the stepchildren of radiology. There is no reason for this. Portable films obtained by modern equipment in the nursery should be as good as those taken in the

radiology department. In older children the capability of portable technology must be properly appreciated and not pushed beyond its limits. The major limitations are patient size and cooperation.

Before the arrival of CT conventional tomography (referred to as tomography hereafter) was a widely used technique in chest radiology. Two of its major functions, however, have been largely taken over by CT. To outline mediastinal masses and search for pulmonary metastases, CT is better than tomography.

Tomography still holds the edge in visualizing the trachea and the major bronchi. When it comes to small parenchymal or rib lesions tomography is probably better then CT (Fig. 19-14). Possibly the same holds true for the diaphragm, although ultrasound is a real competitor in the area of phrenic imaging.

Figures 19-16 and 19-17 are included here, without discussion, to illustrate two of the most common chest diseases in the pediatric age group: acute asthma and cystic fibrosis.

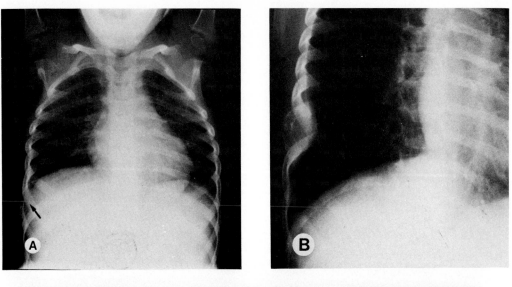

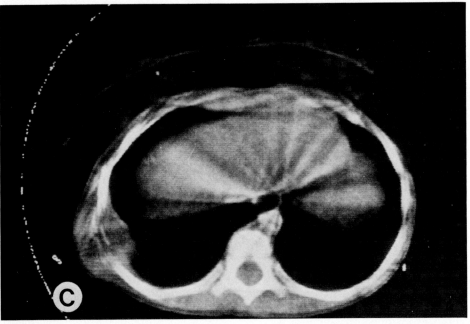

Figure 19-14. Rib lesion. **(A),** The lesion in the right eighth rib was hardly visible even on the original chest film *(arrow).* **(B),** The oblique view in good inspiration clearly shows the distinctive rib lesion and surrounding soft tissue component. **(C),** The CT scan confirms the presence of the lesion and shows its extent. At surgery a localized eosinophilic granuloma was found and excised. There was no systemic involvement.

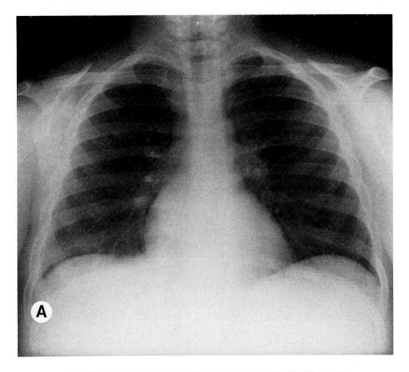

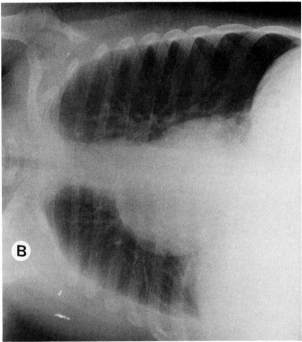

Figure 19-15. Hidden pleural effusion. **(A),** The PA view shows the high position of both hemidiaphragms and just a hint of pleural effusion on the right. **(B),** The right lateral decubitus film shows a large pleural effusion on the right. In the upright position the fluid is situated between the lung and the diaphragm.

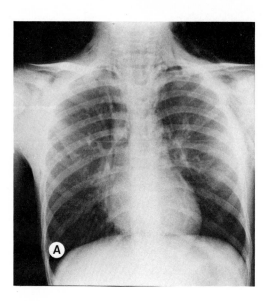
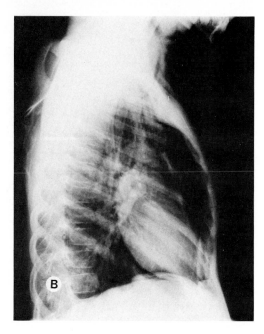

Figure 19-16. Acute asthma. Hyperinflated lungs. (**A**) The air dissected up into the neck and is seen in the soft tissues of both supraclavicular areas. (**B**) Free air in the mediastinum is best seen on lateral view behind the sternum.

COMPUTED TOMOGRAPHY

CT took radiology by a storm during the last decade and permanently altered the world of diagnostic imaging.[29-38] Its initial use was confined to the head. To this date the vast majority of CT examinations in children are performed for intracranial problems.

During the past few years, however, new advanced scanners became available. Exposure times have been drastically reduced, thereby eliminating motion artifacts. At the same time the resolution of the scans improved, and radiation doses decreased sufficiently to make CT imaging of the body an attractive diagnostic modality.

The most important contribution of CT outside of the skull is in tumor diagnosis. In the chest both the mediastinum and lung parenchyma yield themselves excellently to CT examination.

CT scans of mediastinal masses will not only outline the contours of the mass but provide detailed information about the tumor's relationship to surrounding structures (Fig. 19-18). Extension into the spine or vertebral destruction is superbly depicted on CT scans, providing invaluable information for the thoracic surgeon. Rib or sternal involvement also can be detected by CT, at times yielding dramatic pictures. And the variable absorption capacity of different tissues also can be expressed by CT, thereby facilitating specific diagnosis. With the aid of contrast enhancement vascular structures can be differentiated from solid organs or tumors.

The other great usefulness of CT is in visualizing parenchymal lesions, primarily metastases (Fig. 19-19). Small, peripheral, or posterior metastases often escape detection on chest films. CT is used today instead of conventional whole lung tomograms.

LUNG SCANNING

Isotope scanning of the lungs is widely used in adults for a variety of diagnostic purposes[39-44] Perfusion scans, using technetium-labeled macroaggregates and ventilation scans with technetium aerosol permit qualitative evaluation of regional lung function. The addition of the Anger

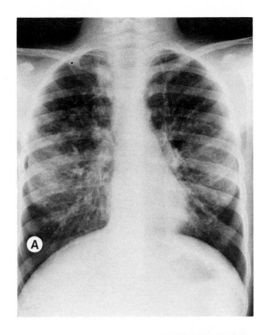

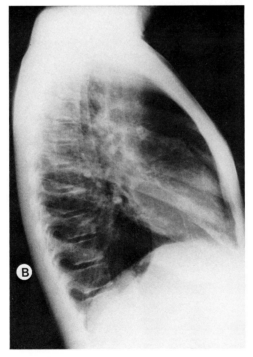

Figure 19-17. (A & B) Cystic fibrosis. Moderately hyperinflated lungs and diffuse peribronchial thickening. Moderately advanced cystic fibrosis in an adolescent. Ventilation and/or perfusion lung scans almost certainly would have showed far more extensive disease than the chest films suggest.

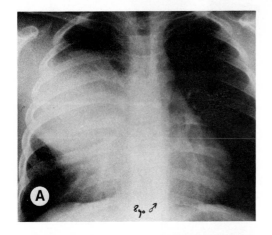

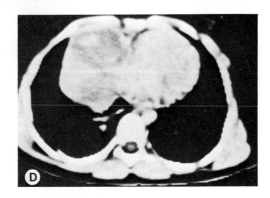

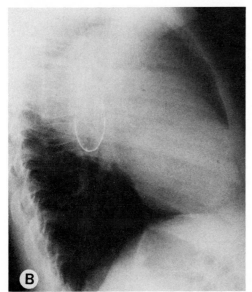

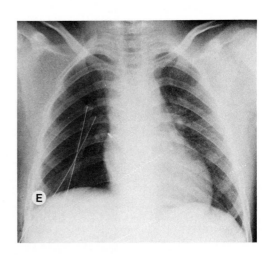

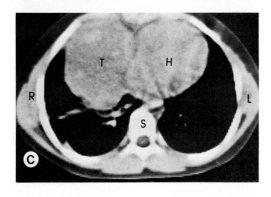

Figure 19-18. Mediastinal mass. (**A** and **B**) The AP and lateral views show the presence of a large, central mass, which is probably mediastinal. (**C**), The CT scan shows the relationship of the mass to the heart and its exact location in the thorax. The calcifications in the mass were not visible on the chest films. *T*, Tumor; *H*; heart; *R*; right; *L*, left; *S*, spine. (**D**), After intravenous contrast injection the repeat scan shows enhancement in its lower portion. (**E**), Postoperative chest. At surgery a small cell sarcoma was completely excised.

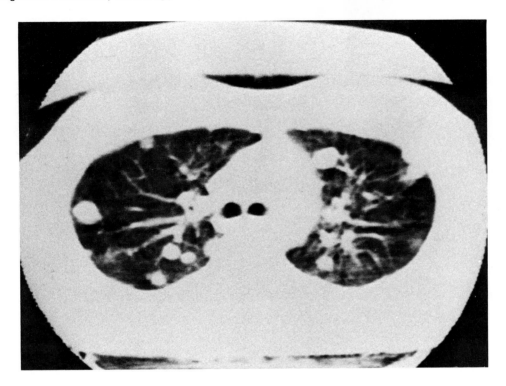

Figure 19-19. Pulmonary metastases on CT scan. Multiple pulmonary metastases from a testicular tumor.

camera and the application of computers made it possible to obtain quantitative measurements as well.

In children lung scanning has relatively few applications. In the early days of lung scanning numerous studies were conducted in children with asthma and cystic fibrosis, and interesting physiologic observations were made. In clinical practice, though, lung scans are used infrequently. Two interesting applications of lung scanning in the pediatric age group are shown in Figures 19-20 and 19-21.

Perfusion/ventilation scans are helpful in evaluating overall lung function in children with localized pulmonary disease such as congenital or acquired bronchiectasis and unilateral or regional hyperlucent lungs. When the pulmonary artery is absent or hypoplastic, the perfusion scan is an elegant way of demonstrating the resulting flow pattern.

It should be mentioned here that the presently used bronchographic contrast agents interfere with the accuracy of lung scans—precisely because they alter regional ventilation. When com-

bining the two procedures, scans should be done *before* bronchography.

BRONCHOGRAPHY

Far fewer bronchograms are requested today than 10–15 years ago.[45–47] There are several reasons for this. First, the procedure acquired a bad reputation in children because often it was done improperly. "Flooding" the lungs with large amounts of contrast material can lead to serious respiratory complications. Second, the presently available contrast agents are not ideal. Unfortunately, the better contrast agents are either unavailable because of FDA regulations or proved to be toxic in the long run. Third, fiberoptic endoscopy replaced bronchography in a number of situations.

It is best to perform bronchography under general anesthesia. With the assistance of the anesthesthiologist, coughing and respirations can be safely controlled, and a small plastic catheter can be advanced to or into the orifice of the

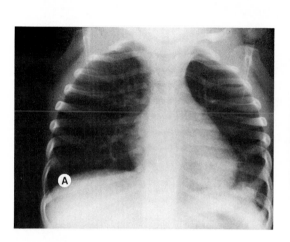

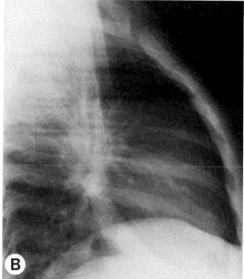

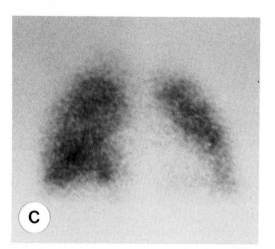

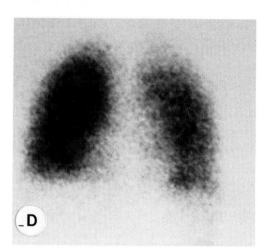

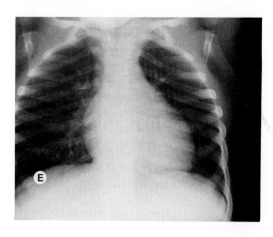

Figure 19-20. Localized atelectasis. (**A** and **B**), The AP and lateral chest films show an area of left lower lobe atelectasis. (**C**), The initial perfusion scan shows significantly decreased perfusion on the left. (**D**), Repeat perfusion scan 4 days later shows equal perfusion of both lungs. (**E**), Normal follow-up chest film. Obstructing vegetable material was removed from the left main bronchus. In small children who are unable to cooperate a perfusion study will often be helpful, although alterations in perfusion do not always mirror changes in ventilation. (See Fig. 19-21.) (Courtesy Dr. M. Hayes.)

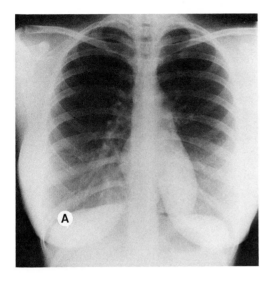

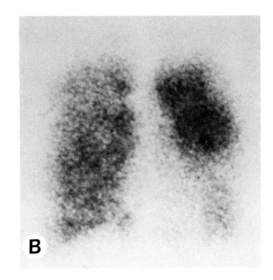

Figure 19-21. Airway disease versus pulmonary emboli. **(A),** Slight hyperinflation on otherwise negative chest film of a 16-year-old girl with chest pain and difficulty breathing. Patient was taking oral contraceptives. **(B),** AP perfusion scan shows multiple, bilateral filling defects. **(C),** Ventilation scan shows far more disturbance of ventilation than perfusion. The diagnosis was asthmatic bronchitis *not* pulmonary emboli. The patient improved with appropriate treatment. (Courtesy Dr. M. Hayes.)

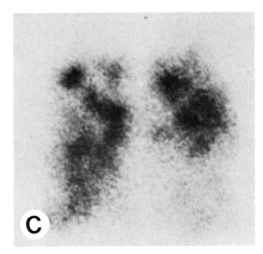

bronchus in question. By depositing a small amount of warm, well-mixed contrast material (1–2 ml) into the bronchus and relying on the anesthesiologist to coat the bronchial wall by "bagging," undesirable overfilling of the airways can be avoided. Bilateral studies are almost never performed in one sitting.

The most important indication for bronchography is suspected bronchiectasis (Fig. 19-22). No other diagnostic modality can compete with contrast bronchography in fully evaluating congenital or acquired bronchiectasis. In chronic, localized atelectasis or infection the purpose of the bronchogram is to visualize the regional bronchus and the smaller bronchi beyond an area of narrowing. Fiberoptic bronchoscopy is a competitive technique in this respect, although the two can be combined into a joint procedure. Whether it will be possible to obtain high-quality, selective bronchograms consistently via the fiberoptic bronchoscopes remains to be seen.

On occasion bronchography has been used to demonstrate or localize a foreign body in terms of segmental anatomy (Fig. 19-23). Such precise localization should permit the thoracic surgeon to perform a bronchotomy and removal, rather than segmental resection.

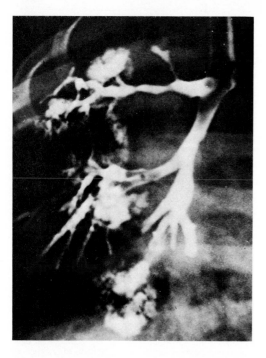

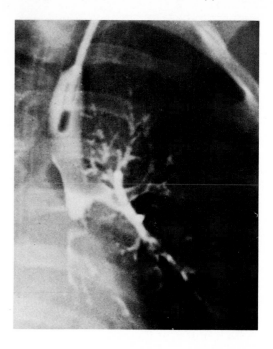

Figure 19-22. Bronchiectasis. Congenital saccular bronchiectasis involving the upper, middle, and lower lobe bronchi. Unilateral bronchogram was obtained under general anesthesia. Patient in oblique position to prevent spilling of contrast material onto the contralateral lungs.

Figure 19-23. Foreign body in the left lower lobe bronchus. Unilateral bronchogram shows incomplete and irregular obstruction of the left lower lobe bronchus. The lobe is atelectatic due to the obstruction. At bronchoscopy a small broken piece of a plastic toy was found and removed.

ANGIOGRAPHY

Angiocardiography[48–50] remains the definitive imaging modality for accurate and detailed anatomic visualization of congenital heart lesions. The author tends to do fewer aortograms for suspected mediastinal tumors than in years past. When it comes to the differentiation of a solid tumor from a vascular anomaly (such as an aneurysm or pseudocoarctation), CT with contrast enhancement is the modality of choice. If the lesion proves to be vascular by CT, then an angiographic study, such as an aortogram or pulmonary arteriogram might be indicated for better anatomic delineation.

On the other hand, a thoracic aortogram is the most direct way to demonstrate a large feeding artery in pulmonary sequestration, thereby also confirming the diagnosis (Fig. 19-24).

Visualization of the pulmonary vascular bed,

that is, pulmonary arteriography, is the modality of choice if a congenital arteriovenous malformation is suspected or for the depiction of anomalous vessels. For example, scimitar syndrome, partial anomalous venous return into the inferioer vena cava, is beautifully demonstrable by pulmonary arteriography.

Bronchial arteriography, performed by selective catheterization of the bronchial vessels, enjoyed a brief period of popularity some years ago. A great deal of interesting pathophysiologic information was obtained through those years about the appearance of these rarely visualized vessels in various congenital heart lesions, cystic fibrosis, etc. The presence of bronchopulmonary anastomoses in vivo was established by bronchial arteriography, in tetralogy of Fallot, for example (Fig. 19-25). Today bronchial arteriograms are rarely performed in children, except perhaps to demonstrate the site of bleeding in

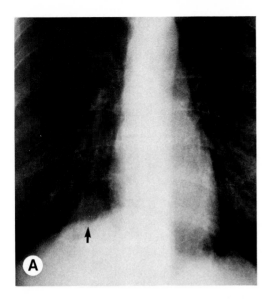

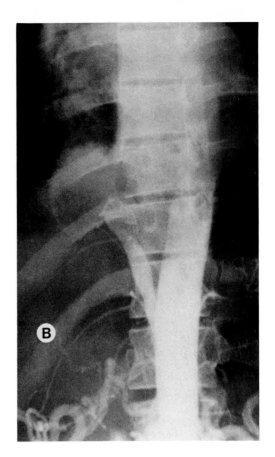

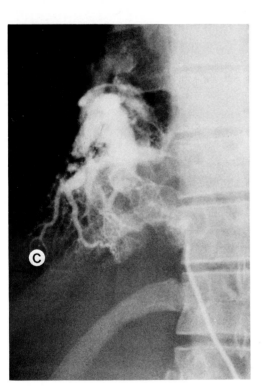

Figure 19-24. Pulmonary sequestration. **(A)**, The chest film shows a barely visible, small round density in the right lower lobe *(arrow)*. **(B)**, the aortogram shows a large feeding artery coursing toward the round density. **(C)**, Selective arteriogram shows the irregular vascularity in the sequestration.

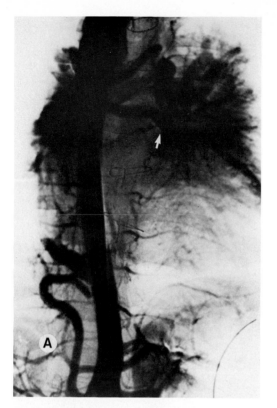

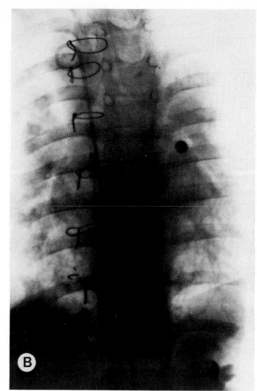

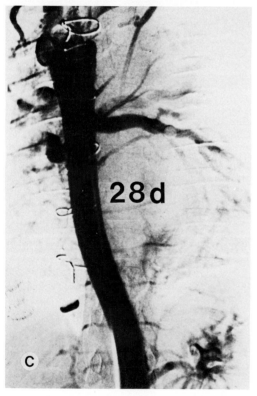

Figure 19-25. Tetralogy of Fallot, huge bronchial arteries, and hemoptysis. **(A),** Huge left bronchial artery *(arrow)* with tortuous branches. **(B),** Two black balloons in situ. The catheter is in the right aortic arch. **(C),** Twenty-eight days after balloon occulusion a repeat aortogram shows almost complete absence of perfusion through the large bronchial artery on the left. Balloonis in situ. The angiograms are subtraction films. (Courtesy Drs. P. Stanley and Mark Mehringer.)

cystic fibrosis. In some cases these enlarged, bleeding arteries have been successfully embolized, thereby bringing interventional techniques to pediatric radiology.

EPILOGUE

By the time this book is published there may well be one or more new imaging modalities on the diagnostic scene.[51-57] Nuclear magnetic resonance (NMR)[52,54,57] could conceivably compete with CT for a role in transverse axial imaging (without ionizing radiation). Digital angiography[51,55,56],could eventually eliminate the need for catheters and selective arteriography in vascular diagnosis. And two-dimensional real-time ultrasound, which is already a functional clinical tool, will probably "invade" the chest (or at least the mediastinum) to compete with CT and NMR.[53]

Increasingly the problem will be how to select the proper imaging modality and in what sequence. Pediatric radiologists cannot possibly be experts in all these new areas. But they are the clinician's best resource in guiding the sick child into the right direction in this era of diagnostic overkill.

REFERENCES

1. Hirsch JH, et al:Ultrasonic evaluation of radiographic opacities of the chest. *AJR* 130:1153, 1978.
2. Kangarloo H, et al: Ultrasonographic evaluation of juxtadiaphragmatic masses in children. *Radiology* 125:785, 1977.
3. Berger PE, Kuhns LR, Poznanski AK: Simple technique for eliminating tracheal buckling in lateral neck roentgenograms. *Pediatri Radiol* 2:69–71, 1974.
4. Capitanio M, Kirkpatrick JA: Upper respiratory obstruction in infants and children. *Radiol Clin North Am* 6:265–277, 1968.
5. Cochran ST, Gyepes MT, Smith LE: Obstruction of the airways by the heart and pulmonary vessels in infants. *Pediatr radiol* 6:81–87, 1977.
6. Dunbar JS: Upper respiratory tract obstruction in infants and children (Caldwell Lecture, 1969). *AJR* 109:227–246, 1970.
7. Gyepes MT, Desilets DT: The submentovertical projection: a new approach to the study of laryngeal and pharyngeal function in infants. *Radiology* 92:758–762, 1969.
8. Joseph PM, Berdon WE, Baker DH et al: Upper airway obstruction in infants and small children: improved radiographic diagnosis by combined filtration, high KV and magnification. *Radiology* 121:143, 1976.
9. Kushner DC, Harris CGB: Obstructing Lesions of the larynx and trachea in infants and children. *Radiol Clin North Am* 16(2):181, 1978.
10. McSwiney PF, Cavanagh NPC, Languth P: Outcome in congenital stridor (laryngomalacia). *Arch Dis Child* 52:215–218, 1977.
11. Wittenborg MH, Gyepes MT, Crocker D: Tracheal dynamics in infants with respiratory distress, stridor, and collapsing trachea. *Radiology* 88:653–662, 1967.
12. Berdon WE, Baker DH: Vascular anomalies in the infant lung: rings, slings and other things. *Semin Roentgenol* 7:39–64, 1972.
13. Cumming WA: Esophageal atresia and tracheoesophageal fistula. *Radiol Clin North Am* 13:277, 1975.
14. Euler AR, et al: Recurrent pulmonary disease in children: a complication of gastroesophageal reflux. *Pediatrics* 63:47, 1979.
15. Frates RC, Cox KL: Cystic fibrosis mistaken for gastroesophageal reflux with aspiration. *Am J Dis Child* 135:719 1981.
16. Gyepes MT, Linde LM: Familial dysautonomia: the mechanism of aspiration. *Radiology* 91:471, 1968.
17. Harris CGB: A special form of disturbed swallowing: one aspect of familial dysautonomia. *Prog Ped Rad: Gastrointestinal Tract* 2:184, 1969.
18. Neuhauser EBD, Griscom NT: Aspiration pneumonitis in children. *Prog Ped Rad: Respir Tract* 1:265–293, 1967.
19. Smith PD, Swischuk LE, Fagan CJ: an elusive and often unsuspected cause of stridor or pneumonia (the esophageal foreign body). *AJR* 1974; 122:178.
20. Gastroesophageal Reflux: *Seventy-Sixth Ross Conference on Pediatric Research,* 1979.
21. Reed MH: Radiology of airway foreign bodies in children. *J Can Assoc Radiol* 28:111–118, 1977.
22. Riggs WW, Jr: *Pediatric Chest Roentgenology: Recognizing The Abnormal,* St Louis, Warren H Green Inc, 1979.
23. Singleton EB, Wagner ML: *Radiologic Atlas of Pulmonary Abnormalities in Children,* Philadelphia, WB Saunders Co, 1971.
24. Swischuk LE: *Emergency Radiology of the Acutely Ill or Injured Child,* Baltimore, The Williams & Wilkins Co, 1979.

25. Wesenberg RL: *The Newborn Chest.* Hagerstown, Md, Harper & Row Publishers Inc. 1973, p 257.
26. Miller WE, Crowe JK, Muhm JR: The Evaluation of pulmonary parenchymal abnormalities. *Radiol Clin North Am* 14(1):85–94, 1976.
27. Muhm JR, Crowe JK: The evaluation of tracheal abnormalities by tomography. *Radiol Clin North Am* 1976; 14(1):95, 1976.
28. Shaner EG, Chang AD, Doppman JL, et al: Comparison of computed and conventional whole lung tomography in detecting pulmonary nodules: a prospective radiologic-pathologic study. *AJR* 131:51, 1978.
29. Arger PH, Mulhern CB Jr, Littman CB PS, et al: Management of solid tumors in children: contribution of computed tomography. *AJR* 137:251, 1981.
30. Bernard J, Sauvegrain J, Nahum H: Tomography of the lungs in infancy and childhood: techniques, indications, and results. *Prog Ped Rad: Respir Tract* 1:59–90, 1967.
31. Brasch RC, Korobkin M, Gooding CA: Computed body tomography in children: evaluation of 45 patients. *AJR* 131:21, 1978.
32. Gouliamos AD, Carter BL, Emami B: Computed tomography of the chest wall. *Radiology* 134:433, 1980.
33. Jost RG, Sagel SS, Stanley RJ, et al: Computed tomography of the thorax. *Radiology* 126:125, 1978.
34. Kollins SA: Computed tomography of the pulmonary parenchyma and chest wall. *Radio Clin North Am* 14:297, 1977.
35. Mink JH, Marshall EB, Sukov R, et al: Computed tomography of the anterior mediastinum in patients with myasthenia gravis and suspected thymoma. *AJR* 130:239, 1978.
36. Muhm JR, Brown LR, Crowe JK, et al: Comparison of whole lung tomography and computed tomography for detecting pulmonary nodules. *AJR* 131:981, 1978.
37. Muhm JR, Brown LR, Crowe JK: Detection of pulmonary nodules by computed tomography. *AJR* 128:267, 1977.
38. Pedersen KD, Jensen J, Hertz H: CT whole-body scanning in pediatric radiology. *Pediatr Radiol* 6:222, 1978.
39. Ciofetta G, Silverman M, Hughes JM: Quantitative approach to the study of regional lung function in children using krypton 81M. *Br J Radiol* 53:950, 1980.
40. Godfrey S, Hambleton G, Winlove P, et al: Unilateral lung disease detected by radioisotopic scanning in children thought to have asthma. *Br J Dis Chest* 71(1)7, 1977.
41. Kassner EG, Solomon NA, Steiner P, et al: Persisting perfusion defects after bronchoscopic removal or spontaneous expulsion of aspirated foreign objects. *Radiology* 121(1):139, 1976.
42. Lull RJ, Anderson JH, Telepak RJ, et al: Radionuclide imaging in the assessment of lung injury. *Semin Nucl Med* 10(3)302, 1980.
43. Mitnick JS, Kutin NS, Braunstein P, et al: Radioisotopic evaluation of congenital lobar emphysema. *Clin Nucl Med* 6(6):266, 1981.
44. Papanicolaou N, Treves S: Pulmonary scintigraphy in pediatrics. *Semin Nucl Med* 10(3):259, 1980.
45. Brunner S: Tracheography and bronchography: techniques and indications during infancy and childhood. *Prog Ped Rad: Respir Tract* 1:45, 1967.
46. Korhola O, Varpela E, Riihimaki E, et al: The effect of bronchography on pulmonary ventilation. *Ann Clin Res* 9(6):342, 1977.
47. Vandevivere J, Spehl M, Dab I, et al: Bronchiectasis in childhood: comparison of chest roentgenograms, bronchography and lung scintigraphy. *Pediatr Radiol* 9(4)193, 1980.
48. Lefebvre JE, Plainfosse MC: Pulmonary angiography in children: methods and indications, *Prog Ped Rad* 1:91, 1967.
49. Moss AJ, Desilets DT, Higashino SM, et al: Intrapulmonary shunts in cystic fibrosis. *Pediatrics* 41:438, 1968.
50. Pinet F, Froment JC: Angiography of the thoracic Systemic arteries. *Radiol Clin North Am* 16(3)441, 1978.
51. Crummy AB, Strother CM, Sackett JF, et al: Computerized fluoroscopy: digital subtraction for intravenous angiocardiography and arteriography. *AJR* 135(6)1131, 1980.
52. Epstein FH: Nuclear magnetic resonance: a new tool in clinical medicine (editorial). *N Engl J Med* 304(22)1360, 1981.
53. Jaffe CC: Sonograms, radiographs, and the mediastinum (editorial). *AJR* 137:422, 1981.
54. Luiten AL: Nuclear magnetic resonance: an introduction. *Medicamundi* 36(2):98, 1981.
55. Mistretta CA, Crummy AB, Strother CM: Digital angiography: a perspective. *Radiology* 139(2):273–276, 1981.
56. Reuter SR: Digital subtraction angiography (editorial). *AJR* 135(6):1316, 1980.
57. The Proceedings of Nuclear Magnetic Resonance (NMR) Imaging Symposium. Nashville, Tenn, Oct 26–27, 1980. *J Comput Assist Tomogr* 5(2):285, 1981.

Index

a
                                                                                b
                                                                            3 c
                                                                            4 d
                                                                            5 e
                                                                            6 f
                                                                            7 g
                                                                            8 h
                                                                            9 i
                                                                            8 0 j